T0329673

Novartis 238: Gastroenteritis Viruses.
Copyright © 2001 John Wiley & Sons Ltd
Print ISBN 0-471-49663-4   eISBN 0-470-84653-4

GASTROENTERITIS VIRUSES

The Novartis Foundation is an international scientific and educational
charity (UK Registered Charity No. 313574). Known until September 1997
as the Ciba Foundation, it was established in 1947 by the CIBA company
of Basle, which merged with Sandoz in 1996, to form Novartis. The
Foundation operates independently in London under English trust
law. It was formally opened on 22 June 1949.

The Foundation promotes the study and general knowledge of
science and in particular encourages international co-operation in
scientific research. To this end, it organizes internationally
acclaimed meetings (typically eight symposia and allied open
meetings and 15–20 discussion meetings each year) and publishes
eight books per year featuring the presented papers and discussions
from the symposia. Although primarily an operational rather than
a grant-making foundation, it awards bursaries to young scientists
to attend the symposia and afterwards work with one of the other
participants.

The Foundation's headquarters at 41 Portland Place, London W1N 4BN,
provide library facilities, open to graduates in science and allied disciplines.
Media relations are fostered by regular press conferences and by articles
prepared by the Foundation's Science Writer in Residence. The Foundation
offers accommodation and meeting facilities to visiting scientists and their
societies.

Information on all Foundation activities can be found at
http://www.novartisfound.org.uk

Novartis Foundation Symposium 238

GASTROENTERITIS VIRUSES

2001

JOHN WILEY & SONS, LTD

Chichester · New York · Weinheim · Brisbane · Singapore · Toronto

Novartis 238: Gastroenteritis Viruses.
Copyright © 2001 John Wiley & Sons Ltd
Print ISBN 0-471-49663-4 eISBN 0-470-84653-4

Other Wiley Editorial Offices

John Wiley & Sons, Inc., 605 Third Avenue,
New York, NY 10158-0012, USA

WILEY-VCH Verlag GmbH, Pappelallee 3,
D-69469 Weinheim, Germany

Jacaranda Wiley Ltd, 33 Park Road, Milton,
Queensland 4064, Australia

John Wiley & Sons (Asia) Pte Ltd, 2 Clementi Loop #02-01,
Jin Xing Distripark, Singapore 129809

John Wiley & Sons (Canada) Ltd, 22 Worcester Road,
Rexdale, Ontario M9W 1L1, Canada

Novartis Foundation Symposium 238
ix+323 pages, 38 figures, 34 tables

Library of Congress Cataloging-in-Publication Data
Gastroenteritis viruses / [Derek Chadwick, Jamie A. Goode, editors].
    p.cm. – (Novartis Foundation symposium ; 238)
    Includes bibliographical references and index.
    ISBN 0-471-49663-4 (alk. paper)
    1. Viral diarrhea–Congresses. 2. Gastroenteritis–Congresses. 3. Virus
diseases–Congresses.   I. Chadwick, Derek.   II. Goode, Jamie.   III. Series.
QR201.V53 G37 2001
616.3'30194–dc21   2001017866

British Library Cataloguing in Publication Data
A catalogue record for this book is available from the British Library

ISBN 978 0 471 49663 2

Typeset in 10$\frac{1}{2}$ on 12$\frac{1}{2}$ pt Garamond by Dobbie Typesetting Limited, Tavistock, Devon.

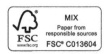

Contents

Symposium on Gastroenteritis Viruses, held at the Novartis Foundation, London, 16–18 May 2000

Editors: Derek Chadwick (Organizer) and Jamie A. Goode

This Symposium is based on a proposal made by Ulrich Desselberger

Participants

Carlos F. Arias   Instituto de Biotecnología, UNAM, Apt. Postal 510-3, Col. Miraval, Cuernavaca, Morelos 62250, Mexico

Ruth Bishop   Department of Gastroenterology and Clinical Nutrition, Royal Children's Hospital, Flemington Road, Melbourne, Victoria 3052, Australia

David Brown   Enteric and Respiratory Virus Laboratory, Central Public Health Laboratory, Public Health Laboratory Service, 61 Colindale Avenue, London NW9 5DF, UK

Mike Carter   School of Biological Sciences, University of Surrey, Guildford GU2 7XH, UK

Ian Clarke   Mailpoint 814, South Block, Southampton General Hospital, Tremona Road, Southampton SO16 6YD, UK

Jean Cohen   Centre de Recherche Moléculaire et d'Immunologie, INRA, 78352 Jouy-en-Josas, Cedex, France

Ulrich Desselberger   Clinical Microbiology and Public Health Laboratory, Level 6, Addenbrooke's Hospital, Hills Road, Cambridge CB2 2QW, UK

Mary K. Estes (*Chair*)   Division of Molecular Virology, Baylor College of Medicine, 1 Baylor Plaza, Houston, TX 77030, USA

Michael J. G. Farthing   Faculty of Medicine, University of Glasgow, 12 South Park Terrace, Glasgow G12 8LG, UK

Roger I. Glass   Viral Gastroenteritis Unit, Centers for Disease Control, 1600 Clifton Road, Atlanta, GA 30333, USA

Kim Y. Green   Epidemiology Section, Laboratory of Infectious Diseases, National Institute of Allergy and Infectious Diseases, National Institutes of Health, 9000 Rockville Pike, Bethesda, MD 20892, USA

Harry B. Greenberg   Stanford University School of Medicine, Office of the Dean, Room M-121, 300 Pasteur Drive, Stanford, CA 94305-5119, USA

Kathryn V. Holmes   Department of Microbiology, Campus Box B175, University of Colorado, Health Sciences Center, 4200 E 9th Avenue, Denver, CO 80262, USA

Albert Z. Kapikian   Epidemiology Section, Laboratory of Infectious Diseases, National Institute of Allergy and Infectious Diseases, National Institutes of Health, 9000 Rockville Pike, Bethesda, MD 20892, USA

Marion P. Koopmans   Virology Division, Research Laboratory for Infectious Diseases, National Institute of Public Health and the Environment, P O Box 2, 3720BA Bilthoven, The Netherlands

Susana López   Instituto de Biotecnología/UNAM, Av. Universidad 2001, Col. Chamilpa, Cuernavaca, Morelos 62210, Mexico

David Matson   Center for Pediatric Research, Eastern Virginia Medical School, 855 W. Brambleton Avenue, Norfolk, VA 23510, USA

Suzanne M. Matsui   Department of Medicine (Gastroenterology), Stanford University School of Medicine, Stanford, CA 94305-5487, USA

Stephan S. Monroe   Viral Gastroenteritis Section, Division of Viral and Rickettsial Diseases, National Center for Infectious Diseases, Centers for Disease Control and Prevention, Atlanta, GA 30333, USA

Paul A. Offit   The Children's Hospital of Philadelphia, 34th St. and Civic Center Blvd., The University of Pennsylvania School of Medicine, Philadelphia, PA 19104, USA

John T. Patton   Laboratory of Infectious Diseases, National Institute of Allergy and Infectious Diseases, National Institutes of Health, 7 Center Drive, MSC 0720, Room 117, Bethesda, MD 20892, USA

Richard Pollok   St Bartholomew's and the Royal London School of Medicine and Dentistry, Digestive Diseases Research Centre, Turner Street, London E1 2AD, UK

B. V. Venkataram Prasad   Department of Biochemistry, Baylor College of Medicine, 1 Baylor Plaza, Houston, TX 77030, USA

Robert F. Ramig   Division of Molecular Virology, Baylor College of Medicine, One Baylor Plaza, Houston, TX 77030, USA

Linda J. Saif   Food and Animal Health Research Programme, Ohio Agricultural Research and Development Center, Ohio State University, 1680 Madison Avenue, Wooster, OH 44691-4096, USA

Timo Vesikari   University of Tampere Medical School, Virology/Vaccine Research, University of Tampere, 33014 Tampere, Finland

Novartis 238: Gastroenteritis Viruses.
Copyright © 2001 John Wiley & Sons Ltd
Print ISBN 0-471-49663-4 eISBN 0-470-84653-4

Introduction

Mary K. Estes

Department of Molecular Virology and Microbiology, Baylor College of Medicine, 1 Baylor Plaza, Houston TX 77030, USA

Gastroenteritis is one of the most common illnesses of humans, and many different viruses have been causally associated with this disease. This symposium on 'Gastroenteritis viruses' is timely because knowledge about these viruses has expanded rapidly in recent years. There have been three previous international meetings that covered various aspects of gastroenteritis (GI) viruses. Two previous symposia were held here at the Novartis Foundation (then the Ciba Foundation) in London, UK. The first on 'Acute diarrhoea in childhood', held in 1975, highlighted the discoveries of rotavirus and Norwalk virus as the first two viruses that cause diarrhoea in humans as well as new information on the pathophysiology of acute diarrhoea (Ciba Foundation 1976). The second symposium (Ciba Foundation 1987), on 'Novel diarrhoea viruses' focused on non-group A rotaviruses, the enteric adenoviruses, astroviruses, small round viruses, caliciviruses and the toroviruses. Since that meeting, the novelty of these agents has been confirmed as illustrated by classification of: (1) the astroviruses within a new virus family called the *Astroviridae*, (2) the small round viruses and caliciviruses in distinct genera within the *Caliciviridae* family, and (3) the toroviruses in a separate genus within the *Coronaviridae* family. An International Symposium on Viral Gastroenteritis, in Sapporo, Japan, in 1995, comprehensively reviewed major molecular breakthroughs that led to characterization of the structure and function of the genes of the GI viruses, changes in understanding the epidemiologic and clinical significance of these pathogens based on the availability of new detection assays, and progress towards making vaccines (Chiba et al 1997). This millennium meeting on a subset of GI viruses is organized to focus on presentation and discussion of new discoveries driven by advances in molecular and cell biology that have resulted in new information about the epidemiology and transmission of disease, virus structure and function, and mechanisms of pathogenesis. Consideration of virus–host interactions and host responses to viral insult are particularly relevant following the rare, but unexpected complication of intussusception in children administered the first live, attenuated rotavirus vaccine. Goals of this meeting are to summarize current knowledge and outline needs and future work.

Acute gastroenteritis continues to be a significant clinical problem throughout the world. In the USA, it is second only to acute viral respiratory disease as a cause of acute illness. Worldwide, more than 700 million cases of acute diarrhoeal disease are estimated to occur annually just in children under the age of 5 years (Snyder & Merson 1982). Gastroenteritis is most commonly manifested clinically as mild diarrhoea, but more severe disease, ranging from upper gastrointestinal symptoms (nausea and vomiting) to profuse diarrhoea leading to dehydration and death, may occur. The annual mortality associated with gastroenteritis has been estimated to be 3.5 to 5 million, with the majority of deaths occurring in developing countries. This is clearly an enormous problem, and while improvements in sanitation have decreased the prevalence of bacterial diarrhoeas, the impact of viral gastroenteritis remains essentially unaffected.

Several viruses cause diarrhoea. Rotaviruses, human caliciviruses, astroviruses and enteric adenoviruses are the major human pathogens, and this meeting focuses on the first three of these pathogens. The rotaviruses, discovered by Ruth Bishop in 1973, are clearly the most important viruses causing life-threatening disease in young children (Bishop et al 1973). Human caliciviruses, which include viruses in two distinct genera: the Norwalk-like viruses, first seen by Albert Kapikian in 1972 (Kapikian et al 1972), and the Sapporo-like viruses, discovered by Madeley & Cosgrove (1976), and Flewett & Davies (1976), are being increasingly recognized as playing an important role in gastroenteritis. The astroviruses, first described by Appleton & Higgins (1975) and subsequently named by Madeley & Cosgrove (1975), are novel agents whose clinical significance continues to be defined. The enteric adenoviruses will not be covered specifically during this meeting but they remain important particularly in causing longer-lasting infections; they should be addressed during the discussions of this meeting. We will also be hearing about coronaviruses that clearly are pathogens in animals and it is likely these are important in humans, but new tests need to be made and applied to confirm this suspicion. Finally, we will discuss a subset of herpes viruses that are not considered gastroenteritis viruses *per se*, but human herpes simplex virus and cytomegalovirus frequently infect cells in the gastrointestinal tract in immunocompromised individuals and cause GI disease as opportunistic infections. A new virus, the Aichi virus, is a picornavirus that we don't know much about yet, but it may be discussed as a new GI pathogen.

Our knowledge of GI viruses has been facilitated by studies of those agents that replicate in cells cultured in the laboratory, but recent analyses have heightened our awareness that the outcome of infection with these viruses is really the consequence of the virus replicating in cells in the intestinal tract. The intestinal villi are composed of multiple cell types and interactions between and among cells within the villi can be quite complex. Cells in the intestinal tract other than the villus epithelial cells need to be considered relative to their roles in responding to infection and in pathogenesis. In the lamina propria, there are T cells that may produce cytokines, neutrophils, B cells, fibroblasts (which can induce mediators such as prostaglandins), macrophages, mast cells and so forth. There are also endothelial cells that can release a range of signalling molecules including cytokines, nitric oxide and hormones. Although this meeting may not discuss all these interactions, it is clear that cross-talk among intestinal cells is quite common and important for proper cell differentiation and functioning. It seems clear that future breakthroughs in understanding the molecular regulation of pathogenesis will require thinking that involves the cell level but moves back to the organ and the organism.

As the chair of this meeting, I think it is worthwhile to outline a few questions that should be discussed during this symposium. These ideas are not an inclusive list of current key questions and surely others will be presented in the meeting. First, what are the cellular receptors that gastroenteritis viruses use to infect cells? Why is it so difficult to cultivate these gastroenteritis viruses? Is it simply because we are unable to grow the highly differentiated cells at the tips of the villus in the laboratory or do we need co-cultures of the diverse cells in the villus to provide the proper cell signalling to support virus replication? The ability of a virus to initiate infection requires that the agent pass through the low pH of the stomach. Then, pathogens are exposed to proteolytic enzymes coming from the pancreas. Some of our gastroenteritis viruses, like many of the mucosal respiratory viruses, actually take advantage of exposure to the pancreatic enzymes and their infectivity is activated through exposure to trypsin and perhaps other enzymes. Can we now explain, either on a structural or molecular basis, what is the mechanism by which infectivity is activated? How do the coronaviruses and other enveloped viruses actually survive the transit through the stomach to infect the gastrointestinal tract? What specific cell functions are required to support GI virus replication? What molecular mechanisms regulate viral replication and why have we been unable to achieve a reverse genetic system for the rotaviruses, the human caliciviruses and the coronaviruses? Once an infection has been initiated, how does the cell and the organism respond immunologically to this virus, and can we use this knowledge to construct new vaccines? Why has it been difficult to identify clear correlates of immunity for these GI viruses? How does the cell response to infection affect pathogenesis? Does virus replication in the GI tract lead to intussusception? This past year, the unexpected, rare complication of intussusception was associated with the tetravalent rhesus rotavirus vaccine. We know that intussusception has been associated with the respiratory adenoviruses. Is the intussusception that is associated with adenovirus and rotavirus infections caused by similar mechanism(s)? Does this involve virus interaction with an integrin that is the receptor for the respiratory adenoviruses and is present in the terminal ileum? Will intussusception be a problem in gene therapy, where people are thinking of using adenovirus vectors to deliver genes? Is intussusception a rare complication associated with many GI viral infections? Molecular epidemiology studies are showing that most GI viruses are not static: they are evolving, and virus is transmitted more frequently than we previously appreciated, often in food. What are the mechanisms driving this evolution and variation, and do we understand them sufficiently to be able to prevent transmission? Will this variation affect vaccination strategies? Will GI infections in immuno-compromised individuals change the recognized patterns of transmission and virus evolution? Should we be more vigilant and concerned about GI infections in settings such as Africa where disease is rampant and spread occurs in increasing numbers in people who are infected with HIV?

My recommendation for our discussion at this meeting is that we share many ideas and also discuss negative data — not poor data, but experiments that we have tried that have not been successful, particularly related to some of the questions that I have addressed above. We should recognize that if we all agree on everything that is presented and discussed, then our knowledge will not move forward. We need to be critical in our thinking, but also open-minded and willing to consider and discuss different approaches and new ideas. I encourage everyone to be provocative, innovative and imaginative; this should lead to a stimulating and productive meeting.

References

Appleton H, Higgins PG 1975 Viruses and gastroenteritis in infants. Lancet 1:1297

Bishop RF, Davidson GP, Holmes IH, Ruck BJ 1973 Virus particles in epithelial cells of duodenal mucosa from children with acute non-bacterial gastroenteritis. Lancet 2:1281–1283

Chiba S, Estes MK, Nakata S, Calisher CH (eds) 1997 Viral Gastroenteritis. Arch Virol 142(supplement 12):1–311

Ciba Foundation 1976 Acute diarrhoea in childhood (Ciba Found Symp 42). Elsevier/Excerpta Medica/North Holland, Amsterdam

Ciba Foundation 1987 Novel diarrhoea viruses (Ciba Found Symp 128). Wiley, Chichester

Flewett TH, Davies H 1976 Caliciviruses in man. Lancet 1:311

Kapikian AA, Wyatt RF, Dolin R, Thornhill TS, Kalica AR, Chanock RM 1972 Visualization by immune electron microscopy of a 27 nm particle associated with acute infectious nonbacterial gastroenteritis. J Virol 10:1075–1081

Madeley CR, Cosgrove BP 1975 28 nm particles in faeces in infantile gastroenteritis. Lancet 2:451–452

Madeley CR, Cosgrove BP 1976 Caliciviruses in man. Lancet 1:199–200

Snyder JD, Merson MH 1982 The magnitude of the global problem of acute diarrhoeal disease: a review of the active surveillance data. Bull World Health Organ 60:605–613

Novartis 238: Gastroenteritis Viruses.
Copyright © 2001 John Wiley & Sons Ltd
Print ISBN 0-471-49663-4   eISBN 0-470-84653-4

Gastroenteritis viruses: an overview

Roger I. Glass, Joseph Bresee, Baoming Jiang, Jon Gentsch, Tamie Ando, Rebecca Fankhauser, Jacqueline Noel, Umesh Parashar, Blair Rosen and Stephan S. Monroe

Viral Gastroenteritis Section, Centers for Disease Control and Prevention, 1600 Clifton Road, Atlanta, GA 30333, USA

Abstract. Acute gastroenteritis is among the most common illnesses of humankind, and its associated morbidity and mortality are greatest among those at the extremes of age, children and the elderly. In developing countries, gastroenteritis is a common cause of death in children <5 years that can be linked to a wide variety of pathogens. In developed countries, while deaths from diarrhoea are less common, much illness leads to hospitalization or doctor visits. Much of the gastroenteritis in children is caused by viruses belonging to four distinct families— rotaviruses, caliciviruses, astroviruses and adenoviruses. Other viruses, such as the toroviruses, picobirnaviruses, picornavirus (the Aichi virus), and enterovirus 22, may play a role as well. Viral gastroenteritis occurs with two epidemiologic patterns, diarrhoea that is endemic in children and outbreaks that affect people of all ages. Viral diarrhoea in children is caused by group A rotaviruses, enteric adenoviruses, astroviruses and the caliciviruses; the illness affects all children worldwide in the first few years of life regardless of their level of hygiene, quality of water, food or sanitation, or type of behaviour. For all but perhaps the caliciviruses, these infections provide immunity from severe disease upon reinfection. Epidemic viral diarrhoea is caused primarily by the Norwalk-like virus genus of the caliciviruses. These viruses affect people of all ages, are often transmitted by faecally contaminated food or water, and are therefore subject to control by public health measures. The tremendous antigenic diversity of caliciviruses and short-lived immunity to infection permit repeated episodes throughout life. In the past decade, the molecular characterization of many of these gastroenteritis viruses has led to advances both in our understanding of the pathogens themselves and in development of a new generation of diagnostics. Application of these more sensitive methods to detect and characterize individual agents is just beginning, but has already opened up new avenues to reassess their disease burden, examine their molecular epidemiology, and consider new directions for their prevention and control through vaccination, improvements in food and water quality and sanitary practices.

2001 Gastroenteritis viruses. Wiley, Chichester (Novartis Foundation Symposium 238) p 5–25

Acute gastroenteritis is among the most common illnesses of humankind and has its greatest impact on people at the extremes of age, children and the elderly. The predominant symptoms of vomiting and diarrhoea are common to infections with a diverse group of more than 20 different microbial agents. The spectrum of disease can range from asymptomatic infections, through mild vomiting or diarrhoea or both, to severe disease leading to dehydration that in some instances can be fatal. In developing countries, children may have repeated episodes of gastroenteritis in their first few years of life, leading to an estimated 2.4–2.8 million deaths each year or nearly one-quarter of all deaths in children under 5 years (Bern et al 1992, Murray & López 1997). In the industrialized world, people of all ages have about one episode of gastroenteritis each year, resulting in many hospitalizations but fewer deaths (Mead et al 1999).

Prior to 1972, the aetiology of most of these episodes was unknown, and illness was attributed to diet and weaning foods, old age, drugs, malnutrition, or unexplained causes referred to as 'idiopathic'. Since then, much of this 'diagnostic gap' has been filled in by the discovery of more than a dozen different pathogens, and we now believe that most of these episodes have an infectious aetiology and are caused by microorganisms (Flewett et al 1987). In many settings, viruses are recognized to be the predominant pathogens. In the 1970s, researchers who turned their electron microscopes to examine faecal specimens from patients with diarrhoea were rewarded with the discovery of the Norwalk virus in 1972 (Kapikian et al 1972), rotaviruses in 1973 (Bishop et al 1973), astroviruses in 1975 (Madeley & Cosgrove 1975, Appleton et al 1975), 'classic human caliciviruses' in 1978 (Chiba et al 2000) and enteric adenoviruses in 1975 (Wadell et al 1987) (Fig. 1). These breakthroughs cleared the way for what has become three decades of scientific advance leading to improvements in our understanding of the role that these viruses play in human disease and in our efforts at their prevention and control. A key recurrent theme in the study of viral gastroenteritis is the observation that, as diagnostic tests have evolved, improved and become more sensitive to detect viral pathogens, our understanding of their epidemiology and associated disease burden has become more fully appreciated (Glass et al 1996, 2000).

This paper reviews the disease burden of gastroenteritis and the role played by the principal viruses. We highlight some distinguishing features of each virus that help explain its particular epidemiologic profile. During the past three decades, a number of other viruses have been discovered whose link to human disease is less well understood, namely, the toroviruses, group B and C rotaviruses, picobirnavirus, enterovirus 22, and a novel picornavirus, the Aichi agent. These agents will be noted in passing with the hope that future investigators will be challenged to assess their importance in human disease. The goal of this effort is to help define public health interventions that can be successfully employed to reduce the morbidity and mortality associated with severe viral gastroenteritis.

Epidemiologic considerations

The disease burden of acute gastroenteritis

Acute gastroenteritis is often considered to be exclusively a problem of children in developing countries. These children have 5–10 episodes of gastroenteritis each

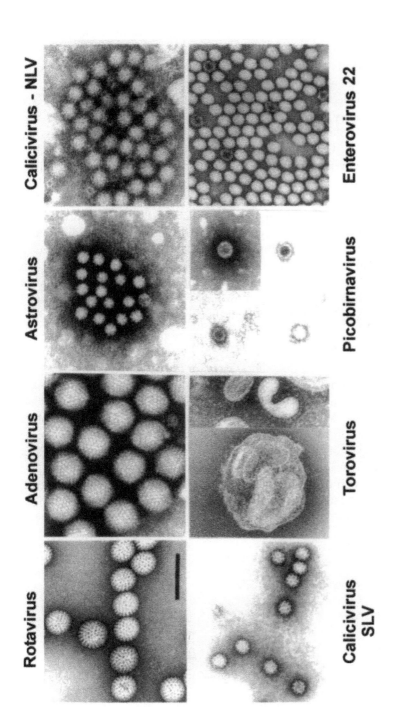

FIG. 1. Viral agents of gastroenteritis as seen by direct electron microscopy. Bar = 100 nm.

year during their first 5 years of life and, though many of these are mild, some episodes can lead to malnutrition, dehydration and death (Bern et al 1992). In the developing world, about one child in 40 will die of diarrhoea, making this the first or second most common cause of death in this age group.

The problem of diarrhoea is not confined to children in developing countries. In the USA, nearly every person experiences an episode of gastroenenteritis each year, but severe and fatal illness is confined to those at the extremes of age, children and the elderly (Fig. 2). Children in the United States will experience only 1.5–2.5 episodes per year, most of which are mild, but each year, an estimated 2 million will visit a doctor or clinic and 160 000 will be hospitalized (Tucker et al 1998). Among adults, about 400 000 are discharged from hospital with diarrhoea reported on their discharge certificates, and about 3000 have diarrhoea reported on their death certificates (Glass et al 2000). For hospitalizations, diarrhoea is reported on discharge diagnoses of 10–12% of all children < 5 years hospitalized in the USA and in about 1.5% of hospitalizations for adults, particularly those > 65 years. For many of these hospitalizations and deaths, diarrhoea is the principal cause, and for others it remains a problem of nosocomial infection or a complication of another severe or chronic disease.

Agents of diarrhoeal illness

In 1970, the causes of diarrhoeal illness were for the most part unknown. A few agents such as salmonella, shigella, *Entamoeba histolytica* and *Giardia lamblia* were commonly sought, but rarely detected, thus, a 'diagnostic void' existed for which the aetiology was attributed to malnutrition, weaning foods, physiologic conditions, drugs or 'idiopathic' (i.e. unknown) causes. The past three decades have seen an explosion in the number of agents identified as causes of diarrhoeal diseases, including many viruses, bacteria, parasites and some toxins.

The discovery of these new agents has filled in this 'diagnostic void' and allowed us to understand the striking differences in the epidemiology of diarrhoea between

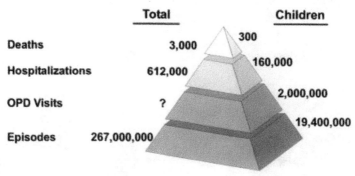

FIG. 2.   The estimated burden of gastroenteritis in the USA.

TABLE 1 Diarrhoeal illnesses among children in the USA and Bangladesh: the role of viruses

	United States	Bangladesh
Episodes/child/year	1–2.5	4–7
Total episodes by age 5	5–7	20–35
Agents		
Viruses		
Rotaviruses	1	1
Astroviruses	1	1
Caliciviruses		
'Norwalk-like viruses'	1	2–5?
'Sapporo-like viruses'	1	
Adenoviruses (enteric)	1	1
Bacteria and parasites	±1	>20
Risk of death	1 in 12 000	1 in 40

children in developed and developing countries. To begin with, children in developing countries experience many more episodes of diarrhoea each year for the first 5 years of life than do US or British children — 4–7 episodes and 1–2.5 episodes per year, respectively (Table 1) (Bern & Glass 1994). The pathogens associated with these illnesses differ markedly, reflecting different levels of sanitation and hygiene. In an industrialized country like Finland, a recent study using the best diagnostics available could identify a virus in 60% of all diarrhoeal episodes in children <2 years, and in 85% that were moderate or severe. Of these pathogens 24% were rotaviruses, 19% caliciviruses, 4% astroviruses and 4% adenoviruses (Pang et al 2000). In developing countries, all of these viruses are also present, but bacteria and parasites transmitted by faecally contaminated food and water play a more prominent role, and no agent can be identified for the remainder of cases. The observation that infection with these gastroenteritis viruses is universal and that all children, rich or poor, are exposed and acquire antibodies in the first few years of life suggests that they may be transmitted by means unrelated to contaminated food or water, perhaps by airborne droplets or person-to-person contact.

Much less is known about the aetiology of diarrhoea that sends adults to the hospital (Fig. 3). Studies in the past have failed to identify an agent in most patients. For example, an investigation of bacterial pathogens that applied the best diagnostic procedures to screen more than 30 000 patients admitted to 10 hospitals in the USA could identify a cause for fewer than 6% of cases, leaving 94% without an aetiology in the 'diagnostic void' (Slutsker et al 1997). Similarly,

A. Hospitalized Patients (N>30,000)

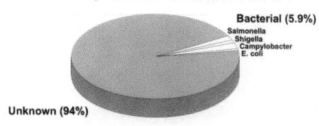

B. CDC Outbreaks 1973-1987 (N=7,458)

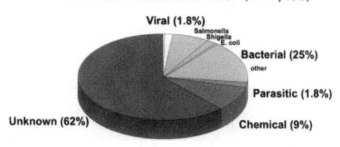

FIG. 3. The diagnostic void for gastroenteritis: aetiology of gastroenteritis among hospitalized patients (A) (Slutsker et al 1997) and outbreaks investigated by CDC, 1973–1987 (B) (Bean & Griffin 1990).

investigation of nearly 7500 outbreaks in the USA by CDC between 1973–1987 identified a viral aetiology in less than 2%. Studies underway may help to clarify the extent to which many of these are due to enteric viruses. Some groups of adults, including those hospitalized or institutionalized, immunocompromised and the elderly, are at particular risk of viral gastroenteritis with caliciviruses, but unlike the situation for children, the proportion of illness caused by viruses has not yet been well defined.

Endemic and epidemic patterns of disease

Viral gastroenteritis occurs in two distinct epidemiologic patterns, endemic childhood diarrhoea and epidemic disease. These patterns reflect differences in the pathogens, the host's response to these infections and their modes of transmission, and all have a direct bearing on strategies for prevention and control (Table 2). Childhood diarrhoea is best exemplified by the group A rotaviruses but the pattern is similar for enteric adenoviruses, astroviruses and the Sapporo-like virus genus of the caliciviruses. Infection with these agents is universal among children during the first few years of life. First infections are

TABLE 2   Epidemiologic patterns of viruses causing acute gastroenteritis

	Endemic childhood disease	Epidemic disease
Viruses	Rotavirus (group A)	Caliciviruses (NLVs & SLVs)
	Astrovirus	Rotavirus (group B)
	Enteric adenoviruses	?astrovirus
	?rotavirus (group C)	
	?caliciviruses (NLVs & SLVs)	
Mode of transmission	Unknown; ?contact; fomites, droplets & aerosols, or person–person	Food, water, ?contact, droplets, and aerosols
Reservoir	Humans	Humans
Antibody	High prevalence by 5 yrs of age	Seroconversion in epidemic
Immunity	Good	Short-term (calicivirus)
Virus variation	Limited discrete serotypes (except caliciviruses)	Many antigenic variants of caliciviruses
Public health control measures	Vaccine — RV (group A)	Outbreak control; improved food safety and handling

symptomatic and usually protect against subsequent severe disease, and therefore disease incidence decreases with increasing age, immunity is relatively good, and the strains have a limited number of specific and distinct serotypes. Since these viruses infect all children — rich or poor — everywhere in the world, improvements in the quality of water, food and sanitation are unlikely to decrease the incidence of disease, and vaccines hold promise for the prevention of severe illness. Epidemic disease is best exemplified by the human caliciviruses, particularly the 'Norwalk-like viruses' (NLVs). These viruses are the most important cause of outbreaks of gastroenteritis in the USA and affect people of all ages from children to adults (Glass et al 2000, Fankhauser et al 1998). This broad age distribution suggests that immunity is not complete or long-lasting and may also reflect the huge genetic and antigenic diversity of strains that is not yet fully understood. Often, these outbreaks are spread by faecally contaminated food or water or person-to-person contact, and therefore the success of control and prevention measures is directly related to the ability to detect their mode of transmission.

A number of agents do not completely fit these paradigms. For the NLV genus of caliciviruses, most children in developed countries and developing countries acquire antibodies in their first years of life, suggesting that childhood infections are universal even though we do not know whether the frequency of infections or the diversity of the infecting strains are comparable (Black et al 1982). Astroviruses have been associated with outbreaks in schools and affect older children and adults, suggesting that immunity to disease may be overcome, perhaps by larger-than-normal inocula of infections spread by atypical vehicles of infection. Finally, two antigenically distinct groups of rotaviruses — group B (Chen et al 1991) and group C (Saif & Jiang 1994) — are unusual. While they are structurally very similar to the common group A rotaviruses, they have been most notably identified in epidemics, and key features of their epidemiology and interactions with their human hosts are unknown.

Biological features of the viruses

The viruses that cause gastroenteritis in humans represent an extraordinary diversity of organisms that have probably evolved over distinct and divergent pathways (Table 3). First, the recognized viruses belong in four different families that have as their most basic building blocks different nucleic acids blueprints — DNA for the adenoviruses, positive sense single-stranded RNA for the caliciviruses and astroviruses, (and toroviruses and enteroviruses [entero 22]), and double-stranded RNA for the rotaviruses (and picobirnaviruses). All have family members that infect other animal species. Consequently, group A rotaviruses are found in most mammalian and avian species, although the serotypes present in humans show limited mixing with those from other animal strains. In no case do animals appear to be a common reservoir for human strains and human disease, but for group A rotaviruses and the NLVs, molecular evidence from sequencing strains suggests that the strains from humans may have evolved through contact with isolates from animals (Bridger 1999, Nakagomi & Nakagomi 1989).

Comparison of these viruses indicates a feature of antigenic diversity that may play a crucial role in their epidemiologic pattern of disease. For those viruses that have been best characterized, some — the rotaviruses, astroviruses, and enteric adenoviruses — have a limited number of very distinct serotypes that yield a good protective immune response in the host. By contrast, the NLVs appear to have a continually growing and changing repertoire of genetic variants and antigenic clusters. These viruses cannot yet be cultivated or serotyped, but the initial genetic observations suggest that the diversity of strains is enormous (Ando et al 2000). This difference may account in part for the different epidemiologic patterns of disease since only the caliciviruses routinely infect humans throughout life, whereas the others primarily cause disease in young children and the elderly while conferring immunity to older children and adults.

Diagnostic advances

In the field of viral gastroenteritis, advances in our understanding of the epidemiology and clinical importance of each virus have required the

TABLE 3   Characteristics of the viruses causing acute gastroenteritis

Virus	Family	Size (nm)	EM Shape	Nucleic acid	Genome organization	Characterization
Rotavirus	Reoviridae	70	Wheel-shaped (rota), triplet capsid	dsRNA	11 segments	Groups A,B,C; Group A has 2 subgroups (I, II); multiple serotypes, classified on the basis of two outer capsid proteins (P and G)
Calicivirus	Caliciviridae	28–35	Small round structured viruses (SRSV) with calices	ss(+)RNA	3 ORFs	Two genogroups: 'Norwalk-like viruses' and 'Sapporo-like viruses', each with multiple distinct antigenic clusters
Astrovirus	Astroviridae	28–33	SRSV star-shaped morphology	ss(+)RNA	2 ORFs	8 serotypes
Adenovirus	Adenoviridae	80	Icosahedral	dsDNA		Enteric serotypes 40, 41, 31, and types 42–48
Other viruses						
Torovirus	Toroviridae		Torus-shaped pleiomorphic	ss(+)RNA		Role in human disease unknown
Picobirnavirus	?		Small round virus	dsRNA	2 segments	Role in human disease unknown
Enterovirus 22	?		Small round virus	ss(+)RNA		Genetically distinct from other enteroviruses
Aichi virus	Picornaviridae		Small round virus	ss(+)RNA		Cause of outbreaks in Japan

ORF, open reading frame.

development of new and sensitive diagnostic assays (Table 4). We know most about the epidemiology of the group A rotaviruses because many simple immunoassays were developed early on, and the virus is shed in such large numbers that detection is simple, sensitive and relatively inexpensive. Yet despite the many recent advances in our understanding of the basic biology of the other gastroenteritis viruses, our ability to establish a viral aetiology for a patient with acute gastroenteritis remains limited. All viruses can be detected by electron microscopy, but this procedure is routinely applied in relatively few laboratories, requires an experienced operator, and can be relatively insensitive for those viruses shed in low titres (10^6–10^7 particles/g) or with faecal specimens not being collected during the acute episode. Besides assays for the group A rotaviruses, commercial immunoassays are available for the enteric adenoviruses (Ad 40 and Ad41) and for astrovirus, but only assays for rotavirus have been routinely used on a wide scale.

In the past decade, many of the enteric viruses have been cloned and sequenced, clearing the way for new molecular methods for detection and characterization of strains. Notable advances have been made for the detection of the caliciviruses by RT-PCR, and these assays are becoming available in public health laboratories in many countries. Problems of genetic diversity of NLVs have led to the use of a cocktail of different primers as well as degenerate primers to detect the wide variety of strains in circulation (Ando et al 2000). Sequence analysis has permitted strains identified in outbreaks to be traced back to their source in faecally contaminated food or water (Beller et al 1997, Dowell et al 1995) and this success has tempted public health laboratories to consider screening suspected food or water for evidence of contamination (Schaub & Oshiro 2000). In addition, mere knowledge of the genetic sequence has permitted outbreaks with identical strains having the same sequence to be linked with a common suspected vehicle of infection.

Our understanding of the epidemiology and causal role of some of the novel agents of viral gastroenteritis, including the group C rotaviruses, toroviruses, picobirnaviruses and the Aichi agent (Yamashita et al 1995, 1998), has been held back because of a lack of adequately sensitive diagnostic assays suitable for their study and inadequate linkages between clinical and laboratory-based studies (Yamashita et al 1991, 1993). Group C strains have been identified in small focal outbreaks and are a recognized pathogen of animals. However, screening assays for Group C rotaviruses based on immunoassays using reagents from animal strains or polyacrylamide gel electrophoresis have underestimated the prevalence of the virus among children hospitalized with diarrhoea (Jiang et al 1995). RT-PCR has improved these estimates but has not yet been simplified or applied on a broader scale. Similarly, toroviruses have been seen by electron microscopy in children with diarrhoea, but confirmation by enzyme immunoassay or molecular methods remains experimental and these latter assays have not yet been more broadly

TABLE 4 Diagnostics available to detect and characterize the gastroenteritis viruses

| Viruses | Quantity in clinical specimens (per gm) | EM[a] | ELA | Molecular Methods | | |
				Detection	Characterization	Typing
Rotavirus Group A	10^{8-12}	++++	++++	Probes RT-PCR	Probes RT-PCR Sequence	Mab–EIA for serotype and subgroup; RT-PCR for genotype
Group B	?	++	(++)	Probes RT-PCR	Probes RT-PCR Sequence	NA
Group C	10^{5-7}	++	(+)			IEM
Caliciviruses NLVs	$\leqslant 10^{7-8}$	+	(specific strains)	RT-PCR	RT-PCR, probes and sequence	RT-PCR probes and sequence
SLVs	$\leqslant 10^{7-8}$	+				
Astrovirus	10^{7-8}	+		RT-PCR	RT-PCR sequence	EIA for serotype RT-PCR for genotype
Adenoviruses (enteric serotypes 40, 41, 31)	10^{7-10}	+++	++++ [hexon] +++ [ad 40/41]	RT-PCR	Restriction digests, immuno assays	Mab–EIA for serotype; restriction enzymes

[a]EM: +, detectable with low sensitivity by skilled microscopist; ++++, easily visible; limit of detection by EM~10^{6-7} virus/gm of stool. ( ) research method.

EIA, enzyme immunoassay; EM, electron microscopy; IEM, immunoelectron microscopy; Mab, monoclonal antibody; NA, not available; NLV, Norwalk-like virus; SLV, Sapporo-like virus.

applied (Koopmans et al 1993). Finally, the picobirnaviruses were first identified by Pereira in faecal specimens from animals with diarrhoea and humans, but their causal relationship to disease in humans has not yet been firmly established (Pereira 1991). Picobirnaviruses have been found in HIV-infected patients with diarrhoea more often than those without diarrhoea, but an immune response, a *sine qua non* of infection, could not be documented by immune electron microscopy (Grohmann et al 1993). The recent cloning and sequencing of the virus should provide the necessary diagnostic advances to examine the epidemiology of this virus more carefully and document a causal role if it exists (Rosen et al 2000).

Prospects for prevention and control

Given the immense disease burden of viral agents of gastroenteritis, our research must be directed toward prevention and control of the resulting disease. For the endemic agents of children, vaccines provide the most likely approach toward prevention. Rotavirus represents the most important virus in this group, and vaccines against rotavirus have already been under development and testing for 15 years (Bresee et al 1999). The enteric adenoviruses and astrovirus pose another challenge, since the disease they cause is less common than rotavirus diarrhoea, and most studies indicate that gastroenteritis associated with astrovirus is less severe than that caused by rotavirus (Pang et al 2000). Consequently, efforts to push for a vaccine would require more data documenting that there was enough severe or fatal disease or hospital or health care costs to justify the massive investment required.

For the epidemic diseases, other challenges remain. The caliciviruses pose the greatest epidemic threats, and investigation often identifies a breach of sanitation with faecal contamination of water or food (either at its source or by a food-handler) that can be corrected. At the same time, the virus can be transmitted by person-to-person contact or perhaps by aerosols, and therefore much disease is not easily prevented (Becker et al 2000). Control of calicivirus disease outbreaks is currently directed at halting those outbreaks where problems of contamination of food or water can be easily corrected. This approach leaves many outbreaks to run their course despite the best public health interventions and intent. Efforts to develop vaccines against the caliciviruses are being pursued with the hope that even mimicking the short-term natural immunity of infection would be a useful preventive measure for travellers and soldiers, provided that the vaccine contained the proper broad mix of antigens or induced immunity to a common immune determinant of many strains (Estes et al 2000).

We know little about the prospects of control of the other novel viruses of epidemic gastroenteritis. Group B rotaviruses that were epidemic in China, affected people of all ages, and were believed to be transmitted by contaminated water have only recently been identified outside of China in India, where they did not cause epidemics (Hung et al 1984). This experience warns us to be on the alert for new viruses that may emerge and spread by novel means and have an impact on health that cannot be assessed in advance.

What the future will hold

The discovery of many novel viral agents of gastroenteritis has allowed us to consider the role that each may play in endemic disease of children and in outbreaks. For children, rotavirus emerges as the most common cause of severe gastroenteritis and has become the target for prevention and control with vaccines. So far, the other common pathogens of children — astroviruses, enteric adenoviruses and caliciviruses — appear to cause illness that is either less common or less severe. Consequently, while vaccines could be developed for prevention, the current approach to control is through improved treatment with oral rehydration and the withholding of antibiotics. For epidemic gastroenteritis, NLVs are the predominant pathogens that are most commonly caused by food faecally contaminated during production (e.g. irrigation with sewage) or preparation (e.g. by an infected food-handler). Prevention will require investigation of outbreaks, identification of the modes of transmission, and interruption of this spread through the use of public health interventions. The recent advances in molecular diagnostics now permit outbreak strains to be compared between patients and traced back to their source in contaminated food and water. Application of the same molecular methods has allowed outbreaks in different settings caused by strains with identical sequences to be linked to a common source and may, in the near future, provide new methods to screen food and water that have become contaminated. Outbreaks with NLVs and the other viruses pose a continuing threat to human health for which expanded surveillance will be required. This surveillance and our further understanding of the full extent of the disease burden of the gastroenteritis viruses will require further advances and simplifications to develop improved, more sensitive detection assays and to make these methods more widely available to physicians and public health laboratories.

Acknowledgements

We thank John O'Connor and Ann Risinger for their help in the preparation of this manuscript.

References

Ando T, Noel JS, Fankhauser RL 2000 Genetic classification of 'Norwalk-like viruses'. J Infect Dis (suppl 2) 181:S336–S348
Appleton H, Buckley M, Thom BT, Cotton JL, Henderson S 1975 Virus-like particles in winter vomiting disease. Lancet i:1297

Bean NH, Griffin PM 1990 Foodborne disease outbreaks in the United States, 1973–1987: pathogens, vehicles, and trends. J Food Protect 53:804–817

Becker K, Moe CL, Southwick K, MacCormack JN 2000 Transmission of Norwalk virus during football game. N Eng J Med 343:1223–1227

Beller M, Ellis A, Lee SH et al 1997 Outbreak of viral gastroenteritis due to a contaminated well. International consequences. JAMA 278:563–568

Bern C, Glass RI 1994 Impact of diarrheal diseases worldwide. In: Kapikian AZ (ed) Viral infections of the gastrointestinal tract, 2nd edn. Dekker, New York, p 1–26

Bern C, Martines J, de Zoysa I, Glass RI 1992 The magnitude of the global problem of diarrhoeal disease: a ten year update. Bull WHO 70:705–714

Bishop RF, Davidson GP, Holmes IH, Ruck BJ 1973 Virus particles in epithelial cells of duodenal mucosa from children with non-acute gastroenteritis. Lancet i:1281–1283

Black RE, Greenberg HB, Kapikian AZ, Brown KH, Becker S 1982 Acquisition of serum antibody to Norwalk virus and rotavirus and relation to diarrhea in a longitudinal study of young children in rural Bangladesh. J Infect Dis 145:483–489

Bresee J, Glass RI, Ivanoff B, Gentsch J 1999 Current status and future priorities for rotavirus vaccine development, evaluation, and implementation in developing countries. Vaccine 17:2207–2222

Chen G-M, Werner-Eckert R, Tao H, Mackow ER 1991 Expression of the major inner capsid protein of the group B rotavirus ADRV: primary characterization of genome segment 5. Virology 182:820–829

Chiba S, Nakata S, Numata-Kinoshita K, Honma S 2000 Sapporo virus: history and recent findings. J Infect Dis (suppl 2) 181:S303–S308

Dastjerdi AM, Green J, Gallimore CI, Brown DW, Bridger J 1999 The bovine Newberry agent-2 is genetically more closely related to human SRSVs than to animal caliciviruses. Virology 254:1–5

Dowell SF, Groves C, Kirkland KB et al 1995 A multistate outbreak of oyster-associated gastroenteritis: implications for interstate tracing of contaminated shellfish. J Infect Dis 171:1497–1503

Estes MK, Ball JM, Guerrero RA et al 2000 Norwalk virus vaccines: challenges and progress. J Infect Dis 181:S367–S373

Fankhauser RL, Noel JS, Monroe SS, Ando TA, Glass RI 1998 Molecular epidemiology of 'Norwalk-like viruses' in outbreaks of gastroenteritis in the United States. J Infect Dis 178:1571–1578

Flewett TH, Beards GM, Brown DW, Sanders RC 1987 The diagnostic gap in diarrhoeal aetiology. In: Novel diarrhoea viruses. Wiley, Chichester (Ciba Found Symp 128) p 238–249

Glass RI, Noel JS, Mitchell D et al 1996 The changing epidemiology of astrovirus-associated gastroenteritis: a review. Arch Virol Suppl 12:287–300

Glass RI, Noel J, Ando T et al 2000 The epidemiology of enteric caliciviruses from humans: a reassessment using new diagnostics. J Infect Dis (suppl 2) 181:S254–S261

Grohmann GS, Glass RI, Pereira HG et al 1993 Enteric viruses and diarrhea in HIV-infected patients. Enteric Opportunistic Infections Working Group. N Engl J Med 329:14–20

Hung T, Chen GM, Wang CG et al 1984 Waterborne outbreak of rotavirus diarrhoea in adults in China caused by a novel rotavirus. Lancet i:1139–1142

Jiang B, Dennehy PH, Spangenberger S, Gentsch JR, Glass RI 1995 First detection of group C rotavirus in fecal specimens of children with diarrhea in the United States. J Infect Dis 172:45–50

Kapikian AZ, Wyatt RG, Dolin R, Thornhill TS, Kalica AR, Chanock RM 1972 Visualization by immune electron microscopy of a 27 nm particle associated with acute infectious nonbacterial gastroenteritis. J Virol 10:1075–1081

Koopmans M, Petric M, Glass RI, Monroe SS 1993 Enzyme-linked immunosorbent assay reactivity of torovirus-like particles in fecal specimens from humans with diarrhea. J Clin Microbiol 31:2738–2744

Madeley CR, Cosgrove BP 1975 28 nm particles in faeces in infantile gastroenteritis. Lancet ii:451–452

Mead PS, Slutsker L, Dietz V et al 1999 Food-related illness and death in the United States. Emerg Infect Dis 5:607–625

Murray CJ, López AD 1997 Global mortality, disability, and the contribution of risk factors: Global Burden of Disease Study. Lancet 349:1436–1442

Nakagomi T, Nakagomi O 1989 RNA–RNA hybridization identifies a human rotavirus that is genetically related to feline rotavirus. J Virol 63:1431–1434

Pang X-L, Honma S, Nakata S, Vesikari T 2000 Human caliciviruses in acute gastroenteritis of young children in the community. J Infect Dis (suppl 2) 181:S288–S294

Pereira HG 1991 Double-stranded RNA viruses. Semin Virol 2:39–53

Rosen BI, Fang Z-Y, Glass RI, Monroe SS 2000 Cloning of human picorbirnavirus gene segments and development of an RT-PCR detection assay. Virology 277:316–329

Saif LJ, Jiang B 1994 Non group A rotaviruses of humans and animals. Curr Top Microbiol Immunol 185:339–371

Schaub SA, Oshiro RK 2000 Public health concerns about caliciviruses as waterborne contaminants. J Infect Dis (suppl 2) 181:S374–S380

Slutsker L, Ries AA, Greene KD, Wells JG, Hutwagner L, Griffin PM 1997 *Escherichia coli* 0157:H7 diarrhea in the United States: clinical and epidemiologic features. Ann Intern Med 126:505–513

Tucker AW, Haddix AC, Bresee JS, Holman RC, Parashar UD, Glass RI 1998 Cost-effectiveness analysis of a rotavirus immunization program for the United States. JAMA 279:1371–1376

Wadell G, Allard A, Johansson M, Svensson L, Uhnoo I 1987 Enteric adenoviruses. In: Novel diarrhoea viruses. Wiley, Chichester (Ciba Found Symp 128) p 63–91

Yamashita T, Kobayashi S, Sakae K et al 1991 Isolation of cytopathic small round viruses with BS-C-1 cells from patients with gastroenteritis. J Infect Dis 164:954–957

Yamashita T, Sakae K, Ishihara Y, Isomura S, Utagawa E 1993 Prevalence of newly isolated, cytopathic small round virus (Aichi strain) in Japan. J Clin Microbiol 31:2938–2943

Yamashita T, Sakae K, Kobayashi S et al 1995 Isolation of cytopathic small round virus (Aichi Virus) from Pakistani children and Japanese travelers from Southeast Asia. Microbiol Immunol 39:433–435

Yamashita T, Sakae K, Tsuzuki H et al 1998 Complete nucleotide sequence and genetic organization of Aichi virus, a distinct member of the *Picornaviridae* associated with acute gastroenteritis in humans. J Virol 72:8408–8412

DISCUSSION

Greenberg: I am confused by the figure you gave of total annual deaths from diarrhoea in children in the USA of 300. What I usually think of is the proportion of severe diarrhoea that is rotavirus related and the numbers you have given are rotavirus deaths. If I remember correctly, the number of rotavirus deaths in the USA is perhaps below 20, and I am having trouble getting from below 20 to 300 for total deaths.

Glass: The number of 300 deaths from diarrhoea is from our mortality death certificate data in children over one month of age. Our estimates of the number of deaths from rotavirus represent the excess of winter over summer deaths in children from 3–24 months of age, and this is in the range of 20–40 deaths a year. This has been one way to assess rotavirus deaths. Since 1993 we have had a new ICD code for rotavirus hospitalizations and can estimate the case fatality rate for rotavirus. Several studies have examined their hospital discharge records for rotavirus. New York State, for example, reports about one death in 800 children with a discharge coded as rotavirus diarrhoea. If you extrapolated these data to the nation, it would suggest that we have 50–60 rotavirus deaths based on the case fatality rate.

Greenberg: The 50 or 60 would be more compatible with the 300 total in my mind. The other question I have is where are we with biliary atresia and group C rotavirus? Do you believe that association?

Glass: We have been trying to reproduce it, and I don't think we have yet done the proper study. Dr Baoming Jiang in our group has obtained sequences of group C rotavirus from liver tissue of patients with biliary atresia; he also found some group C sequences in controls who did not have biliary atresia. He went back to do another study of people who were undergoing liver transplant and these children did not have any virus. We have to look specifically at liver tissue from patients with acute active disease and controls, and test specifically for group C sequences.

Greenberg: Several years ago we did similar studies and could find no group C sequences in our specimens of primary biliary atresia relatively late in the course of the disease.

Matson: With regard to biliary atresia, we used an epidemiological approach, looking at 22 paediatric hospitals. We tried to find correlations of peaks of diagnosis of biliary atresia and peaks of rotavirus illness using a cohort model. We were unable to find any clear correlation. Of course, this was for group A rotavirus and we were not assessing group C, which is far less common than group A.

Desselberger: Bernard Fields looked at this for reoviruses, and stated in his last publication that there was no association between biliary atresia and reoviral infection (Tyler & Fields 1996).

Glass: Rotavirus may cause other severe diseases also. For instance, the Japanese observed seizures in patients with rotavirus diarrhoea (Ushijima et al 1994). This observation was confirmed by others (Pang et al 1996, Yoshida et al 1995, Lynch et al 2001) but we are still uncertain whether this is a causal relationship.

Bishop: We have recently used RT-PCR to detect rotavirus in CSF of two children with rotavirus gastroenteritis associated with neurological abnormalities (Goldwater et al 2000).

Offit: Another mechanism for why you could detect rotavirus by specific RT-PCR in the CSF of a child with pleiocytosis associated with seizures is that if the child is infected with rotavirus, that viral antigen can be taken up in Peyer's patch cells, including macrophages. These are a mobile population of cells that can traffic in the circulation and can enter the CSF yet still not obviously be causative for that disease.

Estes: Roger Glass, you implied that you believe that there really is evidence for direct transmission of rotavirus from animals to humans. It has been my interpretation of the data that there is no direct proof of this. There is evidence that there are similar sequences or similar strains in humans and animals, but I don't know of any study that directly proves transmission.

Glass: The molecular evidence is compelling. When Nakagomi & Nakagomi (1989) found feline rotaviruses in Japanese children, I encouraged them to do a case control study, to see whether those children had cats in their homes, but this was never done. This is the kind of study that we need to confirm this. On the other hand, there are lots of strains in India that are bovine and human reassortants that are in wide circulation. The Brazilians have found many porcine–human reassortants. We don't know whether these represent one key reassortment event and this strain has proliferated, or a few key events, or whether this is happening on a regular basis.

Matson: If you step way back from the epidemiology and do a phylogenetic analysis of rotavirus genes 4, you get about 20 clades. But the key fact is that in almost every clade there is a strain that came from an animal and a strain that came from human. I don't know how this would happen without animal–human transmission.

Estes: I agree that the molecular data look compelling, but there is still no direct proof of virus transmission from animals to humans.

Koopmans: We are doing parallel studies in humans and animals, aimed at a broad range of pathogens, one of which is rotavirus. We have been looking at the diversity of rotaviruses just because of this question. If there is such a thing as interspecies transmission, does it occur? So far we haven't found any evidence for that in a three year study.

Brown: There are many parallels here with influenza A, which infects pigs, avians and humans. For many years, flu virologists have been trying to be in the right pig sty at the right time, but it is not easy to document interspecies transmission if it is rare. This may well be the case for both caliciviruses and rotaviruses.

Saif: I have a comment about the interspecies transmission of rotavirus. We may be looking in the wrong populations. We should be looking at immunodeficient individuals, as in the study from England, where Beards et al (1992) found a bovine-like rotavirus (serotype G10) in an immunodeficient child. There is also the study from Israel where rotaviruses that resembled feline rotaviruses were found in outpatient clinics (Silberstein et al 1995, Nakagomi et al 1990). When the investigators compared a matched rotavirus-infected group from more severely affected hospitalized patients, they didn't find them, suggesting that the feline-like rotaviruses caused milder infections in children. We should be looking in these outpatient clinic and immunodeficient populations for evidence of zoonotic rotavirus infections. It might not be a terribly common event. The interesting aspect would be what then leads to host–host transmission once the virus gets into the new host.

Brown: I agree with many of the observations made by Dr Glass in his presentation. Two points were not clear. First, the distinction between an endemic versus epidemic pattern of NLV infection. It is clear that the incidence of NLVs is highest in young children, and I doubt that the picture of NLVs as an epidemic disease will hold quite as well when more comprehensive information is available. You mentioned the study from Timo Vesikari which showed the importance of human enteric caliciviruses in the general population presenting to their primary care physicians with diarrhoea. In developed countries the role of NLVs is established, but do you know anything about the importance of NLVs in the developing world where the severity and disease burden are much greater? Might there be a different diagnostic gap in these two different situations?

Glass: We are involved in studies looking for caliciviruses in developing countries but do not have a complete answer yet. I think caliciviruses are the one virus type that bridges the endemic/epidemic gap. When I told my daughter that the seasonal peaks of rotavirus were not epidemics but rather seasonal endemics, she looked at me and said that I was no longer an epidemiologist, but an endemiologist!

Desselberger: Some time ago we and others carried out age-related seroprevalence studies using baculovirus recombinant expressed Norwalk virus capsid antigen and found some surprising results (Gray et al 1993, Numata et al 1994, Hinkula et al 1995). There were many probably silent infections during the first two years of life, and there seemed to be statistically significant increases of additional infection at entry into school, and in young adults (aged 20–29) who may become infected from their recently infected young children. Many diarrhoeal episodes which were previously not diagnosed as due to a specific cause may be due to calicivirus infections.

Glass: What distinguishes the study by Pang et al (2000) from previous ones is that if you look at the surveys done by electron microscopists, they rarely found an NLV in a child under 5 years old. Even Gary Grohmann, who looked at 8000 children's specimens, found the Sapporo-like caliciviruses in the younger children, but the NLVs in the older ones (Grohmann et al 1993). This was repeated by many groups. So we never knew whether NLVs in the very young were a pathogen or not. The study in Finland actually found the virus in children with diarrhoea and demonstrated that it is a pathogen.

Greenberg: Just to be slightly provocative, you also mentioned that we still don't know whether long-term immunity exists to caliciviruses. We do know that long-term immunity does not exist in a volunteer setting with a homologous challenge. These experiments have been done by Dr Neil Blacklow. We also know that adults with the antibody can get infected in the community.

Glass: Let me take issue with both of those statements. In all those old volunteer studies, a huge inoculum was given. In natural infection, we know that a virus can be infectious in a small inoculum. We know that mothers who have children with rotavirus infection can get a repeat episode of rotavirus infection even though they have antibody. We assume that this is because they are exposed to an overwhelming inoculum, just as mothers of children with cholera can get cholera even when they are immune. It may well be that some of your long-term immunity has to do with dose. Now that we have begun to sequence all of these caliciviruses and tried to put them into antigenic clusters, we are finding such diversity that we can get one virus today and another tomorrow, and still get sick with a bug that looks exactly the same with a sequence that is not very different. We have a lot to learn about the tremendous variability of that virus.

Desselberger: Roger, could you say more about the mode of transmission of endemic viruses? There are some aspects which are known, starting with neonatal infections in hospitals. There are difficulties in avoiding nosocomial infections despite disinfection and general hygiene measures (careful handwashing, etc.). In this context, it is significant that the infectious dose of transmission is so low. There are studies in rabbits and human volunteers that have shown that only a few infectious units of rotavirus (1–10 PFUs) are required to initiate an infection (Ward et al 1986, Graham et al 1987).

Glass: Nosocomial disease with rotavirus is important. Somewhere between one-fifth to one-third of children who are discharged from hospital with rotavirus had a nosocomial infection. What I don't understand is why children in developing countries get rotavirus year-round, and not just in winter. Winter seasonal disease can be explained by airborne spread or person–person contact. Year-round transmission might reflect different modes of transmission, such as from faecally contaminated water.

Kapikian: I believe, Roger, that your pie charts of aetiological agents of acute gastroenteritis have overestimated what we know. The pie of epidemic gastroenteritis has indeed been filled in substantially, but I disagree with your pie of aetiological agents for severe diarrhoea. In my aetiology pie of severe diarrhoea in developed and developing countries, the astroviruses comprise just a tiny sliver, as do the caliciviruses, whereas the rotaviruses comprise about 45%, leaving a void of about 45% in developed countries and a somewhat lesser void in the developing countries because of the role of bacteria in the latter areas. I believe that the pie of aetiological agents of severe diarrhoea still contains a large void, with rotaviruses clearly being the most important aetiological agents in both developed and developing countries.

Vesikari: There is no question that rotavirus causes more severe disease. If we use the traditional 20-point score in our population of children under the age of 3 years, the median score of rotavirus gastroenteritis in a prospectively followed cohort is 11. The median score of NLV gastroenteritis in the same population is 8. This is clearly number two. Astroviruses and SLVs are around 5 in this scale, so these are comparatively less severe diseases. The reason that NLV-associated enteritis in young children is less severe than rotavirus gastroenteritis is because it has a different clinical picture: rotavirus is both vomiting and diarrhoea, whereas NLV gastroenteritis tends to be more a vomiting disease. SLV is different from NLV in that it is a mild diarrhoeal disease.

I also wanted to comment on the epidemiology. Both NLV and SLV have a winter epidemic season, but they are distinct from each other. In contrast, rotavirus is seen all the year round. In the non-epidemic season it seems that the cases tend to be milder and often the quantity of virus is less, because it is detected by RT-PCR but not ELISA (Ehlken 1999). But the activity remains there. The same was found in Germany: in a hospital-based study there was a clear winter peak and the disease disappeared in the summer, but in the community-based study the winter peak is not that high and the disease did not disappear (Petersen 1999).

Glass: These observations are most interesting. I am thinking of the paper by Velazquez et al (1996) on the natural history of rotavirus. With the first rotavirus infection, most children shed virus in their stool and experienced seroconversion. With the second and third infections they had little shedding in the stool but much seroconversion. What you are saying is that there probably was shedding in the stool but only at a low titre, detectable by RT-PCR. Perhaps this year-round disease is the reservoir of reinfection.

Matson: I want to return to the issue of how much serious gastroenteritis may be calicivirus associated. I have some results from collaborative work in Santiago, Chile with Miguel O'Ryan (O'Ryan et al 2000). When they first looked at a large set of hospital specimens, they found just one calicivirus case using RT-PCR and primers NV35, NV36 and other pairs, out of hundreds of samples. This was a disappointing result. We sequenced the 35/36 product of that single case and aligned it with all the known 35/36 regions that we could find. It turned out that this strain was an SLV in a new clade. We came up with a new primer pair (p289/290). When we applied those new primers, we found by RT-PCR that over a three year period about 8% of hospitalizations for diarrhoea were associated with caliciviruses. In the first year, the detection rate was 16% of hospitalizations and by the third year it was 2%. What this tells me is that there is something about the epidemiology of these strains and how they move throughout a population that is very important to our understanding of burden of disease, and also how important it is to have strain- and locality-specific primers.

References

Beards G, Xu L, Ballard A, Desselberger U, McCrae MA 1992 A serotype 10 human rotavirus. J Clin Microbiol 30:1432–1435

Ehlken B 1999 Community-acquired rotavirus infections in Germany. Abstract book of the 17th annual meeting of the European Society for Paediatric Infectious Diseases, Heraklion, Crete, Greece, May 19–21, 1999, Abstract P-126

Goldwater PN, Rowland K, Power R et al 2000 Rotavirus encephalopathy: pathogenesis reviewed. J Paed Child Health, in press

Graham DY, Dufour GR, Estes MK 1987 Minimal infectious dose of rotavirus. Arch Virol 92:261–271

Gray JJ, Jiang X, Morgan-Capner P, Desselberger U, Estes MK 1993 The prevalence of antibody to Norwalk virus in England. Detection by ELISA using baculovirus-expressed Norwalk virus capsid antigen. J Clin Microbiol 31:1022–1025

Grohmann GS, Glass RI, Pereira HG et al 1993 Enteric viruses and diarrhea in HIV-infected patients. N Engl J Med 329:14–20

Hinkula J, Ball JM, Löfgren S, Estes MK, Svensson L 1995 Antibody prevalence and immunoglobulin IgG subclass pattern to Norwalk virus in Sweden. J Med Virol 47:52–57

Lynch M, Lee B et al 2001 Rotavirus and central nervous system complications: cause or contaminant? Case reports and review. Clin Infect Dis, in press

Nakagomi T, Nakagomi O 1989 RNA–RNA virus hybridisation identifies a human rotavirus that is genetically linked to feline rotavirus. J Virol 63:1431–1434

Nakagomi O, Ohshima A, Aboudy Y et al 1990 Molecular identification by RNA–RNA hybridization of a human rotavirus that is closely related to rotaviruses of feline and canine origin. J Clin Microbiol 28:1198–1203

Numata K, Nakata S, Jiang X, Estes MK, Chiba S 1994 Epidemiological study of Norwalk virus infections in Japan and Southeast Asia by enzyme linked immunosorbent assay with Norwalk virus capsid protein produced by the baculovirus expression system. J Clin Microbiol 32: 121–126

O'Ryan MZ, Mamani N, Gaggero A et al 2000 Human caliciviruses are a significant pathogen of acute sporadic diarrhea in children from Santiago, Chile. J Infect Dis 182:1519–1522

Pang X-L, Joensuu J, Vesikari T 1996 Detection of rotavirus RNA in cerebrospinal fluid in a case of rotavirus gastroenteritis with febrile seizures. Pediatr Infect Dis J 15:543–545

Pang X-L, Honma S, Nakata S, Vesikari T 2000 Human caliciviruses in acute gastroenteritis of young children in the community. J Infect Dis 172:1437–1444

Petersen G 1999 Hospitalizations due to rotavirus infections in Germany. Abstract book of the 17th annual meeting of the European Society for Paediatric Infectious Diseases, Heraklion, Crete, Greece, May 19–21, 1999, Abstract P-127

Silberstein I, Shulman L, Mendelson E, Shif I 1995 Distribution of rotavirus VP4 genotypes and VP7 serotypes among hospitalized and non-hospitalized Israeli children. J Clin Microbiol 33:1421–1422

Tyler KL, Fields BN 1996 Reoviruses. In: Fields BN, Knipe DM, Howley PM et al (eds) Fields Virology, 3rd edition. Lippincott-Raven, Philadelphia, p 1597–1623

Ushijima H, Xin KQ, Nishimura S, Morikawa S, Abe T 1994 Detection and sequencing of rotavirus VP7 gene from human materials (stools, sera, cerebrospinal fluids, and throat swabs) by reverse transcription and PCR. J Clin Microbiol 32:2893–2897

Velazquez FR, Matson DO, Calva JJ et al 1996 Rotavirus infection in infants as protection against subsequent infections. N Engl J Med 335:1022–1028

Ward RL, Bernstein DI, Young EC, Sherwood JR, Knowlton DR, Schiff GM 1986 Human rotavirus studies in volunteers: determination of infectious dose and serological response to infection. J Infect Dis 154:871–880

Yoshida A, Kawamitu T, Tanaka R et al 1995 Rotavirus encephalitis: detection of the virus genomic RNA in the cerebrospinal fluid of a child. Pediatr Infect Dis J 14:914–916

Novartis 238: Gastroenteritis Viruses.
Copyright © 2001 John Wiley & Sons Ltd
Print ISBN 0-471-49663-4 eISBN 0-470-84653-4

Structural studies on gastroenteritis viruses

B. V. Venkataram Prasad*, S. Crawford†, J. A. Lawton*[1], J. Pesavento*, M. Hardy†[2], and M. K. Estes†

Verna and Maars McLean Department of Biochemistry and Molecular Biology, and †Department of Molecular Virology and Microbiology, Baylor College of Medicine, One Baylor Plaza, Houston, TX 77030, USA

Abstract. There are many recent advances in our understanding of the structure-function relationships in rotavirus, a major pathogen of infantile gastroenteritis, and Norwalk virus, a causative agent of epidemic gastroenteritis in humans. Rotavirus is a large (1000 Å) and complex icosahedral assembly formed by three concentric capsid layers that enclose the viral genome of 11 dsRNA segments. Because of its medical relevance, intriguing structural complexity, and several unique strategies in the morphogenesis and replication, this virus has been the subject of extensive biochemical, genetic and structural studies. Using a combination of electron cryomicroscopy and computer image processing together with atomic resolution X-ray structural information, we have been able to provide not only a better description of the rotavirus architecture, but also a better understanding of the structural basis of various biological functions such as trypsin-enhanced infectivity, virus assembly and the dynamic process of endogenous transcription. In contrast to rotavirus, Norwalk virus has a simple architecture with an icosahedral capsid made of 180 copies of a single protein. We have determined the structure of the Norwalk virus capsid to a resolution of 3.4 Å using X-ray crystallographic techniques. These studies have provided valuable information on domain organization in the capsid protein, and residues that may be critical for dimerization, assembly, strain-specificity and antigenicity.

2001 Gastroenteritis viruses. Wiley, Chichester (Novartis Foundation Symposium 238) p 26–46

In recent years electron cryoelectron microscopy coupled with computer image processing (cryo-EM), and X-ray crystallography have provided valuable structural information on gastroenteritis viruses such as rotavirus and Norwalk virus. These studies have provided further insights into the intricate molecular

Present addresses: [1]Department of Chemistry and Biochemistry, 0314, University of California at San Diego, 9500 Gilman Drive, San Diego, CA 92093, USA and [2]Veterinary Molecular Biology, Montana State Univ., Bozeman, MT 59717, USA mechanisms underlying various aspects of the viral life cycle. Here we review recent progress in the structural characterization of these two viruses.

Structural studies on rotavirus

The biochemistry and molecular biology of rotaviruses are well characterized (Estes 1996). Rotaviruses belong to the family of viruses called *Reoviridae*. The rotavirus particle contains multiple protein layers enclosing the genome that consists of 11 segments of double-stranded (ds) RNA. Each segment codes for one protein with the exception of segment 11 that codes for two proteins. Out of the 12 proteins, six are structural and six are non-structural. The outer capsid layer is made of VP7 and VP4. The intermediate layer is composed of VP6. Enclosed within these two layers is the core consisting of VP2, VP1 and VP3. VP1 and VP3 are minor internal proteins present in small quantities. The non-structural proteins participate in various functions during the life cycle of the virus.

To provide a biological perspective to our structural studies, a brief outline of the virus life cycle is given below. The first event in the life cycle of the virus is its interaction with the host cell. It remains unclear as to how rotaviruses enter the cell (see Arias et al 2001, this volume). It is either through an endocytotic pathway or through direct penetration of the cell membrane. The choice of pathway seems to depend upon whether or not the virus is trypsinized. Non-trypsinized viruses may enter the host cell through the rather inefficient endocytotic pathway. On the other hand, the trypsinized viruses may enter by direct penetration (Kaljot et al 1988). During cell entry, mature virions, which are triple-layered particles (TLPs), lose their outer shell and the resulting double-layered particles (DLPs) become transcriptionally active. Endogenous transcription, a common feature of dsRNA viruses, is a dynamic and fascinating process. During this process, the 11 dsRNA segments are transcribed inside the intact DLPs and the mRNA molecules are released. These mRNA molecules act as templates for the progeny RNA and code for all the structural and non-structural proteins (see Patton 2001, this volume). Out of the 12 proteins, 10 are synthesized on the free ribosomes. The other two — VP7, the major outer layer glycoprotein and a non-structural protein, NSP4 — are synthesized on the ribosomes associated with the rough endoplasmic reticulum (RER) where they are co-translationally inserted into the ER membrane. The assembly of progeny DLPs takes place in a specialized compartment called the viroplasm. Newly formed DLPs bud through the ER membrane. NSP4, the non-structural protein localized in the ER membrane, acts as an intracellular receptor and facilitates the budding of the DLPs through the ER membrane. Recently, it has been shown that NSP4 is a viral enterotoxin and by itself can cause diarrhoea in mice (see Estes et al 2001, this volume). One of the unique steps in the morphogenesis of rotavirus is the formation of transiently

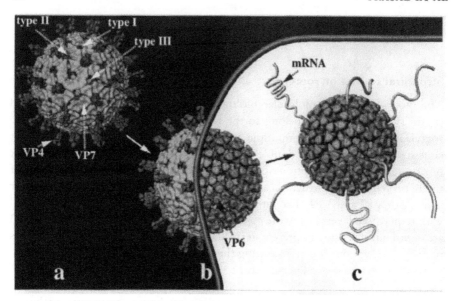

FIG. 1.   Structures of rotavirus TLP (a) and DLP shown in the context of cell entry and removal of the outer layer (b), and transcription (c) inside the cell. Various structural features in the outer layer of the TLP—three types of channels, VP4 spikes, and VP7 trimers are indicated by dashed arrows in (a). In (b) a dashed arrow shows one of the 260 VP6 trimers in the DLP. The nascent mRNA molecules, shown as curvy cylinders in (c) exit through type I channels in the DLP (Lawton et al 1997a). All the structures are shown as viewed along their icosahedral threefold axis. The structures of TLP, DLP and the transcribing particle were determined using cryo-EM techniques.

enveloped particles. Rotavirus particles exit the cells by lysing the cell, or by a non-classical vesicular transport from polarized cells.

We have used the cryo-EM technique to understand the structural basis of trypsin-enhanced infectivity, endogenous transcription, replication, assembly processes, and the budding of the DLPs through the ER membrane (Prasad & Estes 1997, 2000). We review here recent progress on the structure–function relationships in rotavirus.

Overall organization of rotavirus

Rotavirus is an icosahedral particle with an overall diameter of 1000 Å (Fig. 1a). The capsid architecture is built on an icosahedral T=13 lattice (Prasad et al 1988). Two distinct surface features of the structure are spikes, and channels. The channels are located at all the 5- and 6-coordinated positions of the T=13 lattice. Three types of channels are present, depending on their locations with respect to the icosahedral symmetry axes. The type I channels are at the fivefold axes, type II channels surround the icosahedral 5-fold axes, and type III channels neighbour the threefold axes. Each particle has a total of 132 channels — 12 type I, 60 type II and 60 type III channels. VP7, which constitutes the outer layer, clusters into trimers surrounding the channels. Each particle has 260 trimers or 780 molecules of VP7. There are 60 spikes, located at one edge of the type II channels, in each particle.

Our structural analysis using anti-VP4 monoclonal antibodies (MAb) has shown that the spikes are made up of VP4 (Prasad et al 1990). Two molecules of the Fab bind on either side of the bi-lobed head of each spike. VP4 has been implicated in cell entry, neutralization, virulence, and in some animal viruses it is a haemagglutinin (reviewed in Estes 1996). The first MAb that was used in this study is a neutralizing antibody that affects virus binding to cells and prevents internalization of the virus. This MAb binds to the side of the bilobed head of the spike, indicating that this region on the spike is important for neutralization. In addition to interacting with VP7, the outer layer protein, VP4 also interacts with VP6 through a distinct globular domain that is buried inside the type II channels underneath the VP7 layer (Shaw et al 1993, Yeager et al 1994).

During trypsinization, which is known to cause a significant increase in the infectivity of rotavirus (Estes et al 1981), VP4 is cleaved into two fragments VP5* and VP8* that remain associated with the virion (Arias et al 1996). What is the molecular mechanism of trypsin-enhanced infectivity? One answer to this question could come from locating the two proteolytic fragments in the spike structure. Our recent biochemical and structural studies on the TLPs grown in the presence of trypsin and in the absence of trypsin provided some insights into trypsin-enhanced infectivity in rotavirus (S. E. Crawford, M. K. Estes, S. Mukherjee, A. Shaw, J. A. Lawton, R. F. Ramig & B. V. V. Prasad 2000, unpublished results). Based on these studies we have hypothesized that trypsin, by a mechanism that is not yet clear, imparts stability and order to the spike, and such an ordering may be critical not only during the cell entry but also during virus exit, from infected cells.

During the process of cell entry, the mature infectious particle loses its outer layer and becomes a DLP (Fig. 1b). Removal of the outer layer exposes the intermediate layer composed of VP6. This layer also has the same T = 13 icosahedral symmetry as the outer layer and consists of 260 trimers of VP6. These trimers are in register radially with the VP7 trimers such that the channels in the VP7 layer continue into this layer. Recently, the atomic resolution structure of the VP6 protein of rotavirus has been determined by X-ray crystallography (F. Rey, personal communication). The VP6 protein has two domains, the distal domain that interacts with VP7 has an eight-stranded antiparallel β-barrel structure, and the lower domain that interacts with inner VP2 layer is predominantly α-helical. The structure of VP6 bears significant resemblance to the homologous protein (VP7) of blue-tongue virus

(BTV; Grimes et al 1995). Fitting of the X-ray structure of VP6 into the cryo-EM map of the DLP has allowed examination of how this protein adapts to various quasi-equivalent positions of the T = 13 lattice and delineation of the residues that are critical for interactions with VP7, VP4 and VP2.

The outer virion layer consisting of VP7 and VP4 can be removed *in vitro* by treating the TLPs with 10 mM EDTA. The DLPs thus obtained are transcriptionally active and the dsRNA segments are transcribed continuously *in vitro* as long as the precursors necessary for transcription are available in the reaction mixture (Cohen 1977, Cohen & Dobos 1979). Several interesting questions can be asked in connection with the endogenous transcription in rotaviruses. Where are the internal proteins VP1 (the RNA-dependent RNA polymerase; Valenzuela et al 1991) and VP3 (the guanylyl transferase; Liu et al 1992) located? Knowing that the DLPs are capable of repeated cycles of transcription, the question is how are the genome segments organized? Where do the mRNA molecules exit from the intact DLPs? Can blocking the RNA exit channels using ligands arrest transcription?

Internal organization

The strategy that we have used to study the internal organization is as follows (Prasad et al 1996). First, the structures of various recombinant virus-like particles (VLPs) (Crawford et al 1994) were compared between themselves and with the native DLPs to deduce the topographical locations of all the internal structural proteins. Then, higher resolution structural analysis was carried out using a medium high-voltage electron microscope to delineate the internal features, particularly of the RNA, in greater detail. Underlying the VP6 layer, VP2 forms the innermost icosahedral layer between the radii 230 Å and 260 Å (Fig. 2). Apart from VP2, no other rotavirus structural protein has the ability to form native-like icosahedral structures. Thus, VP2 performs the function of the size determinant in rotavirus and provides a platform for the correct assembly of VP6. The diameter and the morphological features of the 2/6 and 1/3/2/6-VLPs match very well with that of the native DLPs indicating that the recombinant particles are in all respects native-like. When the structure of the 1/2/3/6-VLP is compared with that of the 2/6-VLP, flower-shaped structural features attached to the inner surface of the VP2 layer are seen at the fivefold vertices. These flower-shaped structures represent VP1/3 complexes. We think that they represent complexes of VP1 and VP3, because these structures are not seen in either 1/2/6-VLPs or 3/2/6-VLPs. Comparison of the native DLP structure with the structure of 1/2/3/6-VLPs indicates that the genomic RNA forms concentric shells of density surrounding the flower-shaped VP1/3 complexes immediately below the VP2 layer (Fig. 2, bottom panel, right).

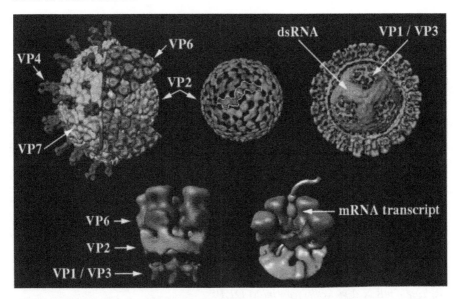

FIG. 2. General architectural features of rotavirus. Top panel: (Left) A cutaway representation of the TLP structure. The outer VP7 layer and the intermediate VP6 layer are partially removed to expose the inner VP2 layer. (Middle) The VP2 layer showing the organization of the 120 molecules as 60 dimers (Lawton et al 1997b). (Right) The RNA layers inside the VP2 layer. The VP6 and VP2 layers are 'opened' to expose the RNA core (Prasad et al 1996). Bottom panel: (Left) A side view of an 'isolated' type I channel showing the VP1/VP3 flower-shaped complex attached to the inside tip of the VP2 layer at the fivefold axis. (Right) Proposed exit pathway of the mRNA molecule through the type I channel (Lawton et al 1997a).

In the higher-resolution structure of the DLP, at a slightly higher threshold the RNA density splits into strand-like features, which are about 20 Å in diameter and separated by 28 Å (Fig. 2, top panel, right). The first layer of RNA immediately below the VP2 layer is icosahedrally ordered. This layer represents about 25% of the genome, or about 5000 base pairs. The remainder of the genome is further inside. The density at the lower radius is not highly reproducible between the independent reconstructions and may not be as well ordered as the first layer of RNA. However, in the near atomic resolution structure of BTV, in which similar features are seen, even the inner layers of RNA are interpreted as being ordered (Grimes et al 1998). The first layer of RNA is well ordered because of its close interactions with VP2, which is icosahedrally ordered and is known to have RNA binding properties (Labbé et al 1994). Since our publication in 1996 (Prasad et al 1996), similar internal structural features including the flower-shaped transcriptase complex and the concentric layers of RNA have been found in several members of *Reoviridae* such as BTV (Grimes et al 1998), aquareovirus

(Shaw et al 1996, Nason et al 2000), and orthoreovirus (Dryden et al 1998, Reinisch et al 2000).

The structural organization of the VP2 layer is unique (Lawton et al 1997a). The thin shell of VP2 is formed by 60 dimers of VP2 (Fig. 2, top panel, middle). Such an organization, which has been described as a T=2 structure, appears to be a common feature in the dsRNA viruses whose structures we know to date. Although the atomic resolution structure of VP2 is not yet available, the structure of homologous VP3 in BTV is known from the X-ray crystallographic studies of the BTV cores (Grimes et al 1998). It is quite likely that the structure of the VP2 will be very similar to that of VP3 in BTV with three domains. It appears that this kind of unique organization in all the dsRNA viruses has evolved because of the requirement for endogenous transcription. Such an organization may be critical for the (1) proper positioning of the transcription enzyme complexes, (2) proper organization of the genomic RNA, and (3) proper organization of the outer VP6 layer.

Release of mRNA molecules from intact DLPs

We have used the cryo-EM technique to visualize the exit pathway of the transcripts in actively transcribing DLPs (Lawton et al 1997b). The cryo-EM pictures of the DLPs in the act of transcription clearly show that the structural integrity of the particles is maintained and as many as four mRNA strands are associated with some of the particles. Based on the 3D structural analysis of the actively transcribing particles (Fig. 1c), a model for the exit pathway of the transcript has been proposed (Fig. 2, bottom panel, right). The mRNA molecule that is being synthesized by the transcription complex (flower-shaped structure), exits through the pores in the VP2 layer that are slightly offset from the fivefold axis and gets into the type 1 channel. Similar cryo-EM analysis on transcribing orthoreovirus particles has shown that channels through the turrets at the icosahedral fivefold axes are used for the extrusion of nascent transcripts (M. Yeager, personal communication). It is quite likely that the exit pathway for the mRNA involves fivefold vertices in other members of the *Reoviridae*.

Although the structural organization of the genome in dsRNA viruses is far from being clear, the existing data appear to support a model in which each genome segment is spooled around a transcription complex. In such a model, consistent with the biochemical data, the segments can be simultaneously and repeatedly transcribed. With such a genomic organization, each dsRNA segment has to move around the transcription-enzyme complex that is anchored to the VP2 layer. What drives such a movement of the template? Are the ends of the dsRNA molecule somehow tethered? What are the interactions that are required in the genomic organization that facilitate such a coordinated movement of the template around the enzyme complexes? Further studies are required to answer these questions. Our recent structural studies to probe further the genomic organization by varying pH and ionic concentrations have shown that hydrogen bond interactions between internal proteins and RNA, and the electrostatic interactions between the RNA strands, are important for proper genome organization (B. Pesavento, J. Lawton, M. K. Estes, B. V. V. Prasad 2000, unpublished results).

Inhibition of transcription by ligands that interact with VP6

Is it possible to arrest transcription by blocking the mRNA exit channels, and can this be exploited to become an antiviral strategy? This question is particularly relevant because it has been shown that 2/6-VLPs can confer protective immunity in mice (O'Neal et al 1998), and also that anti-VP6 IgA molecules can protect mice from rotavirus infection (Burns et al 1996). Can anti-VP6 MAbs inhibit transcription? Earlier biochemical studies with anti-VP6 MAbs showed that some MAbs completely inhibited transcription, while others did not (Ginn et al 1992). A natural ligand to VP6 is VP7. Binding of VP7 to VP6 makes the DLPs transcriptionally incompetent. Why are the TLPs transcriptionally inactive?

Our structural studies have shown that certain ligands (2A11 Fab and VP7) narrow the mRNA exit channels and also cause slight conformational changes in VP6 constricting the exit channels in the interior regions (Lawton et al 1999). A relevant question is whether the narrowing of the channel opening and/or the small but consistent conformational changes in the interior of the exit channels are the reasons for transcriptional inhibition. The process of transcription can be described as having three stages: initiation, elongation and translocation. To determine at which stage transcription is inhibited we have analysed high-resolution RNA gels of transcription reaction mixtures containing transcriptionally competent (DLPs and 8H2 Fab-bound DLPs) and transcriptionally incompetent (TLPs and 2A11 Fab-bound DLPs) particles. These studies have shown that the initiation of transcription is not affected in any of these particles. A consistent feature in all the cases is the presence of a band that corresponds to transcripts of about 6–7 nucleotides in length. Our recent studies have shown that this represents a pause site, and in the case of DLPs the transcription continues past this pause site in an efficient manner to yield full-length transcripts (J. A. Lawton, M. K. Estes & B. V. V Prasad 2000, unpublished results). In the case of 2A11-bound DLPs, only a small number of transcripts of about 70–80 nucleotides in length are made. In TLPs no other transcripts are made past this pause site. It is quite possible that the narrowing of the channel opening is the reason for the transcriptional inhibition in the case of 2A11-bound DLPs. However that is certainly not the reason in the case of TLPs. It is possible that there is a subtle conformational switch that is on when the VP7 layer is removed and off when it is intact. Higher resolution structural analysis may provide some insight into why TLPs are transcriptionally incompetent.

Structural studies on Norwalk virus capsids

Norwalk virus, a member of the *Caliciviridae*, is a prototype human calicivirus that causes epidemic acute gastroenteritis (Kapikian et al 1996). Human caliciviruses have been very difficult to adapt to cell culture systems. The lack of a cell culture system or a practical animal model has to some extent limited the progress in understanding the molecular characteristics of the virus and its replication strategies. However, the successful cloning of the Norwalk virus genome and its expression using the baculovirus system has alleviated this problem and begun to provide a better insight into the epidemiological, immunological, biochemical and other functional properties of the virus (Jiang et al 1990, 1993, Estes & Hardy 1995, Clarke & Lambden 2001 this volume).

In contrast to rotaviruses, Norwalk virus and the other members of the *Caliciviridae* are significantly smaller (diameter ~ 400 Å) and architecturally simpler viruses. The icosahedral capsids of caliciviruses are made of a single structural protein. In these viruses, 180 molecules of the structural protein form a $T=3$ icosahedral capsid (Prasad et al 1994a,b) that contains the viral genome of positive sense single-stranded RNA of approximately 7.5 kb.

Atomic resolution structure of the Norwalk virus capsid

Recently the X-ray crystallographic structure of the recombinant Norwalk virus capsid (Fig. 3) has been determined to 3.4 Å resolution using a low-resolution cryo-EM structure as an initial phasing model (Prasad et al 1999). The structure of the capsid protein exhibits both classical and novel features. The N-terminal 220 residues constitute the S-domain and fold into a classical eight-stranded β-sandwich. The rest of the sequence constitutes the protruding (P) domain and has a fold unlike any other viral protein. The P domain consists of two sub-domains: P2 and P1 (Fig. 3b). An interesting discovery is that the polypeptide fold of the distal P2 domain is similar to that seen in the domain 2 of the EF-Tu protein, an important factor in the biosynthesis of proteins. The functional significance of this structural similarity is still unclear. The distal P2 domain, which exhibits large sequence variation between various Norwalk-like viruses, unlike the S and the P1 domains that are better conserved, may serve as a replaceable module to provide strain specificity. As observed in other $T=3$ viruses (Rossmann & Johnson 1989), there are two distinct conformational dimeric states of the capsid protein: the 'flat' C/C dimers at the icosahedral twofold axes, and the 'bent' A/B dimers at the quasi twofold axes. During the assembly process, the dimer has to switch from one type to the other. Where is

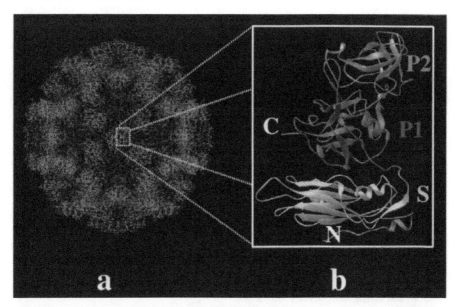

FIG. 3.   Structure of the Norwalk virus capsid. (a) Structure of the recombinant Norwalk virus capsid at 3.4 Å resolution. (b) The ribbon representation of the capsid protein (C subunit) structure. The structure of the capsid protein is shown oriented such that the top is at the exterior of the capsid and the bottom faces the interior. Various domains and subdomains are indicated (Prasad et al 1999).

the switch? We have seen that the N-terminal arm of the B subunit is more ordered than that in the A or C subunits. Based on our structural observations, we have proposed that: (1) the N-terminal 20 residues of the capsid protein may serve as a switch for the capsid assembly, and (2) the hinge region together with the C-terminal residues in the P1 domain that forms hydrogen bonds with the S domain residues are important for conferring the appropriate curvature for the dimers to assemble onto a T=3 icosahedral shell. This atomic resolution model can now allow a systematic mutational analysis, which is in progress, in order to understand the assembly mechanism and other functional properties of Norwalk virus and other caliciviruses.

Acknowledgements

Our work is supported in part by grants from the NIH (AI 36040 and DK 31044, AI46581), and the R. W. Welch Foundation.

References

Arias CF, Guerrero CA, Méndez E et al 2001 Early events of rotavirus infection: the search for the receptor(s). In: Gastroenteritis viruses. Wiley, Chichester (Novartis Found Symp 238) p 47–63

Arias CF, Romero P, Alvarez V, López S 1996 Trypsin activation pathway of rotavirus infectivity. J Virol 70:5832–5839

Burns JW, Siadat-Pajouh M, Krishnaney A, Greenberg HB 1996 Protective effect of rotavirus VP6-specific IgA monoclonal antibodies that lack neutralizing activity. Science 272:104–107

Clarke IN, Lambden PR 2001 The molecular biology of human caliciviruses. In: Gastroenteritis viruses. Wiley, Chichester (Novartis Found Symp 238) p 180–196

Cohen J 1977 Ribonucleic acid polymerase activity associated with purified calf rotavirus. J Gen Virol 36:395–402

Cohen J, Dobos P 1979 Cell free transcription and translation of rotavirus RNA. Biochem Biophys Res Commun 88:791–796

Crawford SE, Labbé M, Cohen J, Burroughs MH, Zhou YJ, Estes MK 1994 Characterization of virus-like particles produced by the expression of rotavirus capsid proteins in insect cells. J Virol 68:5945–5922

Dryden KA, Farsetta DL, Wang G et al 1998 Internal/structures containing transcriptase-related proteins in top component particles of mammalian orthoreovirus. Virology 245:33–46

Estes MK 1996 Rotaviruses and their replication. In: Fields BN, Knipe DM, Howley PM et al (eds) Virology. Raven Press, New York, p 1625–1655

Estes MK, Hardy ME 1995 Norwalk viruses and other enteric caliciviruses. In: Blaser MJ, Smith PD, Ravdin JI, Greenberg HB, Guerrant RL (eds) Infections of the gastrointestinal tract. Raven Press New York, p 1009–1034

Estes MK, Graham DY, Mason BB 1981 Proteolytic enhancement of rotavirus infectivity: molecular mechanisms. J Virol 39:879–888

Estes MK, Kang G, Zeng CQY, Crawford SE, Ciarlet M 2001 Pathogenesis of rotavirus gastroenteritis. In: Gastroenteritis viruses. Wiley, Chichester (Novartis Found Symp 238) p 82–100

Ginn DI, Ward RL, Hamparin VV, Hughes JH 1992 Inhibition of rotavirus *in vitro* transcription by optimal concentrations of monoclonal antibodies specific for rotavirus VP6. J Gen Virol 73:3017–3022

Grimes J, Basak AK, Roy P, Stuart D 1995 The crystal structure of bluetongue virus VP7. Nature 373:167–170

Grimes JM, Burroughs JN, Gouet P et al 1998 The atomic structure of the bluetongue virus core. Nature 395:470–478

Jiang X, Graham DY, Wang K, Estes MK 1990 Norwalk virus genome cloning and characterization. Science 250:1580–1583

Jiang X, Wang M, Wang K, Estes MK 1993 Sequence and genomic organization of Norwalk virus. Virology 195:51–61

Kapikian AZ, Estes MK, Chanock RM 1996 Norwalk group of viruses. In: Fields BN, Knipe DM, Howley PM et al (eds) Virology. Raven Press, New York, p 783–803

Kaljot KT, Shaw RD, Rubin DH, Greenberg HB 1988 Infectious rotavirus enters cells by direct cell membrane penetration, not by endocytosis. J Virol 62:1136–1144

Labbé M, Baudoux P, Charpilienne A, Poncet D, Cohen J 1994 Identification of the nucleic acid binding domain of the rotavirus VP2 protein. J Gen Virol 75:3423–3430

Lawton JA, Estes MK, Prasad BVV 1997a Three-dimensional visualization of mRNA release from actively transcribing rotavirus particles. Nat Struct Biol 4:118–121

Lawton JA, Zeng CQ, Mukherjee SK, Cohen J, Estes MK, Prasad BVV 1997b Three-dimensional structural analysis of recombinant rotavirus-like particles with intact and amino-terminal-deleted VP2: implications for the architecture of the VP2 capsid layer. J Virol 71:7353–7360

Lawton JA, Estes MK, Prasad BVV 1999 Comparative structural analysis of transcriptionally competent and incompetent rotavirus-antibody complexes. Proc Natl Acad Sci USA 96:5428–5433

Liu M, Mattion NM, Estes MK 1992 Rotavirus VP3 expressed in insect cells possesses guanylyltransferase activity. Virology 188:77–84

Nason E, Samal S, Prasad BVV 2000 Trypsin-induced structural transformation in aquareovirus. J Virol 74:6546–6555

O'Neal CE, Clements JD, Estes MK, Conner ME 1998 Rotavirus 2/6 viruslike particles administered intranasally with cholera toxin, Escherichia coli heat-labile toxin (LT), and LT-R192G induce protection from rotavirus challenge. J Virol 72:3390–3393

Patton JT 2001 Rotavirus RNA replication and gene expression. In: Gastroenteritis viruses. Wiley, Chichester (Novartis Found Symp 238) p 64–81

Prasad BVV, Estes MK 1997 Molecular basis of rotavirus replication: structure-function correlations. In: Chiu W, Burnett R, Garcia R, (eds) Structural Biology of Viruses. Oxford University Press, New York, p 239–268

Prasad BVV, Estes MK 2000 On the use of electron cryomicroscopy and computer image processing to study rotavirus. In: Gray J, Desselberger U (eds) Rotaviruses: methods and protocols. Humana Press, New Jersey, p 9–32

Prasad BVV, Wang G J, Clerx JP, Chiu W 1988 Three-dimensional structure of rotavirus. J Mol Biol 199:269–275

Prasad BVV, Burns JW, Marietta E, Estes MK, Chiu W 1990 Localization of VP4 neutralization sites in rotavirus by three-dimensional cryo-electron microscopy. Nature 343:476–479

Prasad BVV, Rothnagel R, Jiang X, Estes MK 1994a Three-dimensional structure of baculovirus-expressed Norwalk virus capsids. J Virol 68:5117–5125

Prasad BVV, Matson DO, Smith AW 1994b Three-dimensional structure of calicivirus. J Mol Biol 240:256–264

Prasad BVV, Rothnagel R, Zeng CQ et al 1996 Visualization of ordered genomic RNA and localization of transcriptional complexes in rotavirus. Nature 382:471–473

Prasad BVV, Hardy M, Dokland T et al 1999 Structure of Norwalk virus at 3.4 Å resolution. Science 286:287–290

Reinisch KM, Nibert ML, Harrison SC 2000 Structure of reovirus core at 3.6 Å resolution. Nature 404:960–967

Rossmann MG, Johnson JE 1989 Icosahedral RNA virus structure. Annu Rev Biochem 58:533–573

Shaw AL, Rothnagel R, Chen D, Ramig RF, Chiu W, Prasad VV 1993 Three-dimensional visualization of the rotavirus hemagglutinin structure. Cell 74:693–701

Shaw AL, Samal SK, Subramanian K, Prasad BVV 1996 The structure of aquareovirus shows how the different geometries of the two layers of the capsid are reconciled to provide symmetrical interactions and stabilization. Structure 4:957–967

Valenzuela S, Pizarro J, Sandino AM et al 1991 Photoaffinity labeling of rotavirus VP1 with 8-azido-ATP: identification of the viral RNA polymerase. J Virol 65:3964–3967

Yeager M, Berriman JA, Baker TS, Bellamy AR 1994 Three-dimensional structure of the rotavirus haemagglutinin VP4 by cryo-electron microscopy and difference map analysis. EMBO J 13:1011–1018

DISCUSSION

Greenberg: I am not sure I understood your trypsin studies with rotavirus. Was the implication that trypsin must enter the cell, because it has a different effect if you grow the virus in the presence of trypsin?

Prasad: There is no evidence that trypsin could enter the cell. Whenever we have grown the viruses in the complete absence of trypsin, we don't see well formed spikes. There has to be some kind of mechanism operating in which trypsin confers proper stability to the spikes.

Greenberg: But it doesn't work as well if you treat the virus after the infection cycle.

Prasad: That's right, you can't get the same effect. But in another experiment where the viruses were grown in the presence of trypsin, the trypsin was present throughout the infection cycle. There was no attempt to remove the trypsin. This is why we did experiments that involved adding the trypsin to viruses grown in its absence. You can see the spikes taking shape, but not to the same extent as we saw in the viruses grown in the continuous presence of trypsin. Trypsin is certainly conferring stability in the spike, but in addition it is probably doing something else as well, particularly in the viruses grown in the presence of trypsin.

Estes: I interpret the trypsin data as showing that there is a previously unrecognized intracellular cleavage event.

Koopmans: How physiological are the two trypsin modifications? You do the observation in the culture system, but how do you go from that to the situation in the gut? I can't envision the trypsin cleavage in the gut on the way out of the cells.

Prasad: The occurrence of trypsinization is natural. When the virus is grown in the absence of trypsin it is not actually physiological. By the time a virus infects the enterocytes, its VP4 is already cleaved. In order to understand what is really happening our strategy was to grow the virus in the presence of trypsin, but then, when we added exogenous trypsin we found that VP4 does not undergo any conformational change. By adding a lot of trypsin it seems that we are introducing conformational changes in the VP7 molecule. We don't know the biological relevance of this.

Arias: The trypsin concentration usually employed to activate the different strains of rotaviruses is $5-10\,\mu g/ml$. Even at $50-100\,\mu g/ml$, we have not found any evidence that VP7 is cleaved.

Prasad: Let me make it clear: VP7 is not cleaved. It is a conformational change that takes place. There is a domain in VP7 that is tucked inside, and when trypsin is added, this domain moves around. If cleavage were to occur, then we would see this in the gel. Sue Crawford has run the gel adding trypsin to VP4, which seems to be further cleaved with the addition of more trypsin. We have also sequenced those bands in gels and found out exactly where the cleavage takes place. Despite the cleavage the structure of VP4 remains the same with added trypsin. The only change we see on adding $25-50\,\mu g/ml$ trypsin is in VP7.

Arias: Do you mean that the trypsin is actually modifying the structure of VP7 without cleaving it? Or might it be that the cleavage in VP4 that is known to occur is inducing the change in VP7?

Prasad: It is quite possible. The change that we have seen in VP7, which is very consistent, is some distance away from where VP4 is. It is surrounding the type 3 channels, whereas VP4 is at the type 2 channel. It is quite likely that changes in VP4 might be propagated because it is a part of the lattice, and VP7 could then loosen up for this domain movement to occur.

Carter: With regard to the use of trypsin, I've always had a slight uneasiness that in a sense it reflects our own lack of imagination that we put trypsin into these cultures. Perhaps it is not the only enzyme that these viruses actually need — it could even be that this is not the main one *in vivo*.

Arias: The protease-induced enhancement of rotavirus infectivity seems to be specific for trypsin or at least for a trypsin-like protease. There seems to be a window in VP4 of about 20 amino acids, the trypsin cleavage region of this protein, that is susceptible to cleavage by proteases with different specificity. However, only cleavage by trypsin at arginine 247 seems to efficiently activate the virus infectivity (Arias et al 1996, Gilbert & Greenberg 1998). Have you tried proteases different from trypsin, which despite cleaving the protein do not activate virus infectivity, to see if these will also induce changes in VP7?

Prasad: No, we haven't done that. We have only been working with the trypsin. This was one of the projects that one of my graduate students took up. Every time, she was coming up with a reconstruction without spikes. I thought she was doing something wrong in growing this virus, but then we realized that viruses grown in the absence of trypsin lacked spikes. We don't know why that happens.

Desselberger: I think we should realize how novel this model is. If you look at well studied systems such as uptake of influenza virus and HIV, these show a conformational change within the cleaved haemagglutinin or glycoprotein after contact with the receptor and at the stage of membrane fusion (e.g. Bullough et al 1994). In contrast, we don't really know yet what is happening here.

Prasad: What we have seen is rather counterintuitive. When we began the study, I thought that trypsinization would confer conformational changes just like in the case of haemagglutinin where there is a massive conformational change. We don't see that. It has something to do with assembly in the complete absence of trypsin. We also wondered whether trypsin inhibitors are making the assembly of VP4 inefficient. We therefore tried to remove these inhibitors, and grow the viruses as much as possible in the absence of trypsin. Even then the spikes are not as well formed as those of viruses grown in the presence of trypsin. We really don't understand why trypsin is so necessary for the proper assembly of VP4.

Arias: With regard to the conformational changes that occur in the influenza virus haemagglutinin, it is not only the cleavage that is needed, but also the low pH of lysosomes. It would not be surprising if the conformational change in rotavirus VP4 requires, in addition to the cleavage of the protein, a second event that will trigger the change. This event, so far unidentified, could be the interaction of the virus with its cellular receptor. Perhaps if the trypsin-treated virus is incubated with sialoglycoproteins or cell membrane extracts then you may find more clear evidence of conformational changes in VP4. I would be surprised if the conformation of VP4 does not change at some point during the early interactions of the virus with the cell surface.

Prasad: Those are difficult experiments to do, from the structure point of view. There could be fusion activity even in the case of rotaviruses: there is a fusion peptide that has been located in the VP5 region, but the necessity for the conformational change is completely different.

Ramig: You showed us a conformational change of VP7 of non-trypsinized virus that was subsequently treated with trypsin.

Prasad: In trypsinized and non-trypsinized virus, when exogenous trypsin is added there is the same conformational change in VP7.

Ramig: This would imply that it is unrelated to the gain of infectivity.

Prasad: We don't know whether conformational change in VP7 is related, but increase in infectivity occurs when we see this change. We were surprised to see extra trypsin causing this change. It is certainly not a cleavage. This may not have anything to do with the enhancement of infectivity, but it shows something about the VP7 structure.

Monroe: There is a lack of reverse genetics for many of these systems. One way perhaps to tackle some of these trypsin questions, where cleavage in one protein may affect another, would be to have a reverse genetics system that would allow us to take out cleavage sites in a protein and to test whether this effect is still seen. From the structure, are there any insights that would help in trying to overcome the problems of developing a reverse genetics system?

Prasad: No.

Greenberg: I have some negative data: early in the 1980s Kaljot and myself tried to look for proteases other than trypsin that would activate rotavirus. We reasoned that the best place to look would be the location of brush border peptidases. We did a whole series of studies isolating intestinal epithelial brush borders under the assumption that it might be some form of the enterocyte brush border protease that cleaved rotaviruses rather than pancreatic trypsin. In fact we had lots of cleavage of VP4 that we could detect on PAGE, but no biologically relevant activation of VP4 as indicated by enhanced viral titre. We never published this, but to us it said that it was in fact trypsin that was responsible for activation.

Estes: David Graham and I did some old studies where we started with pancreatin and elastase and showed that trypsin and elastase can enhance rotavirus infectivity (Graham & Estes 1980). One of the interesting results from these studies was that we took pancreatin and elastase and treated each with acid pH. We lowered the pH to 2.6, which would inhibit elastase activity, and there was a residual acid-stable activity that could activate infectivity of rotavirus. We never characterized what this was, but there may in fact be another enzyme in pancreatin that does have some activity.

Saif: Our experience is that there is a wide variation according to the strain of rotavirus in terms of their sensitivity to trypsin. Did you use a trypsin-sensitive strain?

Prasad: All the work we have done has involved the SA11-4F strain of rotavirus. We have done some preliminary studies on clone 3.

Desselberger: You mentioned that you haven't tried any other proteases, but it is worth looking at the experiences the influenza people have had with a wide variety of different proteases. They found that intercellular proteases such as furin are able to cleave certain influenza haemagglutinins (Klenk & Garten 1994).

Prasad: These are time-consuming experiments, so we have to pick and choose our proteases. That is a good point, but trypsin has been the common protease used all over, and increase of infectivity has been well documented with this.

Greenberg: I am not sure what you mean about the RNA winding around the 1,3 vertices. Do you mean that each vertex has a separate gene, or are all 11 genes wrapped around all 12 vertices?

Prasad: This model was proposed on the basis of several observations. One is that VP1/VP3 is attached to VP2 at all the fivefold vertices. Then there is biochemical evidence that all the genome segments can be transcribed simultaneously in this virus. Also, we have seen in transcribing particles at least four or five transcripts associated with each particle. The reason we only see four or five might be that some of the segments have come out or some of the segments may not have begun being transcribed. This means that at each vertex the transcription complex is acting on a segment, and each segment is near the fivefold axis. This is probably the easiest way to explain the observations that we have had. There is one VP1/VP3 complex acting upon a segment, and then all the segments can be transcribed simultaneously.

Greenberg: So, if you could hybridize and do cryo-EM you would always see a single gene at a single vertex.

Prasad: Yes. This model is very simplistic. In order for repeated cycles of transcription to occur, there has to be some kind of tethering between the 3' and 5' ends of the double-stranded RNA, because it has to re-trace the path and there has to be some connection between the 3' and 5' ends. There is no biochemical evidence so far as to how the 3' and 5' ends are coming together. It is quite clear that they are not covalently linked. Is VP1/VP3 acting as a tether between these ends, or are there some hydrogen bonds involved?

Carter: You show very nicely that type I channels are being used for RNA exit, but you have to make the RNA out of something. Presumably the other channels are for the uptake of raw materials. Is there any difference in those other channels which might explain how that process is done? Do you see it as an active process, or is it simple diffusion through a hole?

Prasad: I think all the precursors enter by simple diffusion, but only one channel is specifically used for the exit of mRNA. It is likely that the others are used for getting in all the precursors necessary for transcription. It makes a lot of sense for the mRNA to exit through the fivefold axis because this is near the VP1/VP3 complex. This is in agreement with the studies done in the reovirus system, although reoviruses are slightly different because there is a turret at the fivefold axis. However, there is a channel in the turret. Old studies showed clearly that this is where the mRNA is coming out. This seems to be a common feature shared by the double-stranded RNA viruses.

Desselberger: We did some studies looking at the characteristics of naked RNA by ultracentrifugation (Kapahnke et al 1986). We found that they were stiff, rigid and stable molecules. You could not imagine how these would be packaged if they were not complexed with protein. You have proposed a very nice model for how this could take place. How many molecules of VP1 and VP3, and possibly VP2, do you actually need to get the RNA packaged into the pre-core structure? What is probably also important is how assembly is controlled. RNA is packaged single-stranded and then double strands are made. The RNA has to be intimately linked to protein in order to be kept packaged.

Prasad: Biochemical studies suggest that there are 12 molecules of VP1 and 12 molecules of VP3 in each particle. The reason why we think that the flower-shaped complex is made up of both VP1 and VP3 is that when we look at particles coexpressing VP1, VP2 and VP6 we don't see that structure. It is seen only when VP1 and VP3 are coexpressed with VP2 and VP6. This is the only reason we think it is a complex of VP1 and VP3. The flower-shaped structure is also an artefact of reconstruction. But reconstructions are clearly indicating that VP1 and VP3 are attaching to the VP2 at the fivefold axis. We use this fivefold symmetrization as a part of an icosahedral symmetrization, and this is what is making VP1/VP3 look as if it has five petals. This would be true only if VP1 and VP3 were to have internal fivefold symmetry, which is very unlikely because you don't see that kind of repeat in the sequence. Also, the VP1 and VP3 we have seen only represent 25% of the total mass of VP1 and VP3. About 75% of the mass we haven't really seen, but it is somewhere in the internal regions. It is difficult to visualize the entire VP1 and VP3, unless we purify them and crystallize the complex.

Patton: Despite their natural tendency to exist as long rigid rods, the dsRNA segments must be organized such that they are flexible and free to move about the core during transcription. Indeed, the interaction of the core proteins with the dsRNA genome may destabilize the duplex, causing the formation of kinks and single-stranded regions that allow the dsRNA to be bent, folded and coiled within the core. The mechanism by which rotavirus genome segments undergo rearrangement in fact suggests that regions of the dsRNA genome are single-stranded within cores. In particular, rearrangements that take place during transcription require the nascent transcript and the RNA polymerase to dissociate from the template and then reassociate at a distant site on the same template, where transcription re-initiates. The reassociation site would be presumably single-stranded, since the RNA polymerase has affinity for single-stranded RNA and not dsRNA and since the nascent transcript would likely need a complementary sequence to which it would anneal. Is it not possible that the effect of salt and pH on the structure of the genome in the core may be due to the existence of extensive regions of single-strandedness within the dsRNA?

Prasad: Actually, that is not true. A minor portion of it could be single-stranded. At pH 11.5 single-stranded RNA would be hydrolysed badly. I was expecting the same thing to happen. I thought it would be completely chewed up, but when the student brought it back to pH 7.5 it was transcriptionally active: it was as efficient as the DLPs. This is remarkable.

Patton: Are you taking into account that the high pH may be impacting the interaction of the dsRNA genome with the core lattice protein, VP2? Given the affinity of VP2 for both ssRNA and dsRNA, VP2 may play a particularly important role in the organization of the genome within the core.

Prasad: My thinking as to why this condensation is occurring is that there are two processes involved. First, disruption of hydrogen bond interactions between VP2 and RNA, and then further charge neutralization because of the presence of ammonium ions. These ions are neutralizing the charges on the RNA, so there is no charge repulsion and that is where the condensation is happening. We are in the process of doing further experiments to address the question of whether it is the hydrogen bond, or the charge neutralization, or both.

Matson: It is an unusual host that has a pH of 11 in the stomach. What do you see at pH 2–4?

Prasad: The reason we used pH 11.5 is that we wanted to understand the interactions between protein and RNA. Of course, we realize that pH 11.5 is quite unphysiological: we have tried using pH 2–3, but we can't do any reconstructions because the viruses make large aggregates. At about pH 3.8 they are OK. We don't have any structural evidence as to what happens at acidic pHs.

Holmes: You presented a fascinating model of a whirling transcription machine. Have you any information about the energy requirements for this process?

Prasad: I have never sat down and calculated this. There is ATP dependence, but we don't know how much energy is required.

Glass: From your beautiful reconstructions of the NLVs can you find some structural reason why these viruses are so diverse, with so many cluster types? Is this genetic, or host-induced? What is it that makes these viruses so diverse?

Prasad: From looking at the structure of the NLVs, all I can say is that the P2 domain, which is an insertion in the P domain, represents the very variable regions in all these strains. This seems to be the only thing that changes between strains and also between NLVs and caliciviruses. We have the structure of the San Miguel sea-lion virus and also primate calicivirus: the top portion of the arch is more elaborate and animal caliciviruses also have a larger diameter.

Clarke: What is the evidence that the ORF3 product is involved in packaging? Why doesn't this product show up in cryoelectron microscopy?

Prasad: When you compare NLVs with other viruses such as tobacco bushy stunt virus (TBSV) or other plant viruses, which all have a very basic internal region that is supposed to be interacting with RNA, NLVs lack this; their interior is quite acidic. But ORF3 is a highly basic protein. This is what prompts us to think that it may be involved in the RNA encapsidation. All the studies from Dr Estes' lab suggest that these are present in small amounts in the capsids (Glass et al 2000). If there are 180 molecules of the capsid protein per particle, perhaps there will be one or two of ORF3. If we have to see the structure of ORF3, we need at least 60, and we don't find that.

Kapikian: I was intrigued by your comments about the rotavirus particles aggregating at acid pH. We have wrestled with the problems of rotavirus inactivation by stomach acid in our studies of live, orally administered rotavirus vaccines. Rotaviruses are acid labile, whereas reoviruses are acid stable. Is this the mechanism for the acid lability of rotaviruses? I thought the virus would disintegrate at low pH.

Prasad: You cannot always believe the results from negative-stain studies because artefacts are introduced. We have also done cryoelectron microscopy, which I think would give a more realistic view of what is happening at acid pH. Between pH 2.4 and 3.8 there is no evidence for large-scale disintegration. It is mainly very bad aggregation. This is probably causing the inactivation. Reoviruses are supposed to be acid stable, but I don't know whether they clump at acid pHs.

Kapikian: In infectivity studies, the sensitivity to acid exposure was a distinguishing feature between rotavirus and reovirus.

Matson: One clump would be counted as one pfu.

Vesikari: Could the absence of trypsin that induced irreversible conformational changes in VP4 be correlated with attenuation of a rotavirus in tissue culture? In other words, if you have a tissue culture-grown rotavirus which we call a vaccine, could this morphologically be more like your absence of trypsin-grown rotavirus?

Prasad: I don't think that I can answer that question. We haven't looked.

Ramig: In this group of viruses, including reoviruses, there are old reports that if you start trypsinization there is a cascade. It is almost as if there is an autoproteolysis. We leaned on that problem fairly hard for a while. We took purified virus, treated it with trypsin, ran it over three sequential CsCl gradients to try to get all of the residual trypsin out, and then added minute amounts of that virus to uncleaved purified ^{35}S-labelled virus. We saw that VP4 was cleaved (D. Chen & R. F. Ramig, unpublished results). This is an issue that floats around with anecdotal observations like these and a few publications in reovirus. Is there some sort of autoproteolysis taking place that could be related to its infectivity or lack thereof?

Prasad: I don't know whether any of our structural studies really address this question, or even support the autocatalytic action of VP4. The structure of VP4 seems quite stable even with exogenous trypsin. There may be some conformational changes taking place when you add exogenous trypsin in VP4. From what we have done so far on the autocatalytic activities of VP4, when one compares this with what is happening in reovirus, it is a completely different story. In reovirus, trypsin reduces it to a core-like structure, taking out the sigma 3 protein and mu 1 proteins. This doesn't happen even with prolonged trypsinization in rotavirus. VP6 and VP7 are completely stable.

Greenberg: Frank Ramig, why did you never publish your data on this? What was wrong with them?

Ramig: We could never inhibit trypsin activity without inhibiting this other activity, so we couldn't prove that we didn't have residual trypsin in the system.

Green: There are certain clinical conditions where people either have depressed levels of trypsin, or they are on soy-rich diets, which has lots of antitrypsin activity. Is there any clinical evidence that kids who either are trypsin deficient or who are taking soy milk diets have less viral gastroenteritis?

Matson: There are many children on soy-rich diets and we have never found any large populations who have escaped rotavirus infection. The ingestion of the soy diet is on a bolus manner through the day so exposures to virus are not likely to coincide temporally. However, the kids who have trypsin deficiency are those with cystic fibrosis: we know that these children suffer from nosocomial rotavirus infections.

Bishop: The presence and/or severity of rotavirus disease in children with cystic fibrosis is almost impossible to study. The disease is now often diagnosed very early in life and then patients receive pancreatic supplements that reverse the trypsin deficiency.

Greenberg: Long ago, Bob Yolken published a mouse study where he attempted to use protease inhibitors to block infectivity. If I remember this study correctly, he had to go to great lengths to find enough protease inhibitor present to have an effect: amounts that would not be seen in a cystic fibrosis patient where there is still residual proteolytic activity in the gut.

Farthing: The pancreas produces at least 10 times the amount of enzyme that any of us need. Clinical malabsorption does not become apparent until 90% of the pancreas is lost. It is likely, therefore, that even in children with cystic fibrosis, there will still be enough trypsin to cleave the virus.

López: We have a variant virus that binds to the cell through VP5. We know that antibodies against VP5 inhibit virus binding. If we grow this variant virus without trypsin, its binding to MA104 cells is not inhibited any more by antibodies to VP8 or VP5. The only way we have been able to inhibit the binding of the untrypsinated variant is by using anti-VP7 antibodies.

Bishop: Within human VP4s, P2A[6] shows a predilection for infecting the neonatal gut. We misinterpreted this originally as showing attenuation: clearly it doesn't. But the original observation still stands: that the P type of rotaviruses endemic among newborn babies in a neonatal nursery is almost always P[6]. Neonates may have less trypsin or their trypsin may be quite different from the more mature infant. It may be interesting to see whether there are any consistent differences, either in initial conformation, in sequence, or cleavage by trypsin between P[6] strains from endemic infections in neonatal nurseries, and P types of strains associated with severe community disease.

Glass: In India P[6] strains are among the most common strains in children with diarrhoea. I don't think the neonatal association is going to be due to trypsin.

Desselberger: It is known from other systems that proteolytic cleavage of viral proteins is necessary for them to interact with cellular receptors or co-receptors. In your pH shift experiments, have you done any studies of the interaction of these changed particles?

Prasad: We haven't. There are studies indicating that the cell entry involves multiple steps. There are several steps which cleavage could be affecting.

References

Arias CF, Romero P, Alvarez V, López S 1996 Trypsin activation pathway of rotavirus infectivity. J Virol 70:5832–5839

Bullough PA, Hughson FM, Shekel JJ, Wiley DC 1994 Structure of influenza haemagglutinin at the pH of membrane fusion. Nature 371:37–43

Gilbert JM, Greenberg HB 1998 Cleavage of rhesus rotavirus VP4 after arginine 247 is essential for rotavirus-like particle-induced fusion from without. J Virol 72:5323–5327

Glass PJ, White LJ, Ball JM, Leparc-Goffart I, Hardy ME, Estes MK 2000 Norwalk virus open reading frame 3 encodes a minor structural protein. J Virol 74:6581–6591

Graham DY, Estes MK 1980 Proteolytic enhancement of rotavirus infectivity: biologic mechanisms. Virology 101:432–439

Kapahnke R, Rappold W, Desselberger U, Riesner D 1986 The stiffness of dsRNA: hydrodynamic studies on fluorescence-labelled RNA segments of bovine rotavirus. Nucleic Acids Res 14:3215–3228

Klenk HD, Garten W 1994 Host cell proteases controlling virus pathogenicity. Trends Microbiol 2:39–43

Novartis 238: Gastroenteritis Viruses.
Copyright © 2001 John Wiley & Sons Ltd
Print ISBN 0-471-49663-4 eISBN 0-470-84653-4

Early events of rotavirus infection: the search for the receptor(s)

Carlos F. Arias, Carlos A. Guerrero[1], Ernesto Méndez, Selene Zárate, Pavel Isa, Rafaela Espinosa, Pedro Romero and Susana López

Departamento de Genética y Fisiología Molecular, Instituto de Biotecnología, Universidad Nacional Autónoma de México, Cuernavaca, Morelos 62250, Mexico

Abstract. The entry of rotaviruses into epithelial cells seems to be a multistep process. Infection competition experiments have suggested that at least three different interactions between the virus and cell surface molecules take place during the early events of infection, and glycolipids as well as glycoproteins have been suggested to be primary attachment receptors for rotaviruses. The infectivity of some rotavirus strains depends on the presence of sialic acid on the cell surface, however, it has been shown that this interaction is not essential, and it has been suggested that there exists a neuraminidase-resistant cell surface molecule with which most rotaviruses interact. The comparative characterization of the sialic acid-dependent rotavirus strain RRV (G3P5[3]), its neuraminidase-resistant variant nar3, and the human rotavirus strain Wa (G1P1A[8]) has allowed us to show that $\alpha 2\beta 1$ integrin is used by nar3 as its primary cell attachment site, and by RRV in a second interaction, subsequent to its initial contact with a sialic acid-containing cell receptor. We have also shown that integrin $\alpha V\beta 3$ is used by all three rotavirus strains as a co-receptor, subsequent to their initial attachment to the cell. We propose that the functional rotavirus receptor is a complex of several cell molecules most likely immersed in glycosphingolipid-enriched plasma membrane microdomains.

2001 Gastroenteritis viruses. Wiley, Chichester (Novartis Foundation Symposium 238) p 47–63

Group A rotaviruses are non-enveloped viruses that possess a genome of 11 segments of double-stranded RNA contained in a triple-layered protein capsid. The outermost layer is composed of two proteins, VP4 and VP7. The smooth external surface of the virus is made up of 780 copies of glycoprotein VP7, while 60 spike-like structures, formed by dimers of VP4, extend from the VP7 surface (Estes 1996).

---

[1]On academic leave from the Departamento de Bioquímica, Facultad de Medicina, Universidad Nacional de Colombia

VP4 has essential functions in the virus life cycle, including receptor binding and cell penetration (Crawford et al 1994, López et al 1985, Ludert et al 1996). The properties of this protein are therefore important determinants of host range, virulence and induction of protective immunity. The role of VP7 during the early interactions of the virus with the cell is not clear, although it has been shown that it can modulate some of the VP4-mediated virus phenotypes, including receptor binding (Beisner et al 1998, Méndez et al 1996), and it has been suggested that it might interact with cell surface molecules after the initial attachment of the virus through the spike protein (Coulson et al 1997, Estes 1996, Méndez et al 1999). For rotaviruses to enter the cell, VP4 has to be cleaved by trypsin into two subunits, VP5 and VP8 (Arias et al 1996, López et al 1985).

Rotaviruses have a very specific cell tropism, infecting only the enterocytes on the tip of villi of the small intestine, suggesting that specific host receptors must exist. In vitro, they also display a strict tropism, binding to a variety of cell lines, but infecting efficiently only those of renal or intestinal epithelium origin.

Different rotavirus strains display different requirements to bind, and thus infect, susceptible cells. The cell attachment of some rotavirus strains isolated from animals (other than humans) is greatly diminished by treatment of cells with neuraminidase (NA), indicating the need for sialic acid (SA) on the cell surface (Ciarlet & Estes 1999, Fukudome et al 1989, Keljo & Smith 1988, Méndez et al 1993). The interaction with a SA-containing receptor, however, does not seem to be essential, since variants which no longer need SA to infect the cells can be isolated from the SA-dependent strains (Ludert et al 1998, Méndez et al 1993). In addition, many animal rotavirus strains are NA-resistant and most, if not all, strains isolated from humans are also NA-resistant (Ciarlet & Estes 1999, Fukudome et al 1989, Méndez et al 1999). Thus, there is a great interest in identifying the NA-resistant cellular receptor(s) for rotavirus, and to determine the role it (they) may have on the narrow tropism observed for this virus. In this context, it is also of importance to define the viral proteins, and their specific domains, involved in contacting the cell receptor(s).

To understand the early events of rotavirus infection we have undertaken the comparative characterization of three rotavirus strains: the SA-dependent simian rotavirus RRV, its NA-resistant variant nar3, and the human rotavirus (HRV) strain Wa, which is naturally resistant to NA. A summary of the advances and approaches we have taken to characterize the early events of infection of these viruses is presented.

The interaction of rotavirus with its host cell is a multistep process

Several lines of evidence suggest that rotaviruses need to interact with more than one cell surface molecule to enter the cell, using during this process different

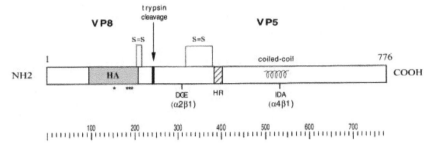

FIG. 1. Distinctive structural features of the outer shell protein VP4. The trypsin cleavage region is indicated by an arrow, which defines the boundary between VP8 and VP5. In VP8, the haemagglutination domain (HA) (aa 93 to 208) is shadowed; the asterisks below this domain indicate aa 155 and 188–190, which are important in the SA binding activity of this protein. The disulfide bridges between Cys203 and Cys216, and between Cys318 and Cys380, are indicated by S=S. In VP5, the position of the DGE and IDA tripeptide sequence binding motifs which might putatively be recognized by integrins $\alpha 2\beta 1$ and $\alpha 4\beta 1$, respectively, are shown. The hydrophobic region (HR), which has been proposed to be a putative fusion domain, and a predicted heptad repeat (coiled-coil) which might form part of a coiled-coil structure are also depicted.

domains of the virus surface protein VP4 (Fig. 1). The following studies, which support these multiple interactions, were carried out in the rhesus monkey kidney epithelial cell line MA104, which is highly susceptible for rotavirus infection.

(a) In an infection assay designed to detect competition for cell surface molecules at both attachment and post-attachment steps (Méndez et al 1999), it was found that HRV Wa efficiently competed with the infectivity of the SA-dependent porcine rotavirus strain YM, and that of the variant nar3 both in untreated, as well as in NA-treated cells. This competition was non-reciprocal since YM and nar3 did not compete with the infectivity of Wa. In contrast, a two-direction competition between the variant nar3 and a SA-dependent strain was found. The fact that the competition between the two NA-resistant strains nar3 and Wa was not reciprocal indicates that they bind to different molecules. In addition, the SA-dependence phenotype clearly differentiates strains, like RRV or YM, from nar3 and Wa. Altogether, these findings suggest the existence of at least three cellular structures involved in rotavirus cell infection, with at least one being shared by human, SA-dependent, and animal, NA-resistant, variant strains.

(b) The comparison of the binding characteristics of wild-type RRV (wtRRV) and nar3 to MA104 cells showed that both the SA-dependent and SA-independent interactions of these viruses with the cell are mediated through two different domains of VP4 (Méndez et al 1993). It was shown that RRV

TABLE 1   Inhibition of binding and infectivity of RRV and nar3 viruses by MAbs to VP4 and by VP8 and VP5 recombinant proteins

		% Binding and infectivity in the presence of the indicated MAbs or recombinant proteins					
	Virus	no MAb	αVP8 (7A12)	αVP5 (2G4)	GST	GST– VP8	GST– VP5
Binding[a]	RRV	100	9	84	102	25	97
	nar3	100	72	9	99	100	24
Infectivity[b]	RRV	100	8	9	87	44	102
	nar3	100	95	16	110	104	50

[a]Expressed as the percentage of virus binding in the absence of antibodies or recombinant proteins.
[b]Expressed as percentage of the virus infectivity obtained in the absence of antibodies or recombinant proteins. The arithmetic means from two independent experiments performed in duplicate are shown.

attaches to the cell through VP8, while nar3 does so through the VP5 domain of VP4 (Zárate et al 2000a). This observation is supported by the fact that neutralizing antibodies to VP8 block the attachment to cells of RRV, but not of its variant nar3, while a monoclonal antibody (MAb) to VP5 (2G4) inhibits the binding of nar3, but not that of RRV. In addition, recombinant VP8 and VP5 proteins produced in bacteria as fusion products with glutathione S-transferase (GST), are capable of inhibiting the binding and infection of wild-type and variant viruses, respectively, when pre-incubated with the cell (Table 1, Zárate et al 2000b). While nar3 only needs to interact (through VP5) with the NA-resistant receptor, wtRRV seems to engage in the two interactions described in a sequential manner, since MAb 2G4, despite selectively blocking the binding of nar3, efficiently neutralizes the infectivity of both viruses (see also below).

(c)   The sequential interaction of RRV with two molecules on the surface of MA104 cells is further supported by the observation that MAb 2D9, which is directed to a cell surface antigen, specifically blocks the infectivity of both wtRRV and nar3, but competes only with the attachment of the variant, indicating that wtRRV is blocked at a post-binding step (López et al 2000). Since MAb 2D9 also blocks the infectivity of nar3 in NA-treated cells, and prevents the cell attachment of the recombinant protein GST–VP5, but does not affect the binding of GST–VP8 (Fig. 3), it would seem to be directed to the NA-resistant receptor used by nar3 to attach to the cell, or to a molecule closely associated with it.

Multiplicity of rotavirus receptors

Despite the advances in the molecular and structural biology of these viruses, little is known about the rotavirus cell receptors. A number of glycoconjugates have been shown to bind to, and to block the infectivity of, SA-dependent animal rotavirus strains, and some of them have been suggested to play a role as possible receptors, like GM3 gangliosides in newborn piglet intestine (Rolsma et al 1998), GM1 in LLC-MK2 cells (Superti & Donelli 1991), and 300–330 kDa glycoproteins in murine enterocytes (Bass et al 1991). It has also been suggested that the NA-resistant ganglioside GM1 may act as a receptor for some HRV strains in MA104 cells (Guo et al 1999). Recently, it was reported that VP4 contains the DGE and IDA tripeptide sequence motifs known to interact with integrins $\alpha2\beta1$ and $\alpha4\beta1$, respectively (Fig. 1), while VP7 contains the $\alpha X\beta2$ integrin ligand site GPR, and the $\alpha4\beta1$ binding motif LDV (Coulson et al 1997, Hewish et al 2000). Antibodies to the integrin subunits $\alpha2$, $\beta2$ and $\alpha4$, as well as peptides that mimic the ligand sites were shown to block the infectivity of the SA-dependent rotavirus SA11 and the HRV strain RV5 (Coulson et al 1997). It was also shown that integrins $\alpha2\beta1$ and $\alpha4\beta1$ can mediate the attachment and entry of rotavirus SA11 into the human myelogenous leukemic cell line K562 (Hewish et al 2000).

As part of the biochemical characterization of the rotavirus cell receptors, we have recently shown that the infectivity of rotaviruses RRV, nar3 and Wa is

TABLE 2 Effect of metabolic inhibitors, cell membrane cholesterol depletion, and octyl-β-glucoside on the infectivity and binding of rotaviruses in MA104 cells

	% Infectivity			*% Binding*		
Inhibitor[a]	*RRV*	*nar3*	*Wa*	*RRV*	*nar 3*	*Wa*
No treatment	100	100	100	100	100	100
PDMP (25 μg/ml)	20	40	23	110	46	104
Tunicamycin (2 μg/ml)	56	48	–	111	101	94
BenzylGalNAc (2 mM)	101	150	147	ND	ND	ND
Octyl-β-glucoside (0.2%)	41	41	39	32	40	33
β-cyclodextrin (10 mM)	9	6	5	112	109	116
OG extract[b] (20 μg/ml)	5	3	4	60	59	57

[a]MA104 cell monolayers were incubated with the indicated concentration of inhibitor for 1 h (β-cyclodextrin), 24 h (tunicamycin), or 72 h (PDMP and BenzylGalNAc) at 37 °C, or for 90 min (octyl-β-glucoside) at room temperature, before virus infection.
[b]Rotaviruses were incubated with either 20 or 400 μg/ml of OG-extracted proteins, for the binding and infectivity inhibition assays, respectively. At 20 μg/ml the binding of all three viruses was inhibited by about 40%.
The mean of at least three independent experiments carried out in duplicate is shown.

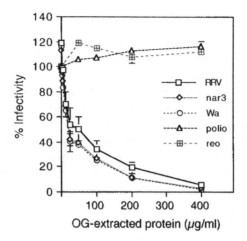

FIG. 2.   Inhibition of rotavirus infectivity by the OG extract. The indicated concentrations of OG-extracted protein were incubated with the viruses for 90 min at 37 °C. The virus–protein mixtures were used to infect MA104 cell monolayers, after an adsorption period at 4 °C, the inoculum was removed and the infection was left to proceed for 14 h at 37 °C. At this time the cells were fixed, and the infectious titre was determined by an immunoperoxidase focus assay. Percentage infectivity is referred to the infectivity of the viruses incubated in 0.2% OG. Error bars represent one standard error of the mean of three independent experiments carried out in duplicate.

partially blocked by metabolic inhibitors of N-glycosylation (tunicamycin), and glycolipid synthesis (PDMP), while it is not affected by the inhibition of the cellular O-glycosylation (Guerrero et al 2000a). In addition, we also showed that depletion of cholesterol from the cell membrane with methyl-β-cyclodextrin reduced the infectivity of the three viruses by more than 90%, while not affecting their binding to the cell (Table 2). The involvement of N-glycosylated proteins, glycolipids, and cholesterol in rotavirus infection suggest that the virus receptor(s) might be forming part of the cell membrane glycosphingolipid-enriched lipid microdomains, termed rafts (Simons & Ikonen 1997).

In a different approach we showed that treatment of MA104 cells with the non-ionic detergent octyl-β-glucoside (OG), under non-lytic conditions, renders the cells largely refractory to binding and infection by rotaviruses (Table 2) (Guerrero et al 2000a), most probably due to the extraction of the rotavirus receptor(s). Accordingly, pre-incubation of the viruses with the OG extract inhibited infectivity by more than 95% (Fig. 2). Five protein bands with the ability to block rotavirus infectivity were purified by preparative electrophoresis from these extracts, and amino acid sequence analysis of the band of 110 kDa, revealed the presence, among other proteins, of the $\beta3$ integrin subunit.

$\alpha 2\beta 1$ integrin mediates the cell attachment of the NA-resistant RRV variant nar3

The initial interaction of nar3 with the cell surface is likely to be with integrin $\alpha 2\beta 1$, through the DGE integrin binding domain present in VP5, since: (i) antibodies to the $\alpha 2$ subunit reduce by 30% the infectivity of both wtRRV and nar3, but only block the cell attachment of nar3; (ii) MAbs to $\alpha 2$ block the attachment of the GST–VP5 fusion protein but not that of GST–VP8 (Fig. 3); (iii) GST–VP5 specifically displaces up to 75% of the cell binding of nar3, while a GST–VP5 mutant polypeptide in which the $\alpha 2$ integrin binding motif DGE was changed to AGE no longer displaces it (Zárate et al 2000b); and (iv) a synthetic VP4 peptide which comprises the $\alpha 2\beta 1$ integrin binding motif DGE efficiently inhibits the attachment of nar3, but not that of RRV (Fig. 3) (Zárate et al 2000b).

Even though the behaviour of MAb 2D9 is similar to that of $\alpha 2\beta 1$ integrin antibodies (Fig. 3), 2D9 is probably not directed to this integrin, since its pattern of staining of mouse small intestinal cells is quite different from that obtained with $\alpha 2\beta 1$ MAbs (R. Espinoza, C. F. Arias & S. López, unpublished data). Nevertheless, the cell structure recognized by 2D9 must be in close proximity to integrin $\alpha 2\beta 1$ on the surface of MA104 cells, since MAb 2D9 displaces the binding of antibodies to $\alpha 2\beta 1$ by flow cytometry (P. Isa, C. F. Arias & S. López, unpublished results). 2D9 might serve as an alternative cell receptor for the variant nar3, since cells that lack $\alpha 2\beta 1$ but are 2D9-positive, like L or CHO, can be infected by this virus, albeit at much lower efficiency (P. Isa, C. F. Arias & S. López, unpublished data).

Integrin $\beta 3$ functions as a co-receptor for rotaviruses

The relevance of $\beta 3$ integrin for rotavirus infection was established by the fact that antibodies to this integrin subunit reduced by 50% the infectivity of RRV, nar3 and Wa rotaviruses. In accordance to this finding, when vitronectin, a $\beta 3$ integrin ligand, was pre-incubated with cells, it specifically blocked rotavirus infectivity up to 70% (Guerrero et al 2000b).

Since integrins $\alpha 2\beta 1$, $\alpha 4\beta 1$ and $\alpha X\beta 2$ have been suggested to play a role during rotavirus entry (Coulson et al 1997), we performed blocking experiments using mixes of antibodies directed to these integrins and to $\alpha V\beta 3$. A clear additive blocking effect was found when antibodies to integrins $\alpha 2\beta 1$ and $\alpha V\beta 3$ were mixed, suggesting that these two integrins might be involved in different stages of rotavirus infection (Guerrero et al 2000b).

The expression of $\beta 3$ integrin into the poorly permissive CHO cells was shown to facilitate the infectivity of rotaviruses. CHO cells stably transfected with the $\beta 3$ integrin gene (Díaz-González et al 1996), overexpressing either

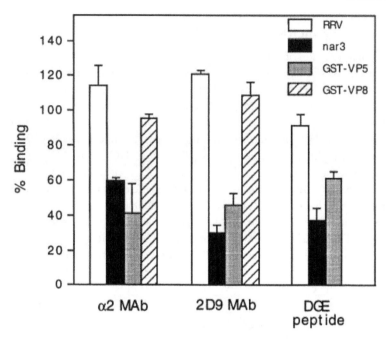

FIG. 3.   Effect of antibodies to the cell surface, and of a VP4 peptide, on the binding of RRV and nar3 viruses. MA104 cells were preincubated for 1 h at 37 °C with a MAb to integrin subunit α2, with MAb 2D9 or with peptide DGE. After incubation, these cells were washed, and purified RRV or nar3 viral particles or affinity purified GST–VP8 and GST–VP5 fusion protein were adsorbed for 60 min at 4 °C with gentle shaking. The amount of cell bound virus, or fusion protein, was determined by an ELISA, as described (Zárate et al 2000a). The VP4 synthetic peptide evaluated comprises amino acid residues 300 to 321 of the protein, and contains the DGE sequence binding motif for integrin α2β1. Data are expressed as the percentage of virus or recombinant protein binding, in the absence of antibodies or peptide. The arithmetic means and standard deviations of two independent experiments are shown.

αIIbβ3 or αVβ3 integrins, were three to four times more susceptible to rotavirus infection than the parental CHO cell line. This increase in infectivity was shown to be blocked by incubation of the cells with either MAbs to β3 or vitronectin (Fig. 4) (Guerrero et al 2000b). Furthermore, it was shown that the interaction of rotaviruses with αVβ3 is at a post-attachment step, probably penetration, since vitronectin and antibodies to β3 do not, or only slightly, inhibit rotavirus cell attachment. Also, the interaction of rotaviruses with β3 integrin was found to be RGD-independent, as expected from the fact that neither VP4 nor VP7 have this integrin binding motif (Guerrero et al 2000b).

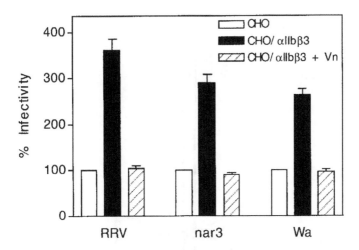

FIG. 4.   The expression of $\beta3$ integrin in CHO cells facilitates rotavirus cell infection. Monolayers of control CHO cells or CHO cells expressing integrin $\alpha IIb\beta3$ (Díaz-González et al 1996), in 96-well plates, were infected with 2×10^3 ffu's of RRV, nar3 or Wa viruses per well. After 60 min adsorption at 37 °C, the infection was left to proceed for 16 h at 37 °C, at which time the cells were fixed and immunostained. In the condition where the cells were preincubated with vitronectin (CHO/$\alpha IIb\beta3$ + Vn), the integrin ligand (1.5 μg/ml) was added for 1 h at 37 °C before virus infection. Data are expressed as percentage of the virus infectivity obtained in the CHO cells. The arithmetic mean from two independent experiments performed in duplicate are shown. The standard error is shown.

A model for the early interactions of rotaviruses with MA104 cells

As a summary of the data presented here, we propose the following working model (Fig. 5), which takes into account the currently available information:

(a)   Wild type RRV interacts primarily with a SA-containing cell receptor through the VP8 domain of VP4. The identity of the SA-containing molecule has not been determined, although good candidates are ganglioside GM3 (Guo et al 1999, Rolsma et al 1998), or the SA present in the integrin molecules (see below). The SA-binding domain of VP8 is located between amino acids 93 to 208, with residues 155, and 188 to 190, having an important role in this function (Fig. 1) (Fiore et al 1991, Fuentes Panana et al 1995, Isa et al 1997).

(b)   Subsequent to the initial interaction with SA, RRV interacts with a second cell receptor, most probably $\alpha2\beta1$ integrin, through the DGE integrin-binding motif located in the VP5 subunit of VP4 (Zárate et al 2000b). The ability of

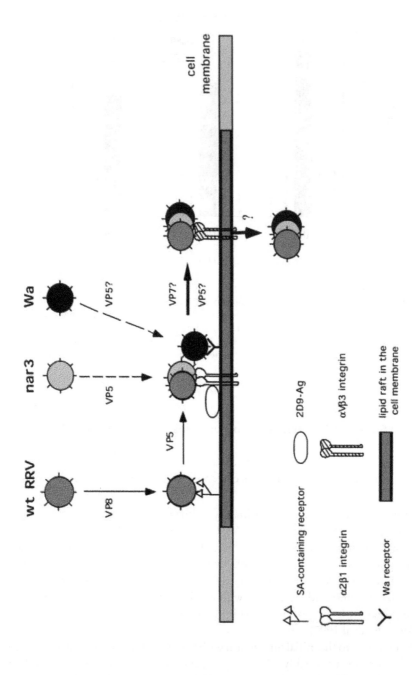

the NA-resistant variant nar3 to interact directly with this integrin is likely to be the result of a slight different conformation of its VP4 protein, compared to that of the wtRRV protein (Méndez et al 1993, 1996). Although the present data clearly indicate the existence of two different interactions between wild-type RRV and the cell surface, it has not yet been established whether two cell molecules, or two sites in the same molecule (e.g. $\alpha 2\beta 1$), interact with VP8 and VP5. The fact that in infection competition assays the wild-type and variant viruses compete with each other reciprocally, suggests that if it is not the same cellular entity, the two cell molecules must be in close proximity.

(c) Integrins $\alpha 4\beta 1$ and $\alpha X\beta 2$ have been implicated in rotavirus cell infection (Coulson et al 1997, Guerrero et al 2000b, Hewish et al 2000). The role of these integrins has not been determined yet, however, given that no additivity was observed when mixes of antibodies to these and other integrins were tested (Guerrero et al 2000b), they may represent alternative interaction sites for rotaviruses.

(d) The results obtained in the infection competition assays described above suggest that HRV Wa initially attaches to a cell surface molecule that is used by RRV and nar3, in a subsequent step after their interaction with $\alpha 2\beta 1$ integrin. It can not be ruled out, however, that the attachment receptor for Wa is not actually used by RRV and nar3, but that HRV Wa interferes with the infectivity of these viruses by binding to a molecule that might be located in close proximity to either $\alpha 2\beta 1$, or to co-receptor $\alpha V\beta 3$. The cellular molecule used by HRV Wa to bind to cells has not yet been characterized, although ganglioside GM1 seems to be a good candidate (Guo et al 1999).

FIG. 5. A model for the early interactions of rotaviruses with MA104 cells. Wild type RRV interacts primarily with a SA-containing cell receptor through the VP8 domain of VP4. Subsequent to this initial interaction, which might induce a conformational change in VP4, the virus interacts with a second, NA-resistant cell receptor, here proposed to be $\alpha 2\beta 1$ integrin. This interaction is through the DGE binding motif of VP5, present at aa 308–310. This second virus–cell interaction might facilitate a third interaction of the virus with $\beta 3$ integrin. The SA-independent variant nar3 is proposed to interact directly, through VP5, with the $\alpha 2\beta 1$ integrin. For the sake of clarity, the SA-containing and NA-resistant cellular receptors are depicted here as two separate entities (the first possibly being ganglioside GM3), however, they could be two domains of the same receptor molecule (see text). The nature of the attachment site for the HRV strain Wa has not been determined, however, we propose that it binds to a molecule that is in close proximity to $\alpha 2\beta 1$, probably GM1 (see text). The antigen recognized by MAb 2D9 (2D9-Ag) has not been identified, but we assume that it should also be close to the $\alpha 2\beta 1$ integrin (see text). After their initial contact with the cell, all three rotavirus strains are proposed to interact with $\beta 3$ integrin, this interaction might mediate the penetration of the viruses into the cell's interior. In this model most, if not all, of the molecules involved in rotavirus binding and entry are proposed to form a complex, probably embedded in glycosphingolipid-enriched lipid microdomains on the cell surface.

Also, the viral protein domain responsible for this interaction has not been determined.

(e) We have found that integrin $\alpha V\beta 3$ plays an important role for infection of all three rotavirus strains at a post-attachment step, most likely penetration; however, the precise function of this protein has yet to be characterized.

(f) The essential components of the glycosphingolipid-enriched membrane domains, termed rafts, are glycoproteins, glycosphingolipids and cholesterol. Since these three components have been found to be important for the initial steps of rotavirus infection (Guerrero et al 2000a), and $\alpha V\beta 3$ integrin has been observed to be present in rafts (C. A. Guerrero, S. López & C. F. Arias, unpublished data, Green et al 1999), we propose that some or all of the various virus–cell interactions described above might take place in these lipid microdomains.

The data presented here are consistent with the existence of several rotavirus receptors which might be tightly organized, maybe forming a complex in glycosphingolipid-enriched rafts. The requirement for several cell molecules to be present and organized in a precise fashion, might explain the exquisite cell and tissue tropism of these viruses. It remains to be established which, if any, of the receptor molecules described so far is indeed non-replaceable, and if in fact there exists a unique pathway of infectivity for rotaviruses, with distinct entry points for different strains.

In conclusion, much remains to be learned about the process of binding and penetration of rotaviruses. The characterization of the nature of the interactions that occur between the cellular and viral partners, and the signal transduction pathways potentially triggered by the early virus–cell contacts, should give insight into the elaborated mechanism used by these viruses to enter cells.

Acknowledgements

This work was partially supported by grants 75197-527106 and 75301-527108 from the Howard Hughes Medical Institute, G0012-N9607 from the National Council for Science and Technology-Mexico, and IN201399 from DGAPA-UNAM.

References

Arias CF, Romero P, Alvarez V, López S 1996 Trypsin activation pathway of rotavirus infectivity. J Virol 70:5832–5839

Bass DM, Mackow ER, Greenberg HB 1991 Identification and partial characterization of a rhesus rotavirus binding glycoprotein on murine enterocytes. Virology 183:602–610

Beisner B, Kool D, Marich A, Holmes IH 1998 Characterisation of G serotype dependent non-antibody inhibitors of rotavirus in normal mouse serum. Arch Virol 143:1277–1294

Ciarlet M, Estes MK 1999 Human and most animal rotavirus strains do not require the presence of sialic acid on the cell surface for efficient infectivity. J Gen Virol 80:943–948

Coulson BS, Londrigan SL, Lee D J 1997 Rotavirus contains integrin ligand sequences and a disintegrin-like domain that are implicated in virus entry into cells. Proc Natl Acad Sci USA 94:5389–5394

Crawford SE, Labbé M, Cohen J, Burroughs MH, Zhou Y J, Estes MK 1994 Characterization of virus-like particles produced by the expression of rotavirus capsid proteins in insect cells. J Virol 68:5945–5922

Díaz-González F, Forsyth J, Steiner B, Ginsberg MH 1996 Trans-dominant inhibition of integrin function. Mol Biol Cell 7:1939–1951

Estes MK 1996 Rotaviruses and their replication. In: Fields BN, Knipe DM, Howley PM et al (eds) Virology. Raven Press, New York, p 1625–1655

Fiore L, Greenberg HB, Mackow ER 1991 The VP8 fragment of VP4 is the rhesus rotavirus hemagglutinin. Virology 181:553–563

Fuentes-Pananá EM, López S, Gorziglia M, Arias CF 1995 Mapping the hemagglutination domain of rotaviruses. J Virol 69:2629–2632

Fukudome K, Yoshie O, Konno T 1989 Comparison of human, simian, and bovine rotaviruses for requirement of sialic acid in hemagglutination and cell adsorption. Virology 172:196–205

Green JM, Zhelesnyak A, Chung J et al 1999 Role of cholesterol in formation and function of a signaling complex involving αVβ3, integrin-associated protein (CD47), and heterotrimeric G proteins. J Cell Biol 146:673–682

Guerrero CA, Zárate S, Corkidi G, López S, Arias CF 2000a Biochemical characterization of rotavirus receptors in MA104 cells. J Virol 74:9362–9371

Guerrero CA, Zárate S, Isa P, Méndez E, López S, Arias CF 2000b Integrin αVβ3 mediates rotavirus cell entry. Proc Natl Acad Sci USA 97:14644–14649

Guo C, Nakagomi O, Mochizuki M et al 1999 Ganglioside GM(1a) on the cell surface is involved in the infection by human rotavirus KUN and MO strains. J Biochem (Tokyo) 126:683–688

Hewish M J, Takada Y, Coulson BS 2000 Integrins α2β1 and α4β1 can mediate SA11 rotavirus attachment and entry into cells. J Virol 74:228–236

Isa P, López S, Segovia L, Arias CF 1997 Functional and structural analysis of the sialic acid-binding domain of rotaviruses. J Virol 71:6749–6756

Keljo D J, Smith AK 1988 Characterization of binding of simian rotavirus SA-11 to cultured epithelial cells. J Pediatr Gastroenterol Nutr 7:249–256

López S, Arias CF, Bell J R, Strauss J H, Espejo RT 1985 Primary structure of the cleavage site associated with trypsin enhancement of rotavirus SA11 infectivity. Virology 144:11–19

López S, Espinosa R, Isa P, Zárate S, Méndez E, Arias CF 2000 Characterization of a monoclonal antibody directed to the surface of MA104 cells that blocks the infectivity of rotaviruses. Virology 273:160–168

Ludert J E, Feng N, Yu J H, Broome RL, Hoshino Y, Greenberg HB 1996 Genetic mapping indicates that VP4 is the rotavirus cell attachment protein *in vitro* and *in vivo*. J Virol 70:487–493

Ludert J E, Mason BB, Angel J et al 1998 Identification of mutations in the rotavirus protein VP4 that alter sialic-acid-dependent infection. J Gen Virol 79:725–729

Méndez E, Arias CF, López S 1993 Binding to sialic acids is not an essential step for the entry of animal rotaviruses to epithelial cells in culture. J Virol 67:5253–5259

Méndez E, Arias CF, López S 1996 Interactions between the two surface proteins of rotavirus may alter the receptor-binding specificity of the virus. J Virol 70:1218–1222

Méndez E, López S, Cuadras MA, Romero P, Arias CF 1999 Entry of rotaviruses is a multistep process. Virology 263:450–459

Rolsma MD, Kuhlenschmidt TB, Gelberg HB, Kuhlenschmidt MS 1998 Structure and function of a ganglioside receptor for porcine rotavirus. J Virol 72:9079–9091

Simons K, Ikonen E 1997 Functional rafts in cell membranes. Nature 387:569–572

Superti F, Donelli G 1991 Gangliosides as binding sites in SA-11 rotavirus infection of LLC-MK2 cells. J Gen Virol 72:2467–2474

Zárate S, Espinosa R, Romero P, Méndez E, Arias CF, López S 2000a The VP5 domain of VP4 can mediate attachment of rotaviruses to cells. J Virol 74:593–599

Zárate S, Espinòsa R, Romera P, Guerrero CA, Arias CF, López S 2000b Integrin α2β1 mediates the cell attachment of the rotavirus neuraminidase-resistant variant nar3. Virology 278:50–54

DISCUSSION

Estes: With all the discussion we have been having about trypsinization and rotavirus entry through receptor-mediated endocytosis versus direct penetration of cells, is the β3 integrin that the virus is binding to as the second step normally endocytosed? Do your data give any insight into this?

Arias: It is known that integrin β3 is endocytosed. However, this does not tell us much about the way rotaviruses enter the cell, since they could enter at the level of the cell membrane, before the β3 integrin is endocytosed, or after it has been endocytosed.

Holmes: I have read some descriptions of rotavirus infections that indicate that there may also be upper respiratory symptoms. I wonder whether the expression of the molecules that you have identified would also occur in respiratory epithelial cells.

Arias: As far as I know, no one has shown directly that the virus can replicate in the respiratory mucosa. However, as you mention, some studies have found an association between rotavirus gastroenteritis and respiratory symptoms. Integrins α2β1 and αVβ3 have been described in respiratory epithelia, although this does not mean, of course, that the sole presence of these two integrins will make the cells susceptible to rotavirus infection.

Greenberg: In the export of VP4 to the cell surface, is the VP4 specifically associated with rafts? This would be a way of bringing VP4 together and might give you a marker.

Cohen: We have some preliminary data suggesting that VP4 could be associated with rafts.

Arias: We also have preliminary data suggesting that rotavirus could be associated with rafts during virus entry.

Greenberg: Integrins are signalling molecules. Have you looked at any signalling events that might occur in conjunction with rotavirus binding?

Arias: We have started to look at this, but we do not have any conclusive information yet. However, it is interesting that the expression of αVβ3 in CHO cells did not increase the susceptibility of the cells by more than fourfold. These findings are similar to those of Barbara Coulson's group (Hewish et al 2000) when they expressed the genes for integrins $\alpha2\beta1$ and $\alpha4\beta1$ in the haematopoietic cell line K562. It seems that we are still far away from reaching the degree of susceptibility of MA104 cells. To find out whether each of the various molecules that have been described might play a role during rotavirus attachment and penetration, we would probably need to take a cell line that is devoid of such molecules and start putting them back. My guess is that the combination of several of these molecules will allow us to increase the susceptibility of those cells to a level close to that of MA104 cells.

Greenberg: Barbara Coulson actually activated her cells; with activation she was able to get quite a bit more infectivity.

Arias: That is true, however, to activate the integrin-transfected K562 cells they used a phorbol ester, and these compounds are known to have pleiotropic effects on cells. In fact, it has been reported that phorbol myristate acetate (PMA), the particular phorbol ester they used, induces a high level expression of the integrin $\alpha V\beta3$ gene in K562 cells (Bruger et al 1992). Thus, it is difficult to ascribe the increase of rotavirus infectivity in PMA-treated K562 cells to the increased expression of a single molecule; it might be the result of a combined increase in the level of synthesis of several of the putative virus receptors.

Desselberger: It is striking to look at the kinetics of your reactions. When you fully saturated with an antibody or peptide you always got only a decrease of 40–50% of receptor binding. It seems that the virus then chooses alternative receptors or co-receptors. Do you have a cell line that would be completely devoid of rotavirus-specific receptors, which you then could transfect with cDNA clones expressing all these different factors?

Arias: It seems that there are indeed alternative molecules for at least one of the virus interactions. We recently isolated monoclonal antibody 2D9, directed to the surface of MA104 cells, which recognises a cell surface molecule different from $\alpha2\beta1$. However, 2D9 behaves very much like antibodies to $\alpha2\beta1$ integrin in that it partially blocks the attachment, and thus the infectivity of the variant virus nar3. This suggests that this virus can bind both to the antigen recognised by 2D9 as well as to integrin $\alpha2\beta1$. With respect to cells that would lack the candidate receptor molecules, perhaps CHO cells or the haematopoietic cell line used by Barbara Coulson could be a good point to start from in rebuilding the receptor complexes.

Bishop: Now that you have identified these cell surface components involved in binding viruses, can you explain the difference in susceptibility between crypt cells and mature epithelial cells in terms of what is or is not present on the two cell surfaces?

Arias: There doesn't seem to be a simple correlation. Integrin $\alpha2\beta1$ is more abundant in crypt cells than in mature enterocytes in humans. The distribution of $\alpha V\beta3$ is not that well characterized in the intestinal epithelium, but it is known to be present in mature enterocytes in humans, and in mice it is known that the concentration of $\beta 3$ integrin is higher in the first three weeks of life than in adult animals. I think a single marker is going to be very difficult to associate with susceptibility to infection. Nonetheless, there seems to be a correlation between the susceptibility to rotavirus infection and the presence of integrin $\alpha v \beta 3$ in some cell lines we have tested, however, analysis of a larger panel of permissive and semi-permissive cells is needed to confirm this observation.

Prasad: In the case of sialic acid-dependent strains, is sialic acid binding or interacting with the receptor in some way, positioning the receptor in the appropriate place for VP4 to interact?

Arias: Although there is no direct proof that sialic acid binds directly to VP4, the available data suggest that sialic-dependent strains do bind to sialic acid through the VP8 domain of the protein. It cannot be ruled out, however, that these viruses may interact simultaneously with both sialic acid and with a protein receptor, whose correct conformation may need the presence of the acidic sugar. The protein and carbohydrate moieties could both form part or not of the same cellular molecule.

Estes: You described the nar mutant. Doesn't this virus still haemagglutinate?

Arias: Yes.

Estes: So what is the mechanism by which you think haemagglutination is occurring? Does that virus still bind some sialic acids?

Arias: Yes, nar3 is able to bind sialic acid in the same manner as wild-type RRV does, as judged by the fact that the haemagglutination activity of both viruses is inhibited by neuraminidase-treatment of erythrocytes and is also blocked by preincubation of the viruses with glycophorin A but not by the asialo form of this glycoprotein. However, nar3 does not seem to bind to sialic acid in MA104 cells, since the cell binding of this virus, but not that of RRV, is prevented by monoclonal antibody 2G4 directed to VP5, by antibodies to $\alpha 2 \beta 1$ integrin, and by monoclonal antibody 2D9.

Monroe: You mentioned that VP4 may be targeted to the rafts. But is it possible that any of these other proteins that you have identified are involved in the virus getting out, rather than getting in, in terms of where they are localized within the cells?

Arias: This does not seem to be the case, since the proteins we have identified as putative receptors have also been shown to be present in the membrane of MA104 cells, and antibodies to them block the virus infectivity. In addition, in MA104 cells rotavirus particles exit cells by lysis after accumulating in the endoplasmic reticulum. However, it is not possible to disregard that in Caco-2 cells, where the virus has been shown to be released by a non-lytic vesicular transport, the virions may interact with the identified molecules while they get out.

Holmes: Is the nar3 variant equally infectious in animals?

Arias: We haven't studied this.

Holmes: I raise this point because with Sindbis virus (Byrnes & Griffin 2000) and foot and mouth disease virus (Sa-Carvalho et al 1997), it has been found that adapting the viruses to cell culture often makes them sialic acid-dependent, even though they use other receptors *in vivo*. I thought this was an interesting point: many of these viruses may have been in culture a long time and have picked up this sialic acid dependence which may not be relevant *in vivo*.

Arias: Many of the rotavirus strains that are known to be sialic acid dependent are those originally isolated about 25 years ago. Perhaps they had a special propensity for binding to sialic acid and that is why they were more easily adapted to grow in culture. Mary Estes' group have tested a large collection of animal rotavirus strains, and most of these do not require sialic acids, so this may well be a character required for growing efficiently in cell culture (Ciarlet & Estes 1999).

Greenberg: Long ago, Linda Saif sent us a whole bunch of bovine faecal specimens containing non-cultivated rotaviruses. There were many wild-type isolates that formed large plaques right out of the stool and had haemagglutinating ability prior to passage in cell culture. There are wild-type viruses that, from the time they are isolated, look just like traditional cell culture adapted viruses: they are haemagglutination positive and form big plaques rapidly.

Estes: Are those both bovine and porcine?

Greenberg: I think they were mostly bovine, although Linda sent both.

Estes: I'd like to compliment Dr Arias' group on making significant progress in an area where many people have been working on for at least a decade. Perhaps we are beginning to see the light of day.

References

Bruger SR, Zutter MM, Sturgill-Koszycki S, Santoro SA 1992 Induced cell surface expression of functional $\alpha2\beta1$ integrin during megakaryocytic differentiation of K562 leukemic cells. Exp Cell Res 202:28–35

Byrnes AP, Griffin DE 2000 Large-plaque mutant of Sindbis virus shows reduced binding to heparan sulfate, heightened viraemia and slower clearance from the circulation. J Virol 74:644–651

Ciarlet M, Estes MK 1999 Human and most animal rotavirus strains do not require the presence of sialic acid on the cell surface for efficient infectivity. J Gen Virol 80:943–948

Hewish MJ, Takada Y, Coulson BS 2000 Integrins $\alpha2\beta1$ and $\alpha4\beta1$ can mediate SA11 rotavirus attachment and entry into cells. J Virol 74:228–236

Sa-Carvalho D, Reider E, Baxt B, Rodarte R, Tanuri A, Mason PW 1997 Tissue culture adaptation of foot and mouth disease virus selects viruses that bind to heparin and are attenuated in cattle. J Virol 71:5115–5123

Novartis 238: Gastroenteritis Viruses.
Copyright © 2001 John Wiley & Sons Ltd
Print ISBN 0-471-49663-4 eISBN 0-470-84653-4

Rotavirus RNA replication and gene expression

John T. Patton

Laboratory of Infectious Diseases, National Institute of Allergy and Infectious Diseases, National Institutes of Health, 7 Center Drive, MSC 0720, Room 117, Bethesda, MD 20892, USA

Abstract. Rotavirus mRNAs are capped but non-polyadenylated and serve as templates for both the synthesis of viral proteins and the segmented dsRNA genome. Viral proteins involved in RNA replication include the RNA polymerase (VP1), the core scaffold protein (VP2) and the non-structural RNA-binding proteins (NSP2 and NSP5). VP2 enhances dsRNA synthesis *in vitro*, possibly by forming platform structures on which VP1 functions. NSP2 octamers have NTPase and helix-destabilizing activity, and in conjunction with the phosphoprotein NSP5, are proposed to facilitate RNA packaging. The structure of the mRNA template contributes importantly to RNA replication. In particular, base-pairing between the 5′ and 3′-ends of viral mRNA generates panhandle structures which promote minus-strand synthesis. For the group A rotaviruses, the 3′-consensus sequence, 5′-UGUGACC-3′, which extends as a 3′-tail from the panhandles, also contributes to efficient minus-strand synthesis. Besides containing *cis*-acting replication signals, the 3′-end of viral mRNAs contains information that stimulates gene expression in infected cells. Specifically, the last four nucleotides of the 3′-consensus sequence, 5′-GACC-3′, operate as a virus-specific translation enhancer (3′TE) via a process thought to involve recognition of the element by NSP3. The NSP3–3′TE complex may mimic the function of complexes formed by eukaryotic poly(A)-tails and poly(A)-binding protein, thereby promoting more efficient translation of viral mRNAs.

2001 Gastroenteritis viruses. Wiley, Chichester (Novartis Foundation Symposium 238) p 64–81

Rotavirions are icosahedral triple-layered particles (TLPs) with genomes consisting of eleven segments of double-stranded (ds)RNA (Prasad et al 1988). During entry, the VP4–VP7 outer layer of the virus is lost, which produces double-layered particles (DLPs). RNA-dependent RNA polymerases associated with DLPs transcribe the dsRNA segments into 11 mRNAs. The mRNAs of group A rotaviruses are capped but non-polyadenylated, and other than the 5′- and 3′-terminal consensus sequences, 5′-GGC-poly(A/U)-3′ and 5′-UGUGACC-3′, respectively, the mRNAs share no sequence homology (Desselberger & McCrae 1994). Translation of the 11 mRNAs yields six structural and six non-structural

TABLE 1 Properties of the rotavirus RNA-binding proteins

Protein	RNA specificity	Site of accumulation*	Enzymatic or other activity	Structural features
VP1	3′-end of viral mRNA	VP **	RNA-dependent RNA polymerase	Located at the vertices of the core ($\sim$ 12 copies per virion)
VP2	ssRNA and dsRNA nonspecific	VP	Stimulates viral RNA replicase activity	Forms T = 1 shell of core (120 copies per virion)
VP3	ssRNA, nonspecific	VP **	Capping enzyme: guanylyltransferase, methyltransferase	Located at the vertices of the core ($\sim$ 12 copies per virion)
NSP1	5′-end of viral mRNA	CySk	Non-essential function in virus propagation	Suspected zinc finger protein
NSP2	ssRNA, nonspecific	VP	NTPase, helix-destabilizing activity; possible molecular motor for packaging	Forms barrel-shaped octamers, interacts with VP1 and NSP5
NSP3	3′-end of viral mRNA	CySk	Enhances viral mRNA translation, possible role in circularization of viral mRNAs	Forms dimers, affinity for eIF4GI
NSP5	ssRNA, nonspecific	VP	Serine autophosphokinase, possible modulator of NSP2 activity	O-glycosylated phospho-protein, forms multimers, complexes with NSP2

* CySk, cytoskeleton; VP, viroplasm.
** Proposed site of assembly into cores; site of initial interaction with viral mRNA is not established.

proteins, of which seven have RNA-binding activity (Table 1). The structural proteins, VP1, VP2 and VP3, the non-structural proteins, NSP2 and NSP5, and the viral mRNAs interact to form core-like replication intermediates (core RIs) that, through an associated replicase activity, catalyse the synthesis of dsRNA (Gallegos & Patton 1989) (Fig. 1). The assembly of core RIs and the synthesis of dsRNA is believed to occur in large cytoplasmic inclusions (viroplasms) present in infected cells. The interaction of VP6 with core RIs generates DLPs which acquire the outer layer proteins in the endoplasmic reticulum, forming TLPs (Estes 1996).

RNA replication

Characterization of subviral particles purified from infected cells has indicated that the synthesis of dsRNA occurs simultaneously with the packaging of mRNA

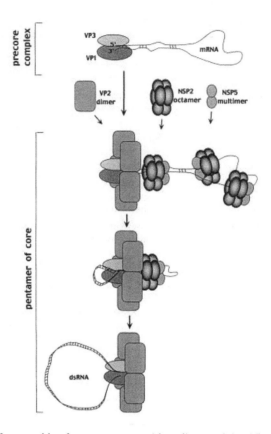

FIG. 1.   Model for assembly of core pentamers with replicase activity. The RNA polymerase, VP1, and capping enzyme, VP3, interact with viral mRNA to form a pre-core complex that lacks replicase activity. In the viroplasm, the complex then interacts with VP2 dimers, NSP2 octamers, and NSP5 multimers producing a structure that represents one of the vertices (pentamers) of the core. In core replication intermediates, the pentamer structures have replicase activity that catalyses the synthesis of dsRNA. The properties of NSP2 and NSP5 suggest that they facilitate the packaging of viral mRNA into cores during RNA replication.

templates into core RIs (Gallegos & Patton 1989). RNase treatment of core RIs with replicase activity prevents further dsRNA synthesis and reduces the size of the intermediates, results that indicate that the mRNAs pass from the exterior to the interior of the RI as dsRNA synthesis takes place (Fig. 2) (Patton & Gallegos 1990). On the basis of rotavirus structure predictions, the mRNA templates may be predicted to pass into cores through channels that exist at the fivefold axes of the VP2 shell (Prasad et al 1996). VP1 is situated at the interior base of these fivefold channels (Lawton et al 1997), which presumably would assure that each mRNA template encounters the RNA polymerase and is replicated as it is packaged.

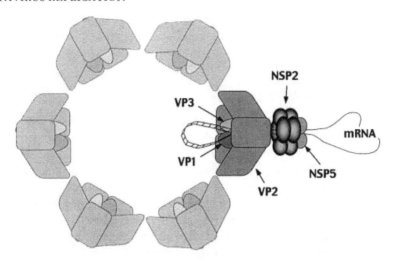

FIG. 2. A possible structure of a core-like replication intermediate. During the synthesis of dsRNA, the viral mRNA is proposed to move through channels present at the 5'-fold axes of the VP2. Whether packaging of the 11 mRNAs proceeds through a common site or eleven separate sites of the core is not known. It is also not resolved whether core assembly occurs before or after the assortment of the 11 viral mRNAs.

Considerable insight into the process of dsRNA synthesis has been gained using the template-dependent cell-free replication system developed by Chen et al (1994). The source of replicase activity in the system consists of cores which have been purified from virions and disrupted ('opened') by incubation in hypotonic buffer. The replicase activity of open cores is specific, catalysing the *de novo* synthesis of minus-strand RNA from exogenous viral mRNA to yield dsRNA.

Initiation complex for minus-strand RNA

The level of dsRNA synthesis in the open core replication system decreases as the concentration of monovalent salt, e.g. NaCl, in the reaction mixtures increases (Chen & Patton 1999). Recent studies have shown that the salt inhibition can be overcome if open cores, the mRNA template and GTP are pre-incubated prior to the addition of salt and the other 3 ribonucleotides (Chen & Patton 1999). Notably, pre-incubation will not overcome salt inhibition if any of these three components are left out or if GTP is replaced with ATP or CTP. When GTP is included in the pre-incubation mixture, the dinucleotides pGpG and ppGpG are made, possibly by a template-independent process (Chen & Patton 2000). When included in replication assays, pGpG can serve as a primer for minus-strand synthesis. Together, the data indicate that during rotavirus genome replication, an initiation complex is formed by the interaction of the viral RNA polymerase, the mRNA template and GTP or (p)pGpG and that this event is salt sensitive. Once formed, the initiation complex is salt resistant, and GTP or a derivative of it, i.e. pGpG or ppGpG, serves as the primer for elongation of the minus-strand.

mRNA structure and dsRNA synthesis

The open core replication system has been used to identify features of viral mRNAs that contribute to the synthesis of dsRNA. By adding viral mRNAs containing deletions of the 3'-consensus sequence, 5'-UGUGACC-3', to the replication system, it was shown that this sequence contains a *cis*-acting signal that is essential for minus-strand synthesis (Patton et al 1996, Wentz et al 1996). Indeed, placement of the 3'-consensus sequence onto the 3'-end of foreign RNAs is sufficient to allow them to serve as templates for the synthesis of dsRNA by open cores. By site-specific mutagenesis of viral mRNA templates, it has also been possible to assess the importance of the individual residues of the 3'-consensus sequence on the synthesis of dsRNA. The results have indicated that the mRNA template must terminate with one or two C residues for efficient RNA replication to occur (Patton et al 1996, Wentz et al 1996).

While nearly all viral mRNAs possess the same 3'-terminal sequence, there are some important exceptions. For instance, instead of the consensus sequence, the gene 5 RNAs of the SA11 and SA11-4F strains of rotavirus terminate with the sequence, 5'-UGUG<u>A</u>ACC-3', and therefore contain an insertion of an A residue (underlined) (Mitchell & Both 1990a, Patton et al 2000). More remarkably, a triple-plaque purified variant of a RRV×DS1 mono-reassortant has been isolated whose gene 5 RNA has the 3'-terminal sequence, 5'-UGU<u>UU</u>CC-3' and therefore differs at both the -3 and -4 position (underlined) from the 3'-consensus sequence (K. Kearney, D. Chen & J. Patton, unpublished results). On the basis of sequence comparisons of all group A rotavirus RNAs, the only strictly conserved sequences at the 5'- and 3'-termini are 5'-GGC-3' and 5'-CC-3', respectively. Given the sequence variations that have been detected in the 3'-consensus sequence, only the 3'-terminal CC residues can be considered as potentially required for packaging or replication of rotavirus mRNAs *in vivo*.

Several studies using the open core replication system have identified *cis*-acting signals in viral mRNAs that will enhance the synthesis of dsRNA, but unlike the *cis*-acting signal of the 3'-consensus sequence, are not essential for the synthesis of dsRNA. Most notably, analysis of viral mRNAs containing deletions of all or parts of their 5'-untranslated region (UTR) revealed that this region contains sequences that stimulate RNA replication (Patton et al 1996, 1999, Wentz et al 1996). Similarly, deletion mutagenesis showed that sequences upstream of the 3'-consensus sequence in the 3'-UTR contribute to efficient synthesis of dsRNA by open cores. Based on the location of *cis*-acting signals and computer modelling, the ends of the viral mRNAs have been proposed to interact in *cis* via complementary terminal sequences to form panhandle structures that promote the synthesis of dsRNA (Fig. 3) (Patton et al 1996, Chen & Patton 1998).

Besides the 5'- and 3'-termini, replacement of the open reading frame (ORF) of rotavirus mRNAs with foreign sequences of equivalent size has also been shown to decrease the efficiency of replication of the mRNA template *in vitro* (Patton et al 1999). However, more recently, an exhaustive analysis performed by deletion mutagenesis of short and overlapping sequences spanning the entire gene 11 mRNA of porcine CN86 rotavirus has determined that not all regions of the ORF play a role in enhancing dsRNA synthesis (J. Patton & M. Jones, unpublished results). Those regions that do play a role are involved in base-pairing between the termini of the mRNA and, thereby, have an impact on the formation and stability of the panhandle structure. From these analyses, it is clear that sequences that contribute to replication can be located both in the UTRs and the ORF of viral mRNAs and that RNA folding is a critical element affecting the ability of the mRNAs to promote minus-strand synthesis.

An important feature of the predicted secondary structures of the rotaviral mRNAs is that within the panhandle structure, the 3'-consensus sequence is either not base-paired or only partially base-paired to the 5'-terminus (Chen & Patton 1998). Mutations introduced into the RNA which increase the extent of complementarity between the 3'-consensus sequence and the 5'-terminus inhibit dsRNA synthesis in the open core replication system. In particular, when the 5'-end of the mRNA is changed so that it is fully complementary to the 3'-consensus sequence, replication of the mRNA *in vitro* is reduced by more than 100-fold. Hence, the single-stranded nature of the 3'-consensus sequence of the mRNA panhandle is essential for efficient dsRNA synthesis.

Rearrangements and deletions within viral RNAs

Several rotavirus variants have been described with atypical genotypes stemming from sequence duplications or deletions occurring within genome segments encoding VP6, NSP1 (gene 5 product), NSP2, NSP4 or NSP5 (Desselberger 1996). The abnormal segments probably result from the viral RNA polymerase and nascent RNA detaching from the RNA template during plus-strand synthesis, then re-attaching at an upstream or a downstream site on the template where transcription re-initiates (Kojima et al 1996). For genes other than gene 5, sequence duplications begin downstream of the ORF and, hence, the genes still encode a wild-type protein. However, rearrangements occurring within gene 5 can alter the ORF such that the NSP1 product contains a C-terminal truncation, a duplication or a deletion (Fig. 4) (Tian et al 1993, Hua & Patton 1994). Such results indicate that NSP1 is not essential for virus replication (Okada et al 1999). The

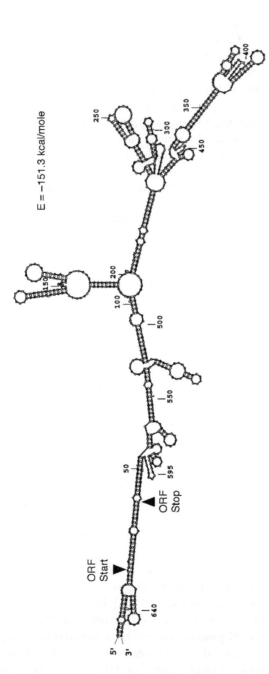

E = −151.3 kcal/mole

FIG. 3. Predicted secondary structure of the gene 11 mRNA of porcine rotavirus CN86 illustrating the interaction of the 5′- and 3′-termini of the mRNA. The structure was generated with the *mfold* program (*http://www.ibc.wustl.edu/~zuker*). Deletion of residues 1–50, 50–100, 500–550, or 650–664 reduces the efficiency of replication of the mRNA *in vitro* by greater than twofold suggesting that sequences within the 5′-UTR, 3′-UTR and ORF of the mRNA all may promote dsRNA synthesis.

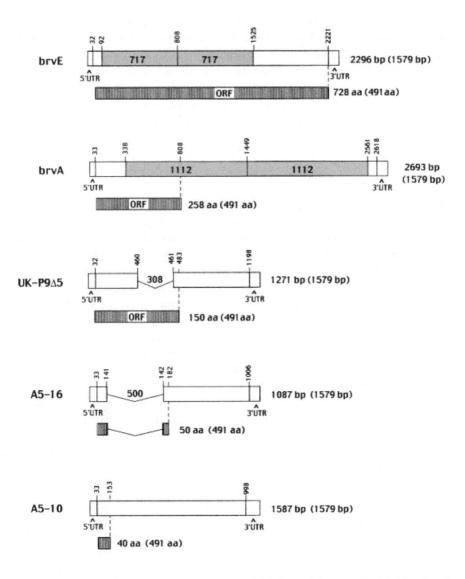

FIG. 4. Schematic illustrating rearrangements and deletions of the gene 5 RNA. The size of each atypical RNA and the NSP1 protein encoded by it are given, and the size of its wild-type counterpart RNA and protein is given in parentheses. Sequence duplications are shaded; the sizes of the duplications and deletions are also shown. The A5-10 RNA does not contain a duplication or deletion, but encodes a truncated NSP1 protein due to a point mutation in the ORF.

largest of the sequence duplications and deletions that have been described occur in gene 5 and are 1112 and 500 nucleotides long, respectively (Hua & Patton 1994, Okada et al 1999). Since these results indicate that the amount of viral RNA present in virion cores can vary by as much as 1600 nucleotides, a headful mechanism may not operate during RNA packaging. Analysis of bovine rotavirus variants with deletions in the normally 1579 nucleotide gene 5 RNA provide evidence that a 600+ nucleotide stretch from residues 141 to 768 is not required for RNA packaging and replication (Okada et al 1999). Isolation and characterization of many such rearranged genes should provide further information about the location of *cis*-acting signals in rotavirus mRNAs that promote packaging and replication.

Viral protein function in RNA synthesis

RIs that have replicase activity contain the structural proteins VP1, VP2 and VP3 and the non-structural proteins NSP2 and NSP5 (Fig. 1) (Gallegos & Patton 1989). As reviewed in Table 1, all these proteins have affinity for single-stranded RNA (Labbé et al 1994, Patton & Chen 1999, Taraporewala et al 1999). As core RIs synthesize dsRNA, they simultaneously undergo maturation into double-layered RIs through the acquisition of VP6 (Gallegos & Patton 1989), a protein that is not required for dsRNA synthesis and, based on *in vitro* assays, has no effect on the activity of the replicase.

Several lines of evidence suggest that VP1 is the viral RNA-dependent RNA polymerase. These include (i) sequence analysis demonstrating that VP1 contains motifs shared among RNA-dependent RNA polymerase (Mitchell & Both 1990b), (ii) experiments showing that VP1 has affinity for nucleotides and that cross-linking of photo-reactable azido-ATP to VP1 inhibits transcription (Valenzuela et al 1991), (iii) electrophoretic gel-shift assays indicating that VP1 has affinity for the 3'-end of viral mRNAs (Patton 1996), and (iv) *in vitro* replication assays showing that VP1 is a common component of RIs and recombinant viral particles with replicase activity (Gallegos & Patton 1989, Zeng et al 1996). By assaying recombinant proteins for enzymatic functions *in vitro*, we found that VP1 only exhibited replicase activity in the presence of VP2, the protein that forms the T=1 shell of the core (Patton et al 1997). Studies with rotavirus *ts* mutants likewise indicate that VP2 plays an essential role in the formation of RIs with replicase activity (Mansell et al 1994). Deletion mutagenesis has shown that the N-terminus of VP2 is necessary for the interaction of the protein with RNA and VP1, and for replicase activity, but not for the assembly of VP2 into cores (Labbé et al 1994, Lawton et al 1997, Patton et al 1997, Zeng et al 1998). While the precise role of VP2 in dsRNA synthesis is not known, it is possible that pentamers formed by VP2 serve as platforms on which the mRNA template binds and VP1 catalyses minus-strand synthesis (Prasad et al 1996). Analysis of VP3 indicates that this protein contains at least two enzymatic activities, guanylyltransferase and methyltransferase, involved in the capping of rotavirus mRNAs (Pizzaro et al 1991, Chen et al 1999). Because VP3 has affinity for GTP, it may be speculated that the protein plays some role in the formation of the initiation complex for minus-strand synthesis.

The non-structural proteins, NSP2 and NSP5, both accumulate in viroplasms, and indeed, the co-expression of these viral proteins in uninfected cells generates viroplasm-like structures (Fabbretti et al 1999). Earlier studies provided evidence that NSP2 forms homo-multimeric complexes *in vivo* and interacts with VP1 (Kattoura et al 1994). More recent work with purified recombinant protein has shown that NSP2 self-assembles into stable barrel-shaped octamers of $\sim$12S, consisting of two tetramers of $\sim$7S (Schuck et al 2001). The NSP2 octamers have strong non-specific affinity for single-stranded RNA, and exhibit Mg^{2+}-dependent NTPase activity (Taraporewala et al 1999) and Mg^{2+}-independent helix-destabilizing activity (Taraporewala & Patton 2001). During hydrolysis of NTP by NSP2, the protein undergoes phosphorylation (Taraporewala et al 1999). Together, these properties suggest that NSP2 octamers may serve as molecular motors, catalyzing the packaging of the mRNA templates into cores as dsRNA synthesis occurs.

The recovery of NSP2–NSP5 complexes from infected cells raises the possibility that NSP5 may modulate the activity of NSP2. NSP5 is an O-glycosylated phosphoprotein that self-assembles into dimers and that has non-specific RNA-binding protein activity (González & Burrone 1991, P. Vende, Z. Taraporewala & J. Patton, unpublished results). The protein has autokinase activity and exists in several phosphorylated isomers in infected cells (Afrikanova et al 1996, Blackhall et al 1997). When co-expressed in uninfected cells, NSP2 induces the hyperphosphorylation of NSP5 (Afrikanova et al 1998). The mechanism of NSP5 hyperphosphorylation is not known but may involve a cascade of events initiated by the NTPase activity of NSP2. Indeed, the interaction of NSP2 and NSP5 may result in the transfer of phosphate groups generated by the NTPase activity of NSP2 to NSP5, causing NSP5 to undergo hyperphosphorylation. In a recent study, NSP5 was shown to form complexes with NSP6, which like NSP5 is a product of gene 11 and accumulates in viroplasms (Torres-Vega et al 2000).

Gene expression

A number of studies have provided evidence that the 5$'$-cap and 3$'$-poly(A) tail of eukaryotic mRNAs work synergistically to stimulate translation through a mechanism that involves interaction of the cap-associated eukaryotic initiation

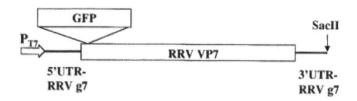

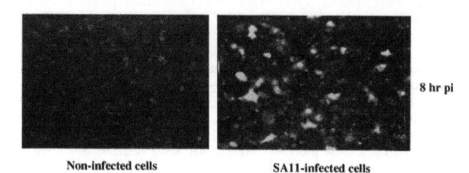

8 hr pi

Non-infected cells   **SA11-infected cells**

FIG. 5.   Stimulation of viral mRNA translation in infected cells. An analogue of the RRV gene 7 mRNA was made that contained the ORF for green fluorescent protein (GFP) inserted in-frame at the N-terminus of the ORF for VP7. The mRNA was transfected in non-infected and rotavirus-infected MA104 cells and, at 8 h post infection, the cells were examined for the expression of GFP by UV light.

factor, eIF-4G, and the poly(A)-binding protein, PABP (Gallie 1998). The interaction of these proteins with the termini of the mRNAs and with each other has been proposed to cause circularization of the mRNAs within polysomes. Circularization is believed to enhance translation by stabilizing the binding of initiation factors to the mRNA and by promoting the recycling of the ribosomes from the 3′ to the 5′ end of the mRNA (Wells et al 1998). Because rotavirus mRNA lack poly(A) tails, the efficient translation of these mRNAs must be accomplished via a process that differs from that of prototypic eukaryotic mRNAs.

*m*RNA *structure and translation*

The location of translation enhancement elements in rotavirus mRNA has been examined by transfection of chimeric reporter mRNAs into infected and uninfected cells (Fig. 5). In one such study, chimeric mRNAs were prepared that contained 5′-caps, the ORF for luciferase and either all or portions of the 5′- and

3′-UTRs of a rotaviral mRNA or of a non-viral mRNA (Chizhikov & Patton 2000). Based on the expression of luciferase from the transfected mRNAs, results were obtained demonstrating that the last four nucleotides of the 3′-consensus sequence of rotaviral mRNAs, 5′-GACC-3′, stimulate translation in infected cells. This translation enhancer (3″TE) does not stimulate translation in uninfected cells, and its activity parallels that of the expression of viral proteins in infected cells. The activity of the 3′-TE also operates independently of the sequence of the 5′-UTR, but efficient translation is cap-dependent (Chizhikov & Patton 2000). Given that the mRNAs of most group A rotaviruses end with the same sequence, 5′-GACC-3′, the 3″TE is likely to represent a common element used to promote viral gene expression in infected cells. In comparison to other enhancers, the 3″TE is remarkable in its small size. Combined with studies defining the location of *cis*-acting replication signals in viral mRNAs, it is apparent that the 3′-consensus sequence has dual and competing functions: to enhance translation of viral mRNAs via the activity of the 3″TE and to promote the use of the mRNAs as a template for minus-strand synthesis.

Viral protein function in translation

The mechanism by which the 3″TE promotes translation is suggested by studies that have been performed on rotavirus NSP3, an RNA-binding protein which specifically recognizes the 3″TE sequence (Poncet et al 1994). NSP3 has been shown by the two hybrid system and by pull down assays to interact with eIF-4GI (Piron et al 1998). Therefore, NSP3 can be considered to be a functional homologue of PABP in that both specifically bind to the 3′-end of mRNAs and both have affinity for a cap-associated initiation factor. Based on these properties, NSP3 has been proposed to catalyse the circularization of rotavirus mRNA within polysomes, thereby increasing translation efficiency.

References

Afrikanova I, Miozzo MC, Giambiagi S, Burrone O 1996 Phosphorylation generates different forms of rotavirus NSP5. J Gen Virol 77:2059–2065

Afrikanova I, Fabbretti E, Miozzo MC, Burrone OR 1998 Rotavirus NSP5 phosphorylation is up-regulated by interaction with NSP2. J Gen Virol 79:2679–2686

Blackhall J, Fuentes A, Hansen K, Magnusson G 1997 Serine protein kinase activity associated with rotavirus phosphoprotein NSP5. J Virol 71:138–144

Chen DY, Patton JT 1998 Rotavirus RNA replication requires a single-stranded 3′-end for efficient minus-strand synthesis. J Virol 72:7387–7396

Chen DY, Patton JT 1999 Requirements for minus-strand initiation in the synthesis of rotavirus double-stranded RNA. Nucleic Acids Res Symp Ser 41:205–207

Chen DY, Patton JT 2000 De novo synthesis of minus-strand RNA by the rotavirus RNA polymerase in a cell-free system involves a novel mechanism of initiation. RNA 6:1455–1467

Chen DY, Zeng CQ-Y, Wentz MJ, Gorziglia M, Estes MK, Ramig RF 1994 Template-dependent, *in vitro* replication of rotavirus RNA. J Virol 68:7030–7039

Chen DY, Luongo CL, Nibert ML, Patton JT 1999 Rotavirus open cores catalyze 5′-capping and methylation of exogenous RNA: evidence that VP3 is a methyltransferase. Virology 265: 120–130

Chizhikov V, Patton JT 2000 A four-nucleotide translation enhancer in the 3′-terminal consensus sequence of the nonpolyadenylated mRNAs of rotavirus. RNA 6:814–825

Desselberger U 1996 Genome rearrangements of rotaviruses. Adv Virus Res 46:69–95

Desselberger U, McCrae MA 1994 The rotavirus genome. Curr Top Microbiol Immunol 185:31–66

Estes MK 1996 Rotaviruses and their replication. In: Fields BN, Knipe D, Howley PM et al (eds) Fundamental virology, 3rd edn. Lippincott-Raven, Philadelphia, PA, p 731–761

Fabbretti E, Afrikanova I, Vascotto F, Burrone OE 1999 Two non-structural rotavirus proteins, NSP2 and NSP5, form viroplasm-like structures *in vivo*. J Gen Virol 80:333–339

Gallie DR 1998 A tale of two termini: a functional interaction between the termini of an mRNA is a prerequisite for efficient translation initiation. Gene 216:1–11

Gallegos CO, Patton JT 1989 Characterization of rotavirus replication intermediates: a model for the assembly of single-shelled particles. Virology 172:616–627

González SA, Burrone OR 1991 Rotavirus NS26 is modified by addition of single O-linked residues of N-acetylglucosamine. Virology 182:8–16

Hua J, Patton JT 1994 The carboxyl-half of the rotavirus nonstructural protein NS53 (NSP1) is not required for virus replication. Virology 198:567–576

Kattoura MD, Chen X, Patton JT 1994 The rotavirus RNA-binding protein NS35 (NSP2) forms 10S multimers and interacts with the viral RNA polymerase. Virology 202:803–813

Kojima K, Taniguichi K, Urasawa T, Urasawa S 1996 Sequence analysis of normal and rearranged NSP5 genes from human rotavirus strains isolated in nature: implications for the occurrence of the rearrangement at the step of plus strand synthesis. Virology 224:446–452

Labbé M, Baudoux P, Charpilienne A, Poncet D, Cohen J 1994 Identification of the nucleic acid binding domain of the rotavirus VP2 protein. J Gen Virol 75:3423–3430

Lawton JA, Zeng CQ, Mukherjee SK, Cohen J, Estes MK, Prasad BV 1997 Three-dimensional structural analysis of recombinant rotavirus-like particles with intact and amino-terminal-deleted VP2: implications for the architecture of the VP2 capsid layer. J Virol 71:7353–7360

Mansell EA, Ramig RF, Patton JT 1994 Temperature-sensitive lesions in the capsid proteins of the rotavirus mutants tsF and tsG that affect virion assembly. Virology 204:69–81

Mitchell DB, Both GW 1990a Conservation of a potential metal binding motif despite extensive sequence diversity in the rotavirus nonstructural protein NS53. Virology 174:618–621

Mitchell DB, Both GW 1990b Completion of the genomic sequence of the simian rotavirus SA11: nucleotide sequences of segments 1, 2, and 3. Virology 177:324–331

Okada J, Kobayashi N, Taniguichi K, Urasawa S 1999 Analysis on reassortment of rotavirus NSP1 genes lacking coding region for cysteine-rich zinc finger motif. Arch Virol 144:345–353

Patton JT 1996 Rotavirus VP1 alone specifically binds to the 3′ end of viral mRNA but the interaction is not sufficient to initiate minus-strand synthesis. J Virol 70:7940–7947

Patton JT, Chen DY 1999 RNA-binding and capping activities of proteins in rotavirus open cores. J Virol 73:1382–1391

Patton JT, Gallegos CO 1990 Rotavirus RNA replication: single-strand RNA extends from the replicase particle. J Gen Virol 71:1087–1094

Patton JT, Wentz M, Xiaobo J, Ramig RF 1996 *cis*-acting signals that promote genome replication in rotavirus mRNA. J Virol 70:3961–3971

Patton JT, Jones MT, Kalbach, AN, He, Y-W, Xiaobo J 1997 Rotavirus RNA polymerase requires the core shell protein to synthesize the double-stranded RNA genome. J Virol 71: 9618–9626

Patton JT, Chnaiderman J, Spencer E 1999 Open reading frame in rotavirus mRNA specifically promotes synthesis of double-stranded RNA: Template size also affects replication efficiency. Virology 264:167–180

Patton JT, Taraporewala Z, Chen D et al 2000 Effect of intragenic rearrangement and changes in the 3'-consensus sequence on NSP1 expression and rotavirus replication. J Virol 75: 2076–2086

Piron M, Vende P, Cohen J, Poncet D 1998 Rotavirus RNA-binding protein NSP3 interacts with eIF4GI and evicts the poly(A) binding protein from eIF4F. EMBO J 17:5811–5821

Pizarro JL, Sandino AM, Pizarro J, Fernandez J, Spencer E 1991 Characterization of rotavirus guanylyltransferase activity associated with polypeptide VP3. J Gen Virol 72:325–332

Poncet D, Laurent S, Cohen J 1994 Four nucleotides are the minimal requirement for RNA recognition by rotavirus non-structural protein NSP3. EMBO J 13:4165–4173

Prasad BVV, Wang GJ, Clerx JPM, Chiu W 1988 Three-dimensional structure of rotavirus. J Mol Biol 199:269–275

Prasad BVV, Rothnagel R, Zeng CQ-Y, Jakana J, Lawton JA, Chiu W, Estes MK 1996 Visualization of ordered genomic RNA and localization of transcriptional complexes in rotavirus. Nature 382:471–473

Schuck P, Taraporewala Z, McPhee P, Patton JT 2001 Rotavirus non structural protein NSP2 self-assembles into octamers that undergo ligand-induced conformational changes. J Biol Chem 276:9679–9687

Taraporewala Z, Patton JT 2001 Identification and characterization of the helix-destabilizing activity of the rotavirus nonstructural protein NSP2. J Virol, in press

Taraporewala Z, Chen C, Patton JT 1999 Multimers formed by the rotavirus nonstructural protein NSP2 bind to RNA and have nucleoside triphosphatase activity. J Virol 73:9934–9943

Tian Y, Tarlow O, Ballard A, Desselberger U, McCrae MA 1993 Genomic concatermerization/ deletion in rotaviruses: a new mechanism for generating rapid genetic change of potential epidemiological importance. J Virol 67:6625–6632

Torres-Vega MA, González RA, Duarte M, Poncet D, López S, Arias CF 2000 The C-terminal domain of rotavirus NSP5 is essential for its multimerization, hyperphosphorylation and interaction with NSP6. J Gen Virol 81:821–830

Valenzuela S, Pizarro J, Sandino AM et al 1991 Photoaffinity labeling of rotavirus VP1 with 8-azido-ATP: identification of the viral RNA polymerase. J Virol 65:3964–3967

Wells SE, Hillner PE, Vale RD, Sachs AB 1998 Circularization of mRNA by eukaryotic translation initiation factors. Mol Cell 2:135–140

Wentz MJ, Patton JT, Ramig RF 1996 The 3'-terminal consensus sequence of rotavirus mRNA is the minimal promoter of negative-strand RNA synthesis. J Virol 70:7833–7841

Zeng CQ-Y, Wentz MJ, Estes MK, Ramig RF 1996 Characterization and replicase activity of double-layered and single-layered rotavirus-like particles expressed from baculovirus recombinants. J Virol 70:2736–2742

Zeng CQ-Y, Estes MK, Charpilienne A, Cohen J 1998 The N terminus of rotavirus VP2 is necessary for encapsidation of VP1 and VP3. J Virol 72:201–208

DISCUSSION

Ramig: I am fascinated by your model. We have added purified NSP3 to the *in vitro* system, and it shuts down the replication reaction. To us, this implies that NSP3 probably binds at the 3' end of the RNA more strongly than VP1. How do you envision any template ever entering into a replication pathway? Our simplistic way of looking at it is that templates might all be shunted towards translation. How do you displace NSP3 to get templates replicated?

Patton: The short answer is that we do not know. However, it may be that there are two populations of viral mRNAs in the cell, of which only one have NSP3 bound to their 3'-ends. Possibly, this population is only translated and never serves as an RNA template for dsRNA synthesis. One would suspect that the second population of mRNA is bound by VP1, and in the viroplasm serves as a substrate for the assembly of cores with replicase activity. If there are two populations, then VP1 would not be required to displace NSP3 from an mRNA.

Greenberg: The original publication from which it looked like this methodology would work (Gorziglia & Collins 1992) showed enhancement of translation and also showed negative strand synthesis, I thought.

Patton: The publication showed that chloramphenicol acetyl transferase (CAT) expression from a viral analogue RNA was greater in infected cells than uninfected cells. The report indicated that this was due to replication of the analogue RNA in the infected cell; unfortunately, no direct evidence was provided that demonstrated the synthesis of dsRNA or minus-sense RNA from the analogue RNA. Instead, more recent studies suggest that the amplification of CAT expression in the infected cells was due to the presence of a viral-specific 3'-terminal translation enhancement element in the analogue RNA that stimulated translation of CAT in the presence of viral proteins.

Desselberger: Your talk reminded me of the RNA fork model which Brownlee's group and others developed for influenza virus transcription (Fodor et al 1994, 1995, Hagen et al 1994). Have you looked at sequence requirements of the terminal sequences of the RNA for optimal polymerase function as these groups did? For example, have you tried changing the ends to get promoters that are stronger than the natural promoters (promoter-up mutations; Flick & Hobom 1999)?

Patton: No, we haven't tried this, although we plan to do so.

Bishop: Is gene 5, or a portion of it, redundant *in vitro*? Do you think it may have a real function *in vivo*?

Patton: Passage of rotaviruses repeatedly in cell culture will characteristically give rise to non-defective variants that do not encode wild-type NSP1 because of rearrangements occurring within gene 5. In cell culture, the rearranged gene 5s are preferentially packaged into progeny indicating that there is selection for variants unable to encode the wild-type protein. The speed at which the NSP1 ORF is lost in cell culture raises the possibility that expression of the protein is indeed selected against in cell culture. However, since viruses recovered from animals almost always contain a functional ORF for wild-type NSP1, presumably the protein does play a role in nature that is essential for the long-term viability of the virus.

Greenberg: If the secondary structure of the RNA is more critical than the coding region, why can't you start trying to get around that by using selectable markers that are smaller and smaller, so you use less and less of your ORF? Why aren't you going in that direction?

Patton: It is a reasonable approach if one could identify small selectable markers that could be used that would not affect the overall long-range secondary structures of the RNAs. Most selectable markers are not small and may not work satisfactorily for a virus with a relatively short life cycle.

Estes: With regard to the interaction of the replicase and the 3' end, the data from all the mutations that were analysed suggested it was more than just the two Cs. Is that right?

Patton: Yes.

Estes: Why is that? Is it because there is no translation in that system?

Patton: The 3'-end of viral mRNAs plays a dual role, promoting both dsRNA synthesis and translation. Based on *in vitro* assays, the two terminal Cs play an essential role in the efficient synthesis of dsRNA, while residues immediately upstream of the two Cs play a less important role in replication. The identification of rotaviruses that are mutated in the 3'-consensus region confirms the importance of the two Cs and indicates that the upstream residues may not be essential for RNA replication. The NSP3 binding site includes the last four to five residues of the 3'-end of the mRNA, and mutation of these residues decreases the ability of NSP3 to bind to the mRNA. If NSP3 does not bind efficiently to the mRNA and thus fails to drive it into polysomes, then it may be that the mRNA is more likely to move to the viroplasm, where it undergoes packaging and then replication. In this scenario, the mutations affect the dual role of the mRNA by shifting it in favour of being used as a template for replication. Hence, despite the fact that the mutation of residues upstream from the two Cs decreases the replication efficiency of the mRNA *in vitro*, in fact the replication of the RNA *in vivo* may not be significantly affected because the mutations have an even greater negative effect on the ability of the mRNA to undergo translation.

Cohen: From your *in vitro* replicase assay you conclude that the two Cs are essential. But you must bear in mind that the *in vitro* replicase assay is a poor one. What is the efficiency of this assay *in vitro*? If you use one template, how many copies do you have? This could be misleading.

Ramig: When we have done careful quantitation, we calculate that we get over 1000 negative strands for each polymerase complex if we assume that there are 12 complexes in one of those particles (M. Wentz & R. F. Ramig, unpublished results). So I think it is quite an efficient reaction.

Patton: I have not done the calculation, so I don't know. I know that this system is probably one of the most powerful systems that exists for the study of RNA replication: it is very specific and works with recombinant proteins, so it is fully definable.

Desselberger: You mentioned in your model the very interesting interaction of NSP2 and NSP5. This reminded me of some of our data, when we analysed over 500 reassortants between bovine rotaviruses and a human rotavirus strain, and found gene linkage between the NSP1, NSP2 and NSP5 genes (Graham et al 1987). Have you looked at this interaction in more detail?

Patton: No. Most of the studies that deal with NSP2/NSP5 interactions have been done outside of our lab. We are working on both of these proteins, but we are still trying to define their activities separately before we put them together to try to find out how their interaction affects each other's activities.

Ramig: The model you presented implied that there was an interaction between your NSP2 octamer and VP2, VP1 or VP3. Do you know anything about this?

Patton: Protein–protein cross-linking studies have shown that NSP2 and VP1 form complexes *in vivo*. Other than that, we have no information regarding the interaction of the structural and non-structural proteins

Ramig: With regard to Ulrich Desselberger's comment on apparent linkage in reassortants, we saw a high degree of linkage between VP3 and NSP1 (Gombold & Ramig 1986). This would almost fit with a VP3–NSP1 interaction.

Arias: Do you have any idea about the possible role of NSP6 in the virus replication pathway?

Patton: We don't.

Ramig: We have also been focusing in on the terminal CC residues as perhaps being important. One thing that was evident from John Patton's paper was that the addition of an extra nucleotide to the end has no effect. If we add a G, replication is about 50% down. We tried adding an A, and it totally killed replication (D. Younker & R. F. Ramig, unpublished results).

Estes: A point of clarification: in your models of secondary structure, is there any direct evidence that this secondary structure exists?

Patton: No, we have yet to demonstrate the accuracy of the secondary structure predictions biochemically. But given the improvements over the last five to 10 years in the algorithms used in these predictions, the structures are probably close to accurate. In particular, the energy value for the computed structure of the gene 11 RNA indicates that the panhandle structure is very stable.

Monroe: One of the improvements in the algorithms is that instead of returning just one answer, you can look at the five or 10 most stable structures.

Patton: In the case of the top 20 most stable structures predicted for gene 11, they all indicate the presence of the same 5′–3′ panhandle.

Ramig: We talked to Dr Zuker last week. For folding, your default and only option is in 1 M salt, which certainly isn't physiological and is inhibitory to this in vitro reaction. I have questions about the relevance of predicted structures to actual structure in replication conditions. We have recently set out to start doing the biochemical probing of structure under replication conditions.

References

Flick R, Hobom G 1999 Interaction of influenzavirus polymerase with viral RNA in the 'corkscrew' conformation. J Gen Virol 80:2565–2572

Fodor E, Pritlove DC, Brownlee GG 1994 The influenza virus panhandle is involved in the initiation of transcription. J Virol 68:4092–4096

Fodor E, Pritlove DC, Brownlee GG 1995 Characterization of the RNA-fork model of virion RNA in the initiation of transcription in influenza A virus. J Virol 69:4012–4019

Gombold JL, Ramig RF 1986 Analysis of reassortment genome segments in mice mixedly infected with rotaviruses SA11 and RRV. J Virol 57:110–116

Gorziglia M, Collins P 1992 Intracellular amplification and expression of a synthetic analog of rotavirus genomic RNA bearing a foreign marker gene: mapping *cis* acting nucleotides in the 3'-noncoding region. Proc Natl Acad Sci USA 89:5784–5788

Graham A, Kudesia G, Allen AM, Desselberger U 1987 Reassortment of human rotavirus possessing genome rearrangements with bovine rotavirus: evidence for host cell selection. J Gen Virol 68:115–122

Hagen M, Chung TDY, Butcher JA, Krystal M 1994 Recombinant influenza virus polymerase: requirement of both 5' and 3' viral ends for endonuclease activity. J Virol 68:1509–1515

Novartis 238: Gastroenteritis Viruses.
Copyright © 2001 John Wiley & Sons Ltd
Print ISBN 0-471-49663-4   eISBN 0-470-84653-4

Pathogenesis of rotavirus gastroenteritis

Mary K. Estes, Gagandeep Kang, Carl Q.-Y. Zeng, Sue E. Crawford and Max Ciarlet

Division of Molecular Virology and Microbiology, Baylor College of Medicine, Houston, TX 77030, USA

Abstract. The outcome of intestinal infection with rotaviruses is more complex than initially appreciated, and it is affected by a complex interplay of host and viral factors. Rotaviruses infect intestinal enterocytes, and the early events in infection are mediated by virus–epithelial cell interactions. Diarrhoea may be caused by several mechanisms including (i) malabsorption that occurs secondary to the destruction of enterocytes, (ii) villus ischaemia and activation of the enteric nervous system that may be evoked by release of a vasoactive agent from infected epithelial cells in the absence of significant pathologic lesions or enterocyte damage, and (iii) intestinal secretion stimulated by the intracellular or extracellular action of the rotavirus non-structural protein, NSP4, a novel enterotoxin and secretory agonist with pleiotropic properties. New studies of rotavirus infection of polarized intestinal epithelial cells show that rotaviruses infect cells differently depending on whether or not they require sialic acid for initial binding, and infection alters epithelial cell functions. NSP4 also affects epithelial cell function and interactions. NSP4 (i) induces an age- and dose-dependent diarrhoeal response in young rodents that is similar to virus-induced disease, (ii) stimulates a Ca^{2+}-dependent cell permeability where the secretory response is age-dependent, and (iii) alters epithelial cell integrity. Antibody to NSP4 protects mouse pups from diarrhoea induced by homotypic and heterotypic viruses. These data support a new mechanism of rotavirus-induced diarrhoea whereby a viral enterotoxin triggers a signal transduction pathway that alters epithelial cell permeability and chloride secretion. This new information about how a gastrointestinal virus causes disease demonstrates common pathogenic mechanisms for viral and bacterial pathogens not previously appreciated. These results also suggest new approaches to prevent or treat rotavirus-induced diarrhoea.

2001 Gastroenteritis viruses. Wiley, Chichester (Novartis Foundation Symposium 238) p 82–100

Acute infectious gastroenteritis is a major cause of infant morbidity in developed countries and of infant mortality in developing areas of the world. Rotavirus is recognized as the most important aetiologic agent of infantile gastroenteritis, and studies of rotavirus serve as models for the complex interactions between enteric viruses and the multifunctional cells of the gastrointestinal tract. Understanding such interactions is significant for microbial pathogenesis because most infections

(> 80%) are initiated at mucosal surfaces. Rotaviruses are pathogens that infect the mature enterocytes of the villi in the small intestine, and infection appears to be limited to these highly differentiated cells in immunologically competent hosts. In such hosts, infections are generally acute, yet diarrhoeal disease can be severe and life threatening. Disease is generally resolved within 2–5 days after infection if affected hosts receive adequate rehydration. In immunocompromised hosts, virus infections persist, the virus can be detected extraintestinally, and virus excretion may be detected for many months.

Rotaviruses infect almost all mammalian and some avian species, and much of our understanding of rotavirus pathogenesis has come from studies in animal models, particularly in small animal models (mice and rabbits), but also in larger animals (cows and piglets). Studies in children are limited due to the difficulty and lack of clinical need for obtaining biopsies from infants, and our inability to determine the precise onset of natural infections. In all animal species where naïve animals can be infected, rotavirus disease is age-dependent. For example, in mice and rabbits, diarrhoeal disease is the outcome of infections that occur only during the first two weeks of life (Ciarlet et al 1998a, Starkey et al 1986), while these animals remain susceptible to viral infection into adulthood, as evidenced by virus antigen shedding and seroconversion (Ward et al 1990, Ciarlet et al 1998a). Rotavirus infections have been reported to occur repeatedly in humans from birth to old age, but the majority of infections after the first 2 years of life are asymptomatic or associated with mild gastrointestinal symptoms. The age-related resistance to rotavirus-induced diarrhoea in humans is thought to be mediated primarily by acquired immunity. The age-dependent resistance to disease could be due to other factors such as intestinal development and maturation, but these cannot be directly tested in humans. Currently, our best understanding of the mechanisms of rotavirus pathogenesis relies on results obtained in animal models.

Results and discussion

Rotavirus pathogenesis is complex and involves several mechanisms

The outcome of an infection with rotavirus is clearly dependent on both host and viral factors, and these factors can affect one or more of the several stages of pathogenesis (Table 1). Host factors have been dissected by analysis of the outcome of infection in animals inoculated with well-defined viral strains. Both natural and experimental rotavirus infections are characterized by viral replication in enterocytes in the small intestine, with subsequent cell lysis and attendant villus blunting, depressed levels of mucosal disaccharidases, watery diarrhoea and dehydration. Many studies have demonstrated malabsorption in

TABLE 1   Stages in enteric virus pathogenesis

Entry into the host

Primary replication

Local or disseminated host cellular responses (signalling)

Spread through host

Host immune response

Cell injury

Stability and survival of virus in the gastrointestinal tract

Adsorption and penetration into enterocytes (receptors)

Uncoating, transcription, translation replication, assembly, release

Effect of viral proteins on cell function (NSP4)

---

enterocytes and correlated this dysfunction with destruction of enterocytes and histopathological changes in the intestine, which are generally seen 24–36 h after infection (Graham et al 1984, Davidson et al 1977). However, malabsorption cannot be the entire basis of rotavirus pathogenesis because it fails to explain the early watery diarrhoea that occurs *prior to* the detection of villus blunting and other histological changes in the intestine (Collins et al 1989, Theil et al 1978, McAdaragh et al 1980, Mebus 1976, Ward et al 1996). In addition, some animals exhibit diarrhoea in the absence of clear histopathological changes (neonatal mice infected with homologous rotavirus strains; Burns et al 1995), and other adult rotavirus-infected animals (rabbits) show typical histological changes in the intestine but do not get diarrhoea (Ciarlet et al 1998a). Finally, oral administration of epidermal growth factor to rotavirus-infected piglets can restore the intestinal mucosa and enzyme activities, but such treatments do not hasten the resolution of diarrhoea (Zijlstra et al 1994). Thus, a clear association of mucosal damage and diarrhoea is lacking. One explanation for this is the fact that the infection is patchy, so one might observe mucosal changes in one part of the intestine but these would be insufficient to cause diarrhoeal disease. In other cases, animals with mucosal damage may release fluid into the intestinal lumen but compensatory physiological mechanisms (colonic reabsorption of fluid) may decrease fluid loss so diarrhoea is not observed. In 1988, Osborne proposed that enteroctye interactions induced a localized response that triggered the production of endogenous, neuroactive, hormonal substances of pathophysiological importance (Osborne et al 1988). Vascular damage due to villus ischaemia was suggested to be involved, possibly being mediated by release of a vasoactive agent from infected epithelial cells. Recent studies are beginning to provide a molecular basis for such new mechanisms of pathogenesis.

The rotavirus particle is composed of three concentric protein layers surrounding the eleven segments of double-stranded RNA which encode the six structural viral proteins VP1–VP4, VP6, and VP7, and six non-structural proteins, NSP1–NSP6. Each genome segment, with the exception of gene 11, which encodes two viral proteins (NSP5 and NSP6), codes for a single viral protein. The innermost core layer is formed by VP2 and encloses the genomic RNA and enzymatic complexes found at the fivefold vertices, which contain VP1 (the RNA-dependent RNA polymerase) and VP3 (a guanylyltransferase and methylase). The intermediate layer is made up of the most abundant rotavirus protein, VP6. The outer layer consists of the glycoprotein VP7 and the haemagglutinin and cell attachment protein VP4.

Viral factors involved in virulence have been dissected by several approaches. Analyses of reassortants that contain a single gene from one 'virulent' parental virus and other genes from another 'avirulent' parental virus have implicated specific viral genes in virulence. These putative virulence genes code for both structural (VP3, VP4, VP7) and non-structural (NSP1, NSP2, NSP4) proteins (reviewed in Burke & Desselberger 1996). The role of some of these proteins (e.g. NSP1) in virulence may vary depending on the host species; for example, NSP1 appears to be a virulence factor for mice but not for rabbits or piglets (Broome et al 1993, Ciarlet et al 1998b, Bridger et al 1998). The genes implicated in virulence that code for the surface proteins of the virus are likely to be involved in virus stability, virus attachment and penetration into cells. The precise roles for the inner capsid protein VP3, which functions as the capping enzyme for viral RNA, and the two non-structural proteins NSP1 and NSP2 in virulence remain unclear. However, these proteins may affect replication efficiency and two of them (VP3 and NSP1) are recognized targets for cytotoxic T lymphocytes. NSP4 is a virulence gene because it functions as an enterotoxin (see below).

Rotaviruses enter polarized intestinal epithelial cells by distinct mechanisms depending on whether or not virus binding to cells is sensitive or resistant to treatment with neuraminidase

A critical initiating event in pathogenesis involves the entry of virus into cells. This process is complex for rotavirus and likely involves two viral proteins and multiple proteins on cells. Recent analyses of the interactions of viruses with polarized intestinal cells, grown on permeable filters, have detected differences in the early steps of viral infection based on whether or not the virus requires interaction with sialic acid or other surface moieties that are sensitive to treatment with neuraminidase (Fig. 1; Ciarlet et al 2000a). Most rotaviruses bind cells in a neuraminidase-independent manner (Ciarlet & Estes 1999). Rotavirus strains (all human strains tested to date, and bovine WC3, porcine Gottfried) that infect cells

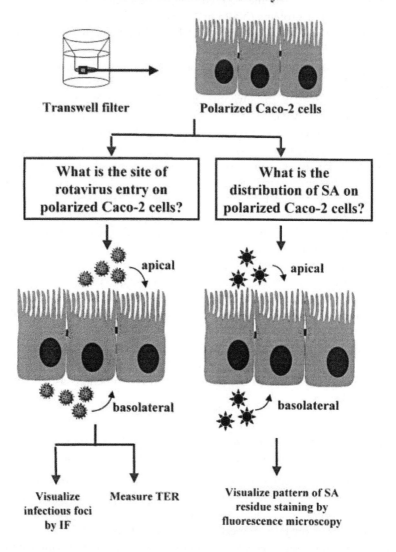

Grow Caco-2 cells on permeable 0.4 µm pore Transwell membrane filters for 15 days

Transwell filter   Polarized Caco-2 cells

What is the site of rotavirus entry on polarized Caco-2 cells?

What is the distribution of SA on polarized Caco-2 cells?

apical

apical

basolateral

basolateral

Visualize infectious foci by IF   Measure TER

Visualize pattern of SA residue staining by fluorescence microscopy

FIG. 1. Experimental design to study rotavirus replication in polarized epithelial cells. Human intestinal Caco-2 cells were grown on permeable 0.4 µm transwell membrane filters until they became polarized. The polarized cells were infected with virus by adding rotavirus to the apical or basolateral surfaces and the infectious process was monitored by immunofluorescence and by measuring the transepithelial cell resistance (TER).

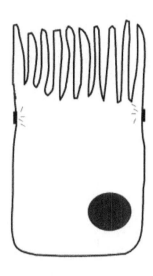

- **Disrupts**
  - **tight junctions**
  - **microvillar, microfilament network**
- **Perturbs protein targeting**
  - **sucrase isomaltase**
- **Induces chemokine responses**
- **Evokes intestinal secretion**
  - **enterotoxin**
  - **enteric nervous system**

FIG. 2.   The effects of rotavirus infection on polarized epithelial cells. Data from Jourdan et al (1998), Brunet et al (2000), Lundgren et al (2000) and Obert et al (2000).

in a neuraminidase-independent fashion infect polarized epithelial cells efficiently through both the apical and basolateral surfaces. Rotavirus strains whose infectivity is reduced by treatment of cells with neuraminidase (e.g. RRV, SA11, bovine NCDV, porcine OSU) only infect polarized epithelial cells efficiently through the apical surface (Ciarlet et al 2000a). These results suggest that distinct rotavirus receptors are present on different cell membranes. Rotavirus infection of polarized cells has other effects including disruption of cell interactions and cell integrity, perturbation of cellular protein trafficking, induction of chemokine responses and induction of intestinal secretion (Fig. 2). These outcomes may be differentially affected depending on whether cells are infected only apically or both apically and basolaterally. These newly recognized differences in virus–cell interactions between neuraminidase-sensitive and -resistant rotaviruses may be important for pathogenesis as well as for selection of virus vaccine strains.

How does the rotavirus enterotoxin NSP4 cause disease?

In 1996, the rotavirus non-structural protein, NSP4 was reported to function as a viral enterotoxin (Ball et al 1996). The discovery that NSP4 functions as an enterotoxin was unexpected because no other viral enterotoxins had been described. The remainder of this article briefly reviews the salient features about

TABLE 2 Properties of Rotavirus NSP4 or NSP4 peptide 114–135

Functions in viral morphogenesis; mediating the acquisition of a transient membrane envelope as subviral particles bud into the ER	Au et al (1989), Meyer et al (1989)
Mobilizes $[Ca^{2+}]_i$ release from internal stores (ER)	Tian et al (1994, 1995), Dong et al (1997)
Associated with virulence based on studies of reassortants	Hoshino et al (1995)
Induces an age-dependent diarrhoea in mice and rats when administered by intraperitoneal or intraluminal routes but not when given intramuscularly	Ball et al (1996)
Does not induce histological changes in the intestine when diarrhoea is present	Ball et al (1996)
Induces age-dependent Cl^- secretion in the intestinal mucosa of young mice	Ball et al (1996)
Alters plasma membrane permeability and is cytotoxic to cells	Tian et al (1994, 1995), Newton et al (1997)
Mutations in NSP4 from virulent/avirulent pairs of virus are associated with altered virus virulence	Kirkwood et al (1996), Zhang et al (1998)
NSP4 induced age-dependent diarrhoea and age-dependent Cl^- permeability changes in mice lacking the CFTR channel	Morris et al (1999)
Children make antibodies and cellular immune responses to NSP4	Richardson et al (1993), Johansen et al (1999)
A cleavage product is secreted into the medium of virus-infected cells	Zhang et al (2000)
NSP4 induces homotypic and heterotypic protection against virus-induced diarrhoea	Zeng et al (2001)
Exogenous NSP4 alters F-actin organizaton and affects transepithelial resistance in polarized epithelial cells	Tafazoli et al (2001)
Used as a agonist to detect novel Ca^{2+}-binding protein in tumour cells	Xu et al (1999)
Is a novel toxin? No primary sequence similarity to other known toxins. Is a novel secretory agonist	Morris et al (1999), Estes & Morris (1999)

this first viral enterotoxin and other pleiotropic properties of NSP4 related to pathogenesis that continue to be discovered (Table 2).

The rotavirus non-structural protein NSP4 was initially identified as a non-structural glycoprotein with a topology that spans the membrane of the endoplasmic reticulum (ER) and which has a distinct role in virus assembly. The functioning of this protein was examined because rotaviruses undergo a unique morphogenesis in which newly made subviral particles bud into the ER, and during this process they obtain a transient membrane envelope that is subsequently lost within the lumen of the ER as particles mature. This process also involves Ca^{2+} to maintain the integrity and specific conformation of the two outer capsid proteins necessary for the correct association of proteins as the virus matures in the ER. NSP4 has multiple domains. NSP4 is a 20 kDa primary translation product, is co-translationally glycosylated to 29 kDa, and oligosaccharide processing yields the mature 28 kDa protein (Ericson et al 1983). The 175 amino acid backbone of NSP4 consists of an uncleaved signal sequence, three N-terminal hydrophobic domains, and a predicted amphipathic α-helix that overlaps a folded coiled-coil region (Chan et al 1988, Taylor et al 1996). The H2 transmembrane domain traverses the ER bilayer and the cytoplasmic C terminus of NSP4 functions as an intracellular receptor in viral morphogenesis (Au et al 1989, Meyer et al 1989, Taylor et al 1993, Bergmann et al 1989). NSP4 mobilizes intracellular Ca^{2+} ($[Ca^{2+}]_i$) release from the ER and this may also affect viral morphogenesis (Tian et al 1994, 1995). NSP4 also possesses a membrane destabilization activity when incubated with liposomes that simulate ER membranes, and it has been hypothesized that this activity may play a role in the removal of the transient envelope from budding particles (Tian et al 1996). Finally, NSP4 may facilitate cell death and virus release from cells (Newton et al 1997), and polarized cells treated with NSP4 undergo reorganization of filamentous actin and lose transepithelial cell resistance due to alterations in tight junctions (Tafazoli et al 2001).

The discovery that NSP4 is an enterotoxin was made serendipitously during studies aimed at dissecting the molecular mechanisms by which NSP4 functions in morphogenesis. A synthetic peptide of NSP4 that contains amino acid residues 114–135 was conjugated to a carrier and injected into mice to produce a new antiserum. Although the mice received peptide (and no virus), they got diarrhoea. Pursuit of this observation showed that both the full-length protein and the 114–135 peptide share several properties that are consistent with NSP4 being an enterotoxin, and recent studies have found novel pleiotropic properties of NSP4 important for pathogenesis.

The protein induces diarrhoea in pups with a DD_{50} of 0.56 nmols while the DD_{50} of the 114–135 peptide is more than 10-fold higher, indicating that this peptide contains only a part of the active domain of the protein. The exact size of the active toxin domain remains unclear. Properties that define bacterial enterotoxins include their ability to stimulate net secretion in intestinal segments in the absence of inducing histological changes. NSP4 possesses these properties, confirming that it functions as an enterotoxin. The early studies and *in vitro* analyses of the response of human intestinal (HT29) cells to exogenously added NSP4 led to a working model for the mechanism of action of this enterotoxin (Ball et al 1996, Estes & Morris 1999). We hypothesized that an extracellular form of NSP4 functions as an enterotoxin after it is released from virus-infected cells. We proposed that extracellular NSP4 binds to an unidentified receptor on secretory intestinal cells, and activates a signalling pathway that mobilizes $[Ca^{2+}]_i$ and leads to Cl^- secretion.

Our model predicted: (i) NSP4 is released from virus-infected cells either by cell lysis or secretion; (ii) avirulent rotaviruses may possess mutant NSP4 genes; (iii) intestinal cells possess a receptor for NSP4; (iv) age-dependent disease results from a change in the signalling pathway; and (v) antibody to NSP4 will reduce rotavirus-induced disease.

Further work has provided evidence for each of these predictions. A cleavage product of NSP4 can be detected in the medium of virus-infected cells and this protein retains enterotoxin activity (Zhang et al 2000). Sequence analyses of virulent/avirulent pairs of viruses detected sequence changes in the NSP4 gene in amino acid residues (aa) 136 and 138, and expressed NSP4 with these mutations shows reduced enterotoxin activity (Zhang et al 1998). These results also indicate that the enterotoxin domain extends beyond aa 114–135 and help explain why the initial NSP4 114–135 peptide was not as active as the full-length protein. A glutathione S-tranferase (GST) fusion protein containing aa 86–175 of the murine NSP4 also causes diarrhoea in mice (Horie et al 1999). Binding experiments of NSP4 to cells has shown that cells possess a receptor for NSP4, but the receptor has not yet been identified (C. Q.-Y. Zeng, M. Zhang & M. K. Estes, unpublished results 1999). Human intestinal cells exposed to exogenously added NSP4 initiate a signalling pathway that involves activation of phospholipase C (PLC), elevation in inositol 1,4,5-trisphosphate (InsP$_3$) and mobilization of $[Ca^{2+}]_i$ (Dong et al 1997). Crypt cells isolated from mice also respond in a similar manner and mobilization of $[Ca^{2+}]_i$ occurs in both young and older mice (Morris et al 1999). Studies in mice lacking the cystic fibrosis transmembrane regulator (CFTR) channel provided evidence that age-dependent disease results from an event downstream of mobilization of $[Ca^{2+}]_i$. Since the CFTR channel is a cAMP-regulated Cl$^-$ channel , it was predicted that such mice should still get diarrhoea based on rotavirus and NSP4 stimulating a Ca^{2+}-activated Cl$^-$ channel. CFTR knockout mice get diarrhoea following rotavirus infection or NSP4 treatment, indicating that a different Cl$^-$ channel than CFTR mediates this effect (Angel et al 1998, Morris et al 1999). CFTR knockout mice do not respond to other classical secretory agonists so the activity of NSP4 in these mice shows that NSP4 is a novel secretory agonist (Morris et al 1999). Cl$^-$ secretion is age-dependent in CFTR knockout mice, indicating that age-dependent disease may result from an age-dependent induction, activation or regulation of this Cl$^-$ channel (Morris et al 1999). This pathway would be one that is activated when NSP4 is released from virus-infected cells, possibly by cell lysis, and the affected cells are hypothesized to be the secretory crypt cells. Other cell types, including villus enterocytes, may also be affected in a similar manner by NSP4. Finally, protection studies using the neonatal mouse model have shown that antibody to NSP4 can induce protection against disease caused by infection with either simian or a highly virulent murine rotavirus (Zeng et al 2001). Protection consists of a reduction in the number of pups that develop diarrhoea, the severity of disease and the duration of the diarrhoea. Exogenous NSP4 has also been shown to alter polarized cell transepithelial cell resistance (Tafazoli et al 2001) and to inhibit the Na^+-D-glucose symporter in brush border membranes (Halaihel et al 2000), two additional properties that may contribute to pathogenesis. An updated model of NSP4 action summarizes these new effects (Fig. 3).

Additional effects of NSP4 most likely occur by alternative pathway(s) that lead to changes in plasma membrane Cl^- permeability or other effects on epithelial cell function that are activated during viral infection when NSP4 is initially expressed as a transmembrane ER-specific glycoprotein within infected enterocytes. Endogenous expression of intracellular NSP4 in cells can also mobilize $[Ca^{2+}]_i$ from internal stores but this is a separate process that is not affected by PLC inhibitors (Tian et al 1995). Changes in plasma membrane permeability are seen in virus-infected cells, but it is unclear whether these effects result from expression of NSP4 or another viral protein (Michelangeli et al 1991, 1995). Future studies of the effects of intracellularly expressed NSP4 may unravel other functions and properties of this multifaceted protein.

Can our new knowledge of the mechanisms of pathogenesis be used to improve methods of treatment and prevention of rotavirus-induced diarrhoeal disease?

The discovery that rotaviruses have multiple effects on polarized epithelial cells and that these viruses produce an enterotoxin that mimics many of the same effects as the virus, raises the possibility that this protein could be useful in the development of new methods to prevent or treat rotavirus-induced disease. Other viral proteins may also be involved and if additional viral proteins play a role in the complex signalling cascades, they might also be useful targets to prevent disease. The discovery of the enterotoxin has stimulated new ideas and work on rotavirus pathogenesis but many questions remain to be answered in greater detail. It is clear that NSP4 is a novel multifunctional virulence factor and secretory agonist that can stimulate several cell signalling pathways, and that this protein has been used to identify novel calcium binding proteins in tumour cells (Xu et al 1999). Recently, involvement of the enteric nervous system in rotavirus diarrhoea has been reported (Lundgren et al 2000), although the mediators that trigger this process remain unknown. NSP4 is one possible factor. Further work is needed to dissect all the targets in the NSP4-induced signalling cascades and to understand the consequences and targets of the different signalling pathways induced by intracellular and extracellular NSP4. Such studies may lead to common mechanisms shared with bacterial pathogens that could lead to development of broadly active drugs to prevent diarrhoea caused by more than one pathogen. Understanding the mechanism of action of NSP4 may lead to new treatments for

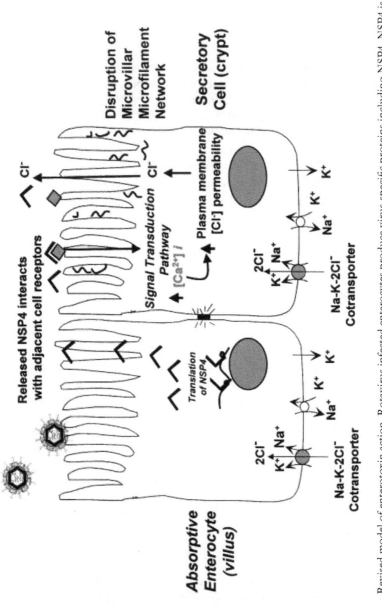

FIG. 3.   Revised model of enterotoxin action. Rotavirus infected enterocytes produce virus-specific proteins including NSP4. NSP4 is released from cells by lysis or secretion and this extracellular NSP4 acts in a paracellular fashion by interacting with a receptor for NSP4 on adjacent cells. These secretory cells are likely to be crypt cells but might also be villus enterocytes. This triggers a rapid response involving a signal transduction pathway that mobilizes intracellular Ca^{2+} and results in increased plasma membrane Cl^- permeability. The plasma membrane permeability is age-dependent based on studies in CFTR knockout mice (Morris et al 1999). Extracellular NSP4 also causes a delayed disruption of the organization of filamentous actin and transepithelial cell resistance (Tafazoli et al 2001). Model modified from Estes & Morris (1999).

rotavirus-induced diarrhoea. For example, it is possible that antibody treatment or new drugs might be developed to treat children or animals with rotavirus infection and diarrhoea, specifically immunocompromised children with chronic rotavirus diarrhoea. Such potential new therapies may require a more detailed understanding of the NSP4 receptor on cells, the NSP4 structure, and whether there are distinct signalling pathways for NSP4 action when the protein is expressed endogenously versus when cells are exposed exogenously to NSP4.

A remaining question is whether this enterotoxin action is important in rotavirus pathogenesis in children. A direct answer is currently not available, but precedents with bacterial toxins indicate that results in animals generally are relevant for humans, so it seems likely that NSP4 plays a role in rotavirus pathogenesis in humans. Future studies can determine if antibody to NSP4 correlates with protective immunity and if vaccination strategies that induce immunity to NSP4 improve vaccine efficacy. Children do make antibody and cellular immune responses to NSP4 (Richardson et al 1993, Johansen et al 1999). Although there is sequence variability in NSP4, and four genetic groups are now known (Ciarlet et al 2000b), the broad immunity induced by NSP4 in mice protects against viruses in at least two distinct NSP4 genogroups (Zeng et al 2001). Whether immunity to NSP4 will provide the long sought after correlate of protection for rotavirus remains an important issue that needs to be investigated.

The discovery of the rotavirus enterotoxin raises interest in knowing whether other viruses code for enterotoxins. This is obviously important for understanding the mechanisms of pathogenesis for other gastroenteritis viruses such as astroviruses, caliciviruses, coronaviruses and enteric adenoviruses. This question is also relevant for viruses such as HIV that cause a devastating enteropathy. Finally, these results emphasize the common mechanisms of pathogenesis shared among microbial pathogens.

Acknowledgements

The work on NSP4 as an enterotoxin summarized in this article includes that of former students, postdoctoral fellows or current collaborators including Kit-Sing Au, Judy Ball, Wai-Kit Chan, Yanjie Dong, Kari Johansen, Andrew P. Morris, Linda J. Saif, J. Scott, L. Svensson, Peng Tian, and Mingdong Zhang. The critical work, friendship and scientific enthusiasm of these colleagues is greatly appreciated.

References

Angel J, Tang B, Feng N, Greenberg HB, Bass D 1998 Studies of the roles for NSP4 in the pathogenesis of homologous murine rotavirus diarrhoea. J Infect Dis 177:455–458
Au KS, Chan WK, Burns JW, Estes MK 1989 Receptor activity of rotavirus nonstructural glycoprotein NS28. J Virol 63:4553–4562

Ball JM, Tian P, Zeng CQ-Y, Morris A, Estes MK 1996 Age-dependent diarrhoea is induced by a viral nonstructural glycoprotein. Science 272:101–104

Bergmann CC, Maass D, Poruchynsky MS, Atkinson PH, Bellamy AR 1989 Topology of the non-structural rotavirus receptor glycoprotein NS28 in the rough endoplasmic reticulum. EMBO J 8:1695–1703

Bridger JC, Dhaliwal W, Adamson MJV, Howard CR 1998 Determinants of rotavirus host range restriction—a heterologous bovine NSP1 gene does not affect replication kinetics in the pig. Virology 245:47–52

Broome RL, Vo PT, Ward RL, Clark HF, Greenberg HB 1993 Murine rotavirus genes encoding outer capsid proteins VP4 and VP7 are not major determinants of host range restriction and virulence. J Virol 67:2448–2455

Brunet J-P, Cotte-Lafitte J, Linxe C, Quero A-M, Géniteau-Legendre M, Servin A 2000 Rotavirus infection induces an increase in intracellular calcium concentration in human intestinal epithelial cells: role in microvillar actin alteration. J Virol 74:2323–2332

Burke B, Desselberger U 1996 Rotavirus pathogenicity. Virology 218:299–305

Burns JW, Krishnaney AA, Vo PT, Rouse RV, Anderson LJ, Greenberg HB 1995 Analyses of homologous rotavirus infection in the mouse model. Virology 207:143–153

Chan WK, Au KS, Estes MK 1988 Topography of the simian rotavirus nonstructural glycoprotein (NS28) in the endoplasmic reticulum membrane. Virology 164:435–442

Ciarlet M, Estes MK 1999 Human and most animal rotavirus strains do not require the presence of sialic acid on the cell surface for efficient infectivity. J Gen Virol 80:943–948

Ciarlet M, Gilger MA, Barone C, McArthur M, Estes MK, Conner ME 1998a Rotavirus disease, but not infection and development of intestinal histopathological lesions, is age restricted in rabbits. Virology 251:343–360

Ciarlet M, Estes MK, Barone C, Ramig RF, Conner ME 1998b Analysis of host range restriction determinants in the rabbit model: comparison of homologous and heterologous rotavirus infections. J Virol 72:2341–2351

Ciarlet M, Crawford SE, Estes MK 2000a Asymmetric infection of polarized epithelial cells by sialic acid-dependent rotaviruses. Gastroenterology 118:A676

Ciarlet M, Liprandi F, Conner ME, Estes MK 2000b Species specificity and interspecies relatedness in NSP4 genetic groups by comparative NSP4 sequence analyses of animal rotaviruses. Arch Virol 145:371–383

Collins JE, Benfield DA, Duimstra JR 1989 Comparative virulence of two porcine group-A rotavirus isolates in gnotobiotic pigs. Am J Vet Res 50:827–835

Davidson GP, Gall DG, Petric M, Butler DG, Hamilton JR 1977 Human rotavirus enteritis induced in conventional piglets. Intestinal structure and transport. J Clin Invest 60:1402–1409

Dong Y, Zeng CQ-Y, Ball JM, Estes MK, Morris AP 1997 The rotavirus enterotoxin NSP4 mobilizes intracellular calcium in human intestinal cells by stimulating phospholipase C-mediated inositol 1,4,5-trisphosphate production. Proc Natl Acad Sci USA 94:3960–3965

Ericson BL, Graham DY, Mason BB, Hanssen HH, Estes MK 1983 Two types of glycoprotein precursors are produced by the simian rotavirus SA11. Virology 127:320–332

Estes MK, Morris AP 1999 A viral enterotoxin: a new mechanism of virus-induced pathogenesis. In: Paul P, Francis D (eds) Mechanisms in the pathogenesis of enteric diseases, 2nd edn. Plenum Press, New York, p 73–82

Graham DY, Sackman JW, Estes MK 1984 Pathogenesis of rotavirus-induced diarrhoea. Preliminary studies in miniature swine piglet. Dig Dis Sci 29:1028–1035

Halaihel N, Lievin V, Ball JM, Estes MK, Alvarado F, Vasseur M 2000 Direct inhibitory effect of rotavirus NSP4 (114-135) peptide on the Na^+-D-glucose symporter of rabbit intestinal brush border membranes. J Virol 74:9464–9470

Horie Y, Nakagomi O, Koshimura Y et al 1999 Diarrhoea induction by rotavirus NSP4 in the homologous mouse model system. Virology 262:398–407

Hoshino Y, Saif LJ, Kang SY, Sereno MM, Chen WK, Kapikian AZ 1995 Identification of group A rotavirus genes associated with virulence of a porcine rotavirus and host range restriction of a human rotavirus in the gnotobiotic piglet model. Virology 209:274–280

Johansen K, Hinkula J, Espinoza F et al 1999 Humoral and cell-mediated immune responses to the NSP4 enterotoxin of rotavirus J Med Virol 59:369–377

Jourdan N, Brunet J-P, Sapin C et al 1998 Rotavirus infection reduces sucrase-isomaltase expression in human intestinal epithelial cells by perturbing protein targeting and organization of microvillar cytoskeleton. J Virol 72:7228–7236

Kirkwood CD, Coulson BS, Bishop RF 1996 G3P2 rotaviruses causing diarrhoeal disease in neonates differ in VP4, VP7 and NSP4 sequence from G3P2 strains causing asymptomatic neonatal infection. Arch Virol 141:1661–1676

Lundgren O, Peregrin AT, Persson K, Kordasti S, Uhnoo I, Svensson L 2000 Role of the enteric nervous system in the fluid and electrolyte secretion of rotavirus diarrhoea. Science 287: 491–495

McAdaragh JP, Bergeland ME, Meyer RC et al 1980 Pathogenesis of rotaviral enteritis in gnotobiotic pigs: a microscopic study. Am J Vet Res 41:1572–1581

Mebus CA 1976 Reovirus-like calf enteritis. Am Dig Dis 21:592–598

Meyer JC, Bergmann CC, Bellamy AR 1989 Interaction of rotavirus cores with the nonstructural glycoprotein NS28. Virology 171:98–107

Michelangeli F, Ruiz MC, del Castillo JR, Ludert JE, Liprandi F 1991 Effect of rotavirus infection on intracellular calcium homeostasis in cultured cells. Virology 181:520–527

Michelangeli F, Liprandi F, Chemello ME, Ciarlet M, Ruiz MC 1995 Selective depletion of stored calcium by thapsigargin blocks rotavirus maturation but not the cytopathic effect. J Virol 69:3838–3847

Morris AP, Scott JK, Ball JM, Zeng Q-Y, O'Neal WK, Estes MK 1999 NSP4 elicits age-dependent diarrhea and Ca^{2+}-mediated I^- influx into intestinal crypts of CF mice. Am J Physiol 277:G431–G444

Newton K, Meyer JC, Bellamy AR, Taylor JA 1997 Rotavirus nonstructural glycoprotein NSP4 alters plasma membrane permeability in mammalian cells. J Virol 71:9458–9465

Obert G, Peiffer I, Servin AL 2000 Rotavirus-induced structural and functional alterations in tight junctions of polarized intestinal Caco-2 cell monolayers. J Virol 74:4645–4651

Osborne M, Haddon SJ, Spencer AJ et al 1988 An electron microscopic investigation of time-related changes in the intestine of neonatal mice infected with murine rotavirus. J Pediatr Gastroenterol Nutr 7:236–248

Richardson SC, Grimwood K, Bishop RF 1993 Analysis of homotypic and heterotypic serum immune responses to rotavirus proteins following primary rotavirus infection by using the radioimmunoprecipitation technique. J Clin Microbiol 31:377–385

Starkey WG, Collins J, Wallis TS et al 1986 Kinetics, tissue specificity and pathological changes in murine rotavirus infection of mice. J Gen Virol 67:2625–2634

Tafazoli F, Zeng CQ, Estes MK, Magnusson KE, Svensson L 2001 NSP4 enterotoxin of rotavirus induces paracellular leakage in polarized epithelial cells. J Virol 75:1540–1546

Taylor JA, O'Brien JA, Lord VJ, Meyer JC, Bellamy AR 1993 The RER-localized rotavirus intracellular receptor: a truncated purified soluble form is multivalent and binds virus particles. Virology 194:807–814

Taylor JA, O'Brien JA, Yeager M 1996 The cytoplasmic tail of NSP4, the endoplasmic reticulum-localized non-structural glycoprotein of rotavirus, contains distinct virus binding and coiled coil domains. EMBO J 15:4469–4476

Theil KW, Bohl EH, Cross RF, Kohler EM, Agnes AG 1978 Pathogenesis of porcine rotaviral infection in experimentally inoculated gnotobiotic pigs. Am J Vet Res 39:213–220

Tian P, Hu Y, Schilling WP, Lindsay DA, Eiden J, Estes MK 1994 The nonstructural glycoprotein of rotavirus affects intracellular calcium levels. J Virol 68:251–257

Tian P, Estes MK, Hu Y, Ball JM, Zeng CQ-Y, Schilling WP 1995 The rotavirus nonstructural glycoprotein NSP4 mobilizes Ca^{2+} from the endoplasmic reticulum. J Virol 69:5763–5772

Tian P, Ball JM, Zeng CQ-Y, Estes MK 1996 The rotavirus nonstructural glycoprotein NSP4 possesses membrane destabilization activity. J Virol 70:6973–6981

Ward LA, Rosen BI, Yuan L, Saif L 1996 Pathogenesis of an attenuated and a virulent strain of group A human rotavirus in neonatal gnotobiotic pigs. J Gen Virol 77:1431–1441

Ward RL, McNeal MM, Sheridan JF 1990 Development of an adult mouse model for studies on protection against rotavirus. J Virol 64:5070–5075

Xu A, Bellamy AR, Taylor JA 1999 Expression of translationally controlled tumour protein is regulated by calcium at both the transcriptional and post-transcriptional level. Biochem J 342:683–689

Zeng CQ-Y, Zhang M, Conner ME, Estes MK 2000 Homotypic and heterotypic protection against rotavirus by immunization with the rotavirus enterotoxin. Submitted

Zhang M, Zeng CQ-Y, Dong Y et al 1998 Mutations in rotavirus nonstructural glycoprotein NSP4 are associated with altered virus virulence. J Virol 72:3666–3672

Zhang M, Zeng CQ-Y, Morris AP, Estes MK 2000 A functional NSP4 enterotoxin peptide secreted from rotavirus-infected cells. J Virol 74:11663–11670

Zijlstra RT, Odle J, Hall WF, Petschow BW, Gelberg HB, Litov RE 1994 Effect of orally administered epidermal growth factor on intestinal recovery of neonatal pigs infected with rotavirus. J Pediatr Gastroenterol Nutr 19:382–390

DISCUSSION

Green: Every time there has been a new discovery on pathogenesis, the article ends with the conclusion that drugs are close at hand that will counteract this mechanism. Are there any developments based on these pathogenic mechanisms that would lead to a miracle drug?

Estes: There is nothing at this point. We don't have a structure, and I think this would be important here. What has been exciting about this is that if NSP4 is involved in activating enteric nerves, this is a common mechanism for both viral and bacterial-induced diarrhoeas. In this case, there might be more interest to try to develop some drugs to stop disease. My understanding is that some of the pharmaceutical companies didn't think the market would be big enough. There has also been some resistance by people to accept this story. We have tried to build evidence to convince people, and this resistance is slowly disappearing.

Offit: If one is to have hope for antiviral drugs that inhibit transcription and translation, there is a problem to be overcome: by the time clinical symptoms are seen, most of the replication that is going to occur has already occurred. By the time that you see clinical diarrhoea, has most of the NSP4 that is going to be made already been made? Would an anti-NSP4 specific agent have any effect at this stage?

Estes: I can't answer that question. With any antiviral for an acute viral disease, the question is how you are going to use it. It may be used prophylactically in a hospital or daycare setting where there is a wave of viral infection and the agent is known.

Greenberg: Neuraminidase inhibitors work for flu.

Offit: But they don't work very well.

Mary Estes, Could you speculate on what biological or clinical differences for rotavirus infections you could imagine being determined by sialic acid-independent or dependent mechanisms of replication?

Estes: I don't understand completely how this might affect pathogenesis. It is possible that a virus that has the potential to infect cells by both routes, when coming down the gastrointestinal tract might begin infecting apically. If transepithelial resistance goes down, the virus that is then being produced by cells might be available to pass through the altered tight junctions and perhaps infect other cells basolaterally. I don't know whether this virus will cause less infection or replicate in a different way.

Offit: Do you think that the reason some viruses, specifically RRV, have the capacity to replicate or cause diarrhoea across species could be determined by sialic acid dependence?

Estes: I can't answer that. We were surprised when we found that WC3 was a sialic acid-independent virus.

Greenberg: I was very impressed by the protection against the murine rotavirus. Did you have the opportunity to look at shedding as well as diarrhoea in those animals? I would assume in this replication-independent anti-diarrhoea effect that shedding would be the same in both the protected and non-protected animals.

Estes: We did not look at this in the murine rotavirus-infected animals, but we did in the SA11-infected animals. This was because we could do plaque assays and we could quantitate the virus as opposed to just doing ELISAs. The surprising thing was that there seems to be less replicating virus in the animals that have antibody against NSP4.

Greenberg: There is very little replication with SA11 in the mouse.

Estes: I wouldn't have expected *any* difference in shedding; I was surprised that we did see an apparent reduction in shedding.

Greenberg: Would your expectation in a human vaccinated with NSP4, for example, be that there is not only less diarrhoea, but also less shedding?

Estes: Possibly.

Greenberg: Have you had the opportunity to look in any homologous system for less shedding with NSP4 immunization?

Estes: No.

Farthing: Intuitively, I would have thought that the major effect of NSP4 would be by intracellular delivery. However, you think that it is released and that there is a surface membrane receptor. Is there any evidence that there is a direct intracellular effect?

Estes: That is an important question, and one that has been difficult to address. We know that if you express NSP4 in insect cells intracellularly, it also mobilizes intracellular Ca^{2+}, but through a different pathway. This event does not involve the activation of phospholipase C. At this point, I can't tell you whether that activation of Ca^{2+} may then be part of changing the transepithelial resistance of a virus-infected cell. One of the things that we hope to do in the next several years is to begin to look at the intracellular effects and what these do to the architecture of the cell. Again, the problem has been that without a reverse genetics system, it has been difficult to knock the gene out, which makes it hard to do experiments to examine intracellular effects in the context of a viral infection.

Green: I am intrigued by this 7 kDa cleavage product. What are the sites for the cleavage, which proteinase do you think is doing this, and is this a site that is conserved in all the strains?

Estes: One of the things that people have been concerned about in connection with this story is that there is significant variation in NSP4 starting at about aa 133, which is part of the sequence in which we had originally identified the toxic peptide. The place where we are seeing the cleavage is at aa 112. This is a methionine that is conserved in every sequenced strain, and the cleavage takes place between this residue and the one to the left, which is variable. We don't know which protease is involved: it is not something that is obvious, in that it is not a trypsin cleavage site.

Green: How do you know it is cleavage and not an internal initiation?

Estes: Because if we treat cells with protease inhibitors we don't see the cleavage product.

Greenberg: Is the cleavage occurring extracellularly or intracellularly?

Estes: Intracellularly. The protease inhibitors will go into cells; some of them are small molecules.

López: What is the advantage of having this toxin for rotavirus? Is there an obvious gain during the infection process for the virus?

Estes: I think it is important for spread of the virus. If a good secretory mechanism exists there will be movement of the virus down the intestinal tract and then spread. This is probably true with bacterial diarrhoeas too. The purpose is to get the organism out into the environment.

López: It seems that this toxin is killing the neighbouring cells; thus it is likely that the virus is not able to replicate any more in the surrounding cells.

Estes: This killing takes quite a while. In the meantime the virus is still replicating.

López: The increase in Ca^{2+} that occurs in the surrounding cells caused by the secreted NSP4 does not seem to be good for virus replication.

Estes: Ultimately, it will kill those cells, but in the short-term the viruses will still replicate and I suspect overall that this helps in the spread of the virus.

Carter: If you pretreat cells with NSP4, do they still support virus replication to the same extent as other pre-treated cells?

Estes: That is a good question; we haven't done that experiment.

López: Is the susceptibility of MDCK cells also different between sialic acid-dependent and -independent viruses?

Estes: We are just doing those experiments now.

Holmes: Can you introduce this diarrhoea by intraperitoneal inoculation of NSP4?

Estes: Yes.

Holmes: How do you think this occurs?

Estes: We did this in very small mice, and we actually thought we were probably inoculating it into the intestine. It works much more efficiently if you do surgery and put it into the lumen of the intestine.

Greenberg: You can determine that by putting a dye in.

Estes: We did, but as fast as we could open the animal up the dye was everywhere because it diffuses so fast.

Saif: Have you done any experiments in which you have tried to infect with the sialic acid-independent strains and block the infectivity of the sialic acid-dependent strains?

Estes: We haven't done those experiments yet.

Saif: With regard to rotavirus pathogenesis, it is my understanding from the literature that there is hardly any villous atrophy in the mouse model with rotavirus infections (Little & Shadduck 1982, Ward et al 1990). Is the diarrhoea then all related to NSP4 and secretory diarrhoea? Or, if you get a malabsorptive diarrhoea in mice, is this caused by apoptosis of villus enterocytes that would be different in other animal models where there is villous atrophy?

Estes: We don't see villous atrophy in mice. We do see vacuolated cells. I wouldn't claim that all the diarrhoea in the mouse is due to NSP4. I think that there are probably changes in the transepithelial resistance and other mechanisms that could result in the diarrhoea. There is clearly no correlation between histological changes and diarrhoea. In rabbits, we see histological changes and there is no diarrhoea. There are also other examples of this.

Saif: My understanding was that in the rabbit models, diarrhoea doesn't occur because of colonic compensation.

Estes: That is not the case. Margaret Conner has done experiments where she has excluded the colon, and these animals still don't get diarrhoea.

Koopmans: Is the sialic acid-independent entry dependent on cell polarization?

Estes: The only thing we have done on this is to look at polarized cells. In this case the sialic acid-independent viruses go in either way.

López: NSP4 doesn't cause diarrhoea in adult mice, so the process is therefore age dependent. Do you think this is because the receptor for NSP4 is not present in the adult mice?

Estes: We think the receptor is probably there in both young and old mice, but we haven't done that experiment directly. We know that in the adult CFTR knockout mice there is Ca^{2+} mobilization, suggesting that the signalling pathway is activated, which suggests that the receptor is there.

López: Then what is missing?

Estes: We think it is either the activation or the regulation of the Cl^- channel. It could be something else, but it is downstream of Ca^{2+} mobilization.

Koopmans: Mary Estes, from the pathogenesis and neurology studies, do you have a hypothesis about what is going on with the intussusception story?

Estes: I don't think we understand the pathogenesis of intussusception. I mentioned earlier that there could be lymphoid hyperplasia that may have to do with the efficiency of virus replication in cells. There could also be changes in intestinal motility; this could be altered by secondary mediators stimulated by virus infection in the intestine or some of the responses of other cells present.

References

Little LM, Shadduck JA 1982 Pathogenesis of rotavirus infection in mice. Infect Immun 38: 755–763

Ward RL, McNeal MM, Sheridan JF 1990 Development of an adult mouse model for studies on protection against rotavirus. J Virol 64:5070–5075

Novartis 238: Gastroenteritis Viruses.
Copyright © 2001 John Wiley & Sons Ltd
Print ISBN 0-471-49663-4   eISBN 0-470-84653-4

General discussion I

Desselberger: It has already been mentioned that there is no reverse genetics system for rotaviruses. On the other hand, we have had fascinating insights from John Patton into the replication of rotavirus. Why do you think that a reverse genetics system for rotaviruses has not yet been established?

Patton: Development of a reverse genetics system has been complicated by both the lack of fundamental information on how rotaviruses package and replicate their genomes and technical difficulties in introducing functional recombinant RNAs into the viral replication cycle. Despite several years of effort, we have as yet been unsuccessful in using the vaccinia virus vTF7.3 system as a tool for generating a reverse genetics system. We have noted two technical problems with this system. First, cleavage of the 3'-end of viral mRNAs transcribed from viral cDNAs with an HDV ribosome leaves a 3' phosphate. This may interfere with the recognition of the 3'-end of the viral mRNAs by the viral RNA polymerase or by NSP3 and therefore may interfere with the entry of the mRNAs into the replication cycle. Second, T7 RNA polymerase does not transcribe RNA efficiently in the cell from vectors in which the T7 promoter is positioned immediately upstream from the 5'-end of a viral cDNA. Despite these problems, we have attempted to replace the VP7 gene of one strain of rotavirus with that of another, derived from a cDNA, using the vTF7.3 system and a combination of neutralizing antibodies for selection. We have also attempted such monogene replacement experiments by directly transfecting cDNA derived from VP7 mRNA into infected cells, instead of using the vTF7.3 system. Neither of these approaches has yet been successful, although in both cases it is clear that the mRNAs were translated, and at least by that measure, could be considered to be biologically active.

Desselberger: Naked RNA transfection hasn't worked in other systems. People have also made RNA–protein complexes and transfected those, e.g. for reoviruses (Roner et al 1990). Have you tried this?

Patton: We have tried a few such experiments. Incubation of core proteins with cDNA-derived mRNAs will form complexes that can synthesize double-stranded (ds)RNA *in vitro*. But transfection of these complexes into cells does not generate infectious virus. Perhaps the addition of these non-structural proteins to the complexes and other modifications will eventually yield infectious RNA–protein complexes.

Greenberg: Have you done positive selection as well as negative selection?

Patton: What are you going to use for positive selection?

Greenberg: Puromycin.

Patton: There are rather convincing data that the secondary structure of rotavirus mRNAs plays a critical role in its ability to serve as an efficient template for the synthesis of dsRNA. This has to be considered when making chimeric RNAs which contain the 5′- and 3′-UTRs of a viral gene and the open reading frame (ORF) of a reporter gene such as green fluorescent protein (GFP), luciferase or chloramphenicol acetyl transferase (CAT). Such chimeric RNAs probably lack the *cis*-acting signals that promote the synthesis of dsRNA in an effective way. Generally, we have tried to replace the VP7 gene of a mono-reassortant such as DxRRV with a cDNA-derived VP7 mRNA that could change the reassortant back to wild-type RRV. In this case, the positive selection comes from the fact that the wild-type RRV grows much better than the reassortant. Negative selection comes from using neutralizing antibodies to inactivate parental virus containing D VP7.

Desselberger: Did you use the plasmid cDNA transcription and plasmid expression approach?

Patton: To some extent, but we haven't been successful with that. The possible combinations and permutations in designing such experiments go on and on. To say that we have reached the end of the road on that approach is not true.

Matson: In the cryoelectron microscopy experiments, VP1, VP2 and VP3 appear to be foci for RNA organization. Is there anything that organizes rotavirus RNA in the test-tube? What organizes the RNA, and will knowing this be crucial to recovering viable virus?

Prasad: If you mix all these particles you will not be able to incorporate the dsRNA which is outside. Somehow, the dsRNAs must be threaded through the virus-like particles (VLPs), which have VP1, VP3 and VP2 and VP6. This may not be possible. The packaging could be concomitant with the assembly of the VP1/VP2/VP3 complex.

Matson: If you start with a VLP and have to thread RNAs into it, this would be difficult.

Prasad: It probably wouldn't be possible.

Matson: What if you start with something else? Can you organize around that?

Desselberger: Frank Ramig, I believe you have tried to package heterologous RNA into the open cores?

Ramig: We tried to do that thinking that perhaps these dsRNA viruses are a degenerate negative-strand virus, because they have their own enzymes. We thought we would try to reconstitute the nucleocapsid. We were never able to do this with soluble proteins. Furthermore, we were not able to replicate and get the ds product packaged in the replicase particle. If we could get it packaged it might transcribe. John Patton talked about using an antibody selection. We have done the same using an anti-VP7 antibody. We made, by old-fashioned means, the reassortant that we were trying to reconstruct and found that it existed and neutralized as predicted with the antibodies we wanted to use for selection. We still couldn't select what we were looking for. It is a problem that is becoming frustrating enough that we don't want to pursue it.

Monroe: In a sense we are talking about reverse genetic systems that don't work. We are missing some of the fundamental biology of how these viruses work.

Green: Frank Ramig mentioned that NSP3 down-regulated replication in *in vitro* systems. Is there any way of up-regulating replication *in vitro?*

Ramig: Not that we have looked at.

Patton: It seems that anything you add is more likely to inhibit than to enhance it.

Ramig: What happens if you add NSP2?

Patton: It will inhibit dsRNA synthesis through a mechanism that is not known to us.

Arias: In the absence of a reverse genetics system, has anyone tried complementing a missing or defective protein function by expression of a functional transplanted gene?

Cohen: We have a cell line constitutively expressing NSP3 and this therefore facilitates the translation of viral messages. These cells have been transfected with viral mRNA, but after three passages no infectious virus was detected.

Ramig: Did you screen the unmapped temperature-sensitive (ts) mutants against that cell line to see whether they would complement?

Cohen: No.

Ramig: We are currently making and characterizing cell lines expressing several proteins for which we do not have ts mutants mapped. We want to determine which ts mutants identify and group those genes by complementation.

Prasad: John Patton, in the model that you proposed with a complex of NSP2, NSP5 and VP1–3, where is the selectivity coming from for packaging each of the 11 dsRNAs into each particle?

Patton: I have no idea. This is a mystery for all of us working on the *Reoviridae.*

Prasad: How much do we know about the role of host cell proteins in either assortment or for bringing correct mRNAs to the proper place?

Patton: The role of host proteins in assortment or trafficking has not been documented. But it would seem reasonable to suspect that the cytoskeletal components of the infected cell would play an important role in moving viral mRNAs and proteins to the viroplasm.

López: Dr Prasad, in your model, do you suppose that there might be 12 genes in each viral particle?

Prasad: We have made it look like 12 because of the icosahedral symmetry implicitly used in our reconstructions. We had to have 12, but this will not be true in real life. In the case of the reoviruses there would be 10 genes and 10 transcription complexes, and in rotaviruses there will be 11. Eleven sites are occupied and one site is empty. As far as structural analysis is concerned we have 95% occupancy. It is the same question with the VP4: that it is an idealized structure showing 60 spikes, but in reality, each particle may only have 30 or 40. In each particle there are 11 corners and 11 transcription complexes acting upon 11 genes. One of the sites is empty. Some of the particles may not even have all 11 segments. Even with the biochemistry, all the experiments suggest that on average every particle has 11 segments.

Desselberger: I disagree. It has been shown by several people that when one takes a highly purified particle suspension and measures the infectivity, one can obtain an infectivity/number of virus particles ratio of almost one particle per plaque-forming unit (e.g. Hundley et al 1985). If you then estimate the concentration of the genomic RNA segments on gels and measure according to size, they are present in equimolar amounts. This strongly suggests that particles package exactly 11 segments per particle with a great degree of precision.

Ramig: I don't think that you can exclude the virus packaging 12. You can argue that it doesn't package less than 11.

Prasad: The structural results from rotaviruses, bluetongue viruses and reoviruses all indicate why we have never seen more than 12 segments in any of these dsRNA viruses. It is probably a structural constraint.

Patton: The analysis of rotavirus variants containing genome segments with rearrangements and deletions indicates that the headful mechanism of packaging does not apply in the case of the rotaviruses. For example, non-defective variants have been described in which the gene 5 segment contains an extra 1000 nucleotides or lacks 500 nucleotides, indicating that RNA size is not a factor in packaging of the core. This differs from the segmented dsRNA bacteriophage phi6 for which data have been obtained that successful packaging occurs by a headful mechanism.

Arias: In our experience with animal strains there is one infectious particle for about every hundred physical particles, and in human viruses this ratio can be 1 in 10 000. Could you speculate about why there are so many defective virus particles?

Prasad: This could be for several reasons. One is that VP4 assembly may be a factor. I don't think a ratio of one to one has been reported; it is more like one infectious particle per hundred particles.

Desselberger: It depends on the system. Low infectious particle to actual particle ratios were found for highly cell-culture adapted viruses.

Matson: What is it for SA11/4F?

Ramig: The plaque-forming unit to particle ratio for SA11/4F was 1:2.4 (Burns et al 1989).

Matson: So Dr Prasad's structures are of viable viruses?

Prasad: Those are the two factors that I can think of: VP4 and not having the correct number of segments in each particle. Perhaps there are more.

References

Burns JW, Chen D, Estes MK, Ramig RF 1989 Biological and immunological characterization of a similar rotavirus SA11 variant with an altered gene segment 4. Virology 169:427–435

Hundley F, Biryahwaho B, Gow M, Desselberger U 1985 Genome rearrangements of bovine rotavirus after serial passage at high multiplicity of infection. Virology 143:88–103

Roner MR, Sutphin LA, Joklik WK 1990 Reovirus RNA is infectious. Virology 179: 845–852

Novartis 238: Gastroenteritis Viruses.
Copyright © 2001 John Wiley & Sons Ltd
Print ISBN 0-471-49663-4 eISBN 0-470-84653-4

Correlates of protection against rotavirus infection and disease

Paul A. Offit

The Children's Hospital of Philadelphia, 34th St. and Civic Center Blvd., The University of Pennsylvania School of Medicine, Philadelphia, PA 19104, and The Wistar Institute of Anatomy and Biology, 36th and Spruce Sts, Philadelphia, PA 19103, USA

Abstract. Repeated infections with the 'mucosal' pathogen rotavirus are common in children. Subsequent rotavirus infections usually cause milder symptoms than first-time infections. Therefore, although natural rotavirus infection attenuates the severity of subsequent infections, it does not prevent reinfection or mild disease. On the other hand, natural infection with 'systemic' viruses such as measles, mumps, rubella, or varicella often confers life-long protection against mild disease associated with reinfection. The degree to which differences in the pathogenesis of systemic and mucosal pathogens determines differences in the capacity of natural infection to induce life-long protective immunity will be discussed. This paradigm will be used to explore the immunological effector functions associated with protection against rotavirus challenge.

2001 Gastroenteritis viruses. Wiley, Chichester (Novartis Foundation Symposium 238) p 106–124

Rotaviruses were first discovered to be a pathogen in humans more than 25 years ago (Bishop et al 1973). Since that time, they have been found to be the most important cause of acute gastroenteritis in infants and young children throughout the world (Black et al 1981, Ho et al 1988). Because of the worldwide impact of rotavirus infections, immunological correlates of protection against rotavirus infection and disease have been extensively studied. What has emerged from these studies is a clear picture of how natural rotavirus infection protects against disease caused by subsequent infections, and why it will be difficult to develop a vaccine that confers lifelong protection against mild rotavirus disease.

Natural rotavirus infection induces protection against disease caused by reinfection, but protection is often incomplete

Natural infection of newborns causes protection against moderate-to-severe, but not mild, disease caused by reinfection

Evidence that natural rotavirus infection induces protection against disease caused by reinfection was provided first by Ruth Bishop and colleagues (Bishop et al

TABLE 1   Capacity of rotavirus infection of newborns (<1 month of age) to protect against rotavirus disease associated with subsequent infection during childhood

Infected as newborn (n)	Severity of disease (%)			
	Asymptomatic	Mild	Moderate	Severe
No (20)	15	15	30	40
Yes (24)	63	13	25	0

1983). Newborns in Melbourne, Australia were screened in the first two weeks of life for the presence of rotavirus in stools by electron microscopy. Twenty infants who did not excrete rotavirus and 24 infants who did excrete rotavirus were followed prospectively for 3 years. The incidence of reinfection was indistinguishable in the two groups (55% in infants infected as newborns and 54% in infants not infected as newborns). Therefore, rotavirus infection did not protect against reinfection.

However, rotavirus infection during the first 2 weeks of life did protect against moderate-to-severe disease associated with reinfection (Table 1). Whereas 70% of children with first-time rotavirus infections had moderate-to-severe disease associated with reinfection, only 25% of children with subsequent rotavirus infections had moderate-to-severe disease.

Natural infection of infants causes protection against moderate-to-severe disease independent of the severity of the primary infection

David Bernstein and co-workers (Bernstein et al 1991) studied children 2–12 months of age prospectively for two years (Table 2). Similar to studies done by Bishop and co-workers (Bishop et al 1983), the percentage of infants infected

TABLE 2   Capacity of symptomatic or asymptomatic rotavirus infection of infants (<1 year of age) to protect against rotavirus disease associated with subsequent infection during childhood

Infected as infant (n)	Presence or severity of reinfection (%)		
	Uninfected	Asymptomatic	Symptomatic
No (82)	65	24	11
Yes (60)	93	3	3
Asymptomatic (20)	95	5	0
Symptomatic (40)	93	3	5

with rotavirus between 2 and 12 months of age that were protected against symptomatic disease was lower than that found in infants who were *not* infected in the first year of life (3% vs. 11%). This study extended the findings of Bishop in two important ways. First, protection was afforded by natural infection that occurred anytime in the first year of life. Second, protection caused by a first-time natural infection occurred independent of the severity of that infection. The percent of children with symptomatic reinfection following asymptomatic or symptomatic primary infection was similar (0% vs. 5%).

Taken together, the studies described above showed that an asymptomatic infection of newborns or infants could protect against symptomatic disease associated with reinfection. Because the goal of a rotavirus vaccine would be to mimic an asymptomatic infection of infants, these initial findings were encouraging for the development of a successful rotavirus vaccine.

Protection against moderate-to-severe disease results
from two natural rotavirus infections

Velázquez and co-workers (Velázquez et al 1996) studied 200 Mexican infants from birth to 2 years of age (Table 3). Similar to previous studies, they found that (1) independent of the severity of the first infection, protection was afforded against disease associated with reinfection and, (2) a single natural infection protected against moderate-to-severe disease (87% efficacy) as compared with protection against mild disease (73% efficacy) or asymptomatic reinfection (38% efficacy). Investigators extended previous studies by showing that all children (100%) were protected against moderate-to-severe rotavirus disease subsequent to two natural rotavirus infections.

Natural rotavirus infection induces protection against disease caused by reinfection, but protection is often short-lived

Whereas children commonly develop symptomatic rotavirus infections with the same rotavirus serotype one year after a primary rotavirus infection, it is

TABLE 3   Capacity of one, two or three natural rotavirus infections to protect against symptomatic reinfection

	Protection against infection or disease (%)		
No. of previous infections	*Asymptomatic*	*Mild*	*Moderate-to-severe*
1	38	73	87
2	62	75	100
3	74	99	—

uncommon for children to be symptomatically infected with the same rotavirus serotype twice within the same season (a rotavirus season in temperate climates is about 4 months long) (reviewed in Offit 1996). Therefore, complete protection against disease (i.e. protection against mild, moderate and severe rotavirus disease) associated with rotavirus reinfection is relatively short-lived. A number of investigators have determined why complete protection following natural rotavirus infection is short-lived.

Protection against symptomatic rotavirus infection is mediated by virus-specific secretory IgA present at the intestinal mucosal surface

Barbara Coulson and co-workers (Coulson et al 1992) studied 35 infants and young children acutely infected with rotavirus. Faecal specimens were collected every 7–10 days for 1–2 years and tested for the presence of rotavirus-specific IgA. Faecal virus-specific IgA was presumed to correlate with the presence of virus-specific IgA at the small intestinal mucosal surface. Two groups of children were defined; one group had persistently high levels of virus-specific IgA (12 children) and the other did not (23 children). The investigators found that during intervals when virus-specific IgA was detected in the faeces months after acute rotavirus infection, the mean annual rate of symptomatic rotavirus reinfections was significantly less than that found in children who did have virus-specific IgA in the faeces (0.51 vs. 2.14).

Matson et al (1993) extended the findings of Coulson et al (1992) by showing that the level of virus-specific IgA detected in the faeces correlated with the severity of disease associated with reinfection. One hundred and twenty nine children in daycare centres between 10 and 18 months of age were tested weekly for the presence of rotavirus-specific IgA in faeces and studied for approximately 1 year. Children with high levels of rotavirus-specific IgA (geometric mean of 1:1290) in faeces were significantly less likely to be infected than children with lower levels of virus-specific IgA (geometic mean of 1:438). Similarly, children with even lower levels of virus-specific IgA in faeces (geometric mean of 1:139) were more likely to develop symptomatic rotavirus infection than children in either of the other two groups.

Complete protection against rotavirus disease following natural infection is short-lived because production of virus-specific IgA at the intestinal mucosal surface is often short-lived

In the studies of Coulson and Matson (Coulson et al 1992, Matson et al 1993), many children no longer had detectable virus-specific IgA in faeces one year after natural rotavirus infection. These studies are consistent with those of Grimwood et al (1988) who found that rotavirus-specific sIgA was not detected in either the faeces or duodenal fluids obtained from infants 75 days after acute rotavirus infection.

Whereas complete protection against rotavirus disease following natural infection is mediated by high levels of virus-specific IgA present at the intestinal mucosal surface, modification of rotavirus disease is likely mediated by the differentiation of virus-specific intestinal memory B cells to antibody-secreting cells

Protection against subsequent infection following natural rotavirus infection is similar to that caused by infection with 'mucosal' viruses such as influenza virus and respiratory syncytial virus (RSV). Similar to rotaviruses, protection following infection with influenza or RSV is often short-lived (lasting less than 1 year) and incomplete (protection against moderate-to-severe, but not mild disease). These findings are in contrast to protection following infection with 'systemic' viruses such as measles, mumps, rubella or varicella. Protection following infection with 'systemic' viruses is often long-lived and complete.

Differences in the capacity of 'mucosal' and 'systemic' viruses to induce long-lived and complete protection against disease caused by reinfection are explained by differences in the pathogenesis of natural infection. 'Mucosal' viruses replicate solely at mucosal surfaces at the site of entry into the host. Because the pathogenesis of mucosal viral infection does not involve replication of virus at sites distant to the mucosal surface, incubation periods are short (usually lasting between 1–4 days). In contrast, viraemia is an important component of 'systemic' viral infections. 'Systemic' viruses replicate at sites distant to the mucosal surface of entry, and usually undergo primary, secondary and occasionally tertiary sites of replication. Spread to and replication in sites distant to mucosal surfaces takes time, so that incubation periods following infection with 'systemic' viruses are usually long (lasting between 8 and 14 days).

Both 'mucosal' and 'systemic' viral infections induce virus-specific memory B cells following natural infection. Following reinfection, these B cells differentiate to antibody-secreting cells — a process that takes about 3–5 days. However, 3–5 days is outside the incubation period of most 'mucosal' viral infections. Therefore, following reinfection with 'mucosal' viruses, symptoms of the disease will appear before B cells in the mucosal lamina propria differentiate to IgA-secreting cells. The consequence is that memory B cell responses following reinfection with 'mucosal' viruses results in a modification of disease associated with reinfection (protection against moderate-to-severe disease), but not complete protection against disease (protection against mild, moderate and severe disease). In contrast, differentiation of virus-specific memory B cells to antibody-secreting cells following reinfection with 'systemic' viruses occurs before symptoms begin. Therefore, protection following reinfection with 'systemic' viruses is often complete.

Animal model studies support the hypothesis that complete protection against rotavirus disease following reinfection is mediated by virus-specific sIgA present at the intestinal mucosal surface

Studies of the immunological correlates of protection against rotavirus disease in infants and children are limited to coproantibodies. The presence of rotavirus-specific IgA in faeces presumably reflects production of antibodies by small intestinal lamina propria lymphocytes. However, direct detection of virus-specific IgA-secreting cells in the intestinal lamina propria, or a more definitive comparison of the relative importance of virus-specific IgA and virus-specific cytotoxic T lymphocytes, requires studies of experimental animals.

Protection against disease caused by rotavirus reinfection is predicted by the frequency of rotavirus-specific IgA-secreting cells in the small intestinal lamina propria

Yuan, Saif and co-workers (Yuan et al 1996) determined the immunological correlates of protection against rotavirus disease in neonatal gnotobiotic pigs. They found that pigs orally inoculated with a virulent human rotavirus (strain Wa) developed diarrhoea and were completely protected against challenge 21 days later with virulent Wa rotavirus. In contrast, pigs orally inoculated with an avirulent strain of Wa were only partially protected against challenge with virulent Wa virus. Protection against challenge correlated with the frequency of virus-specific IgA-secreting but not IgG-secreting cells in the small intestinal lamina propria, mesenteric lymph nodes and blood as detected by ELISpot assay.

Protection against rotavirus disease caused by reinfection is mediated by virus-specific antibodies, not virus-specific cytotoxic T lymphocytes

To determine the relative importance of virus-specific antibodies and virus-specific cytotoxic T lymphocytes in protection against disease caused by rotavirus reinfection, mice lacking B cells ($J_H D$ knockout mice) or T cells (β_2-microglobulin-knockout mice) were studied. Both McNeal, Ward and co-workers (McNeal et al 1995) and Franco & Greenberg (1995) found that $J_H D$-knockout mice were not protected against viral shedding caused by murine rotavirus challenge following immunization with murine rotavirus. In addition, Franco & Greenberg (1995) found that β_2-microglobulin-knockout mice were fully protected against reinfection with murine rotavirus. Therefore, protection against shedding caused by rotavirus reinfection was mediated by virus-specific antibodies and not virus-specific cytotoxic T lymphocytes.

Animal model studies support the hypothesis that modification of rotavirus disease is mediated by the differentiation of virus-specific memory B cells to IgA-secreting cells in the intestinal lamina propria

To determine the capacity of IgA generated from intestinal virus-specific memory B cells to protect against challenge, Moser, Offit and co-workers (Moser et al 1998) examined mice orally inoculated with simian strain RRV. They found that 16 weeks after immunization with RRV, virus-specific IgA was not produced by small intestinal B cells located in the lamina propria as determined by fragment culture. However, approximately 4 days after EDIM challenge, virus-specific IgA was produced by lamina propria B cells at a level significantly greater than that found in unimmunized mice. Production of virus-specific IgA 4–6 days after EDIM challenge correlated with ablation of viral shedding observed 4–6 days after challenge. Therefore, following immunization with RRV, mice were partially, but not completely, protected against shedding following challenge; ablation of viral shedding occurred several days, but not immediately, after challenge. This model is consistent with the hypothesis that virus-specific IgA generated from memory B cells is associated with amelioration, but not complete protection against challenge.

In contrast, several investigators found that immunization of mice with murine rotavirus strain EDIM induces long-lived production of virus-specific IgA at the intestinal mucosal surface and complete protection against challenge. McNeal & Ward (1995) found that mice orally immunized with a dose of EDIM continued to produce intestinal virus-specific IgA, and were completely protected against challenge. Therefore, murine rotavirus strain EDIM might induce an immune response in mice that is very different from that found in humans naturally infected with human strains. Whereas many infants naturally infected with rotavirus no longer produce virus-specific IgA at the intestinal mucosal surface one-year after infection, mice continue to produce virus-specific IgA for at least one-half of the total life of the animal. Long-lived production of virus-specific IgA following EDIM immunization is associated with long-lived complete protection against challenge.

Summary

The best rotavirus vaccines will be those that induce long-lived, complete protection against subsequent challenge. Complete protection can only be accomplished by long-lived production of virus-specific IgA at the intestinal mucosal surface. However, even following natural infection with rotavirus, production of virus-specific IgA by intestinal B cells is often short-lived. Therefore, the challenge to rotavirus vaccines will be to produce a vaccine that induces an immune response that is longer-lived than that which occurs after natural infection. It might be of value to explore the characteristics of EDIM infection in mice to determine why this particular infection induces long-lived virus-specific IgA responses that result in long-lived complete protection against challenge.

References

Bernstein DI, Sander DS, Smith VE, Schiff GM, Ward RL 1991 Protection from rotavirus reinfection: 2-year prospective study. J Infect Dis 164:277–283

Bishop RF, Davidson GP, Holmes IH, Ruck BJ 1973 Virus particles in epithelial cells of duodenal mucosa from children with acute non-bacterial gastroenteritis. Lancet 2:1281–1283

Bishop RF, Barnes GL, Cipriani E, Lund JS 1983 Clinical immunity after neonatal rotavirus infection. A prospective longitudinal study in young children. N Engl J Med 309:72–76

Black RE, Merson MH, Huq I, Alim A, Yunus MD 1981 Incidence and severity of rotavirus and *Escherichia coli* diarrhea in rural Bangladesh. Implications for vaccine development. Lancet 1:141–143

Coulson BS, Grimwood K, Hudson IL, Barnes GL, Bishop RF 1992 Role of coproantibody in clinical protection of children during reinfection with rotavirus. J Clin Microbiol 30:1678–1684

Franco MA, Greenberg HB 1995 Role of B cells and cytotoxic T lymphocytes in clearance of and immunity to rotavirus infection in mice. J Virol 69:7800–7806

Grimwood K, Lund JC, Coulson BS, Hudson IL, Bishop RF, Barnes GL 1988 Comparison of serum and mucosal antibody responses following severe acute rotavirus gastroenteritis in young children. J Clin Microbiol 26:732–738

Ho MS, Glass RI, Pinsky PF, Anderson LJ 1988 Rotavirus as a cause of diarrheal morbidity and mortality in the United States. J Infect Dis 158:1112–1116

McNeal MM, Ward RL 1995 Long-term production of rotavirus antibody and protection against reinfection following a single infection of neonatal mice with murine rotavirus. Virology 211:474–480

McNeal MM, Barone KS, Rae MN, Ward RL 1995 Effector functions of antibody and CD8+ cells in resolution of rotavirus infection and protection against reinfection in mice. Virology 214:387–397

Matson DO, O'Ryan ML, Herrera I, Pickering LK, Estes MK 1993 Fecal antibody responses to symptomatic and asymptomatic rotavirus infections. J Infect Dis 167:577–583

Moser CA, Cookinham S, Coffin SE, Clark HF, Offit PA 1998 Relative importance of rotavirus-specific effector and memory B cells in protection against challenge. J Virol 72:1108–1114 (erratum: 1998 J Virol 72:2564)

Offit PA 1996 Host factors associated with protection against rotavirus disease: the skies are clearing. J Infect Dis 174:S59–S64

Velázquez FR, Matson DO, Calva JJ et al 1996 Rotavirus infection in infants as protection against subsequent infection. N Engl J Med 335:1022–1028

Yuan L, Ward LA, Rosen BI, To TL, Saif L 1996 Systemic and intestinal antibody-secreting cell responses and correlates of protective immunity to human rotavirus in a gnotobiotic pig model of disease. J Virol 70:3075–3083

DISCUSSION

Vesikari: A simple question: as much as you talked about IgA, you did not mention what the target antigens of this IgA are. What are they?

Offit: There are a number of studies that have looked at the relative capacity of the different rotavirus proteins to induce virus-specific antibodies. The most compelling of these show that VP4 or VP7, or both, appear to invoke antibodies which neutralize virus infectivity *in vitro* and appear to protect against challenge *in vivo*.

Vesikari: I appreciate that answer, but my question was specifically about this IgA known to be protective in many systems.

Saif: A summary of our findings for human rotavirus (human Wa strain infection of gnotobiotic pigs) may shed a bit of light on this. Paul Offit has already presented the first part. If we give virulent human rotavirus orally to pigs, we can induce a high degree of protection against virus shedding and diarrhoea (Saif et al 1996, Ward et al 1996, Yuan et al 1996). This correlates with the high IgA antibody-secreting cell numbers in the duodenum; we see very low numbers in the systemic lymphoid system such as the spleen (Yuan et al 1996). After oral inoculation of pigs with the attenuated Wa rotavirus, one can see that we get similar protection rates against diarrhoea to those obtained in the oral rotavirus human clinical trials. Three doses (63% protection) are better than two doses (36% protection), and these protection data also correlate with IgA antibody-secreting numbers in the duodenum of the small intestine compared with the results in the spleen where we get more IgG antibody-secreting cells (Saif et al 1996, Yuan et al 1996). If we give the inactivated virus to pigs parenterally with adjuvant or orally without adjuvant, we get low numbers of IgA antibody-secreting cells in the intestine and low protection against diarrhoea and virus shedding (Yuan et al 1998). What we have done lately, to address your question about which proteins might be important, is to inoculate the 2/6 Wa rotavirus-like particles (VLPs) intranasally three times with mutant *Escherichia coli* heat-labile toxin (LT), because we wanted to compare these responses in pigs with the responses generated in mice to these same types of 2/6 VLPs (Yuan et al 2000). We got low numbers of IgA antibody-secreting cells in the small intestine and higher numbers of IgG antibody-secreting cells. In the pig model we could not induce protection against rotavirus diarrhoea or shedding by the intranasal route with mutant LT toxin and 2/6 VLPs. We think that VP6 alone, in terms of the experimental model of antibody-induced protection against diarrhoea, was not effective. However, because of the intussusception reports in terms of the attenuated, live rotavirus vaccine, we tried a combination vaccine (L. Yuan & L.F. Saif, unpublished results). Our first approach was to try the 2/6 Wa VLPs given intranasally twice, followed by attenuated Wa virus given once orally. This did induce some protection against diarrhoea. There were some IgA antibody-secreting cells in the intestinal tract and more IgG antibody-secreting cells in the spleen. This was not optimally protective, but it was a little better than giving the VLPs alone. Our recent studies suggest that if we give one dose of attenuated Wa orally followed by two doses of 2/6 VLPs plus mutant LT intranasally, we get a high degree of protection against virus shedding and diarrhoea and a moderate-to-high number of IgA antibody-secreting cells in the intestinal tract. This suggests to us that we probably need to prime with an intact virus that has VP4 and VP7 but for some reason we can come back via a different mucosal route, intranasally, and boost effectively only with 2/6 VLPs. The mechanisms involved are unclear, but may involve cross-reactive, primed CD4$^+$ T cells.

Koopmans: In connection with the data that Linda Saif described, we have some experience with work on polio virus. In The Netherlands we use an inactivated polio vaccine whereas almost all other countries use the oral live poliovirus vaccine (OPV). We have shown in human volunteers that people who had prior mucosal infection either with wild-type or OPV, get a very prominent booster IgA response with the injectable vaccine given later. We have shown from sorting circulating lymphocytes, that they are on their way to mucosal surfaces (Herremans et al 1997, 1999).

Saif: Was this in children?

Koopmans: This was in adults.

Offit: The notion that one can boost a mucosal immune response by giving a parenteral vaccine only if there has already been a mucosal priming has also been shown for influenza. One of the reasons that the inactivated influenza works so poorly in children less than two years of age is that they haven't already been primed. It is hard to prime the immune system by giving a parenteral vaccine, but the vaccine does have some efficacy in older people because it acts as a booster.

Desselberger: With regard to the antigen against which protection might be directed, of course antibodies against VP4 and VP7 would be neutralizing, but there are data from Harry Greenberg's lab (Burns et al 1996), in which they showed that the VP6-specific IgA in the mouse 'backpack' model produced protection from shedding. There are also data from John Herrmann's group who tested a VP6-specific DNA vaccine and produced partial protection (Herrmann et al 1996, Chen et al 1997). The possible mechanism is that VP6-specific IgA antibodies transcytose as shown in Fig. 1 (*Desselberger*), interact with bilayered particles in the viroplasm and aggregate them. There are some good data from the influenza field by Mazanec et al (1992), who showed that influenza-virus-infected cells that were grown on a semipermeable membrane and were transcytosed with a nucleoprotein-specific IgA produced a significantly decreased titre of virus. I also remember that Harry Greenberg's group produced some data at a recent meeting trying to elucidate this model for rotaviruses.

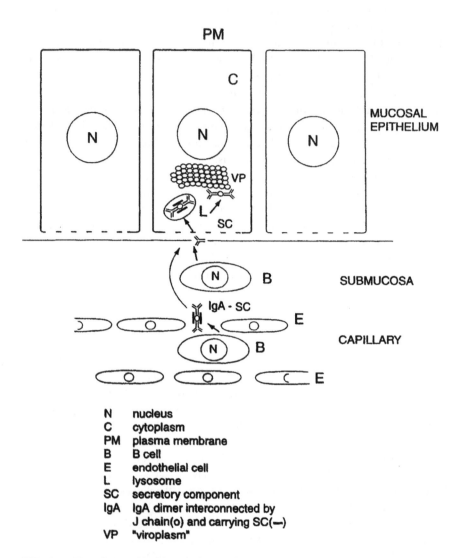

FIG. 1. *(Desselberger)* Model of IgA transport and possible intracellular neutralization of rotavirus single-shelled particles in viroplasm by transcytosed VP6-specific IgA. IgA dimers are secreted from B cells located in capillaries or in the submucosa. IgA–SC dimers then bind to the basal plasma membrane of epithelial cells which express SC acting as a polymeric IgA receptor. IgA-SC is endocytosed and found in lysosomal compartments where it loses SC. It can then bind to specific proteins intracellularly; rotavirus VP6-specific IgA is thought to bind to single-shelled subviral particles which are often arranged in paracrystalline arrays in the viroplasm. (Reproduced from Desselberger 1998.)

Estes: We have to be careful when we are interpreting these data as to whether we are talking about model systems where people are measuring protection from infection, or model systems where people are measuring protection from disease.

Bishop: The IgA response in the intestinal tract must be at least partly due to VP6 because it can be measured by ELISA. There is neutralizing antibody there as well which can be measured in a neutralizing antibody assay (Coulson & Masendycz 1990). It is still difficult to identify the components of the intestinal tract response to individual viral proteins, even though it is possible to show a full range of responses in serum to viral proteins (Richardson et al 1993, Johansen et al 1994).

Greenberg: It seems that the number of memory B cells is also relevant to protection. Paul Offit, you are correct that it takes time for memory cells to become effector cells; the more memory cells you have, the faster this appears to occur, because the rate at which IgA is generated increases. In effect, the more memory cells you have in the gut, the better off you are after infection. How memory cells get into the gut and stay in the gut would be another fruitful research direction.

Offit: We have data which I didn't show that are relevant here. We did an *in vitro* analysis in which we tried to identify the frequency of memory B cells within gut-associated lymphoid tissue at various intervals after immunization with RRV. We found that 16 weeks after immunization, the principal location of virus-specific memory B cells was in the lamina propria. They were much less commonly present in the Peyer's patch, in the spleen, or in the mesenteric node. In fact, both the number and the site of memory B cells determined protection against shedding associated with reinfection. You are right; it is not just memory B cell number, it is also where they are. I would say, though, that even in the best of immunization schemes, it still took a number of days to elicit antibody-secreting cells from memory B cells. Once we had infected and allowed that infection to become quiescent in terms of production of IgA in the lamina propria, it still took at least four days in order to detect virus-specific antibody secreting cells derived from memory B cells in the lamina propria.

Greenberg: If the number was five times higher, it might have been three days.

Offit: It is possible; we could never do that.

Greenberg: That in part happens with wild-type infection.

Offit: Even with wild-type virus, we could never get to a point of quiescence; there was always production of IgA in the lamina propria.

Greenberg: It becomes a little bit of an 'apples and oranges' scenario. It has to do with numbers. You also have a hugely increased number of memory cells with wild-type.

Offit: Absolutely. The problem is that it is hard to sort out memory from effector cells if there is an ongoing effector cell response.

Greenberg: Cells become enteric memory cells because they have molecules on their surface that allow them to go to the gut. These molecules have classically been the integrin α4β7, but there is a whole set of new chemokines being found that also mediate intestinal trafficking. The most widely studied of these to date is CCR9 and its counter-receptor TECK. The ability to manipulate the way in which B or T cells develop those molecules on their surface would be another mechanism by which you could influence mucosal immunity. At the moment the only way we know how to do this is to immunize at the mucosal surface, but this simply means that there is some form of signalling that occurs at the mucosal surface that doesn't happen when you immunize parenterally. Presumably one could figure this out and induce memory cells that think they want to travel to the gut after systemic immunization. Nelly Koklin and I have asked the question, what is more important: the ability of B cells to secrete IgA antibody, or the ability of B cells to home to the intestine? We have looked at this in a combination of knockout mice in which we can delete either IgA or β7. We asked, if you had to have one phenotype, which would rather have after a natural infection? The answer was interesting: mice that had IgG-producing cells that could home to the intestine were better protected than mice that had IgA-producing memory B cells that could not home to the intestine.

Offit: One always has to insert some level of caution in work with knockout mice. Margaret Connor recently published a paper in which she stated that IgG could be protective against challenge with rotavirus, in what was essentially an IgA knockout mouse (O'Neal et al 2000). What was interesting was that in her normal animals that were not IgA knockout mice, she was unable to detect virus-specific IgG at the intestinal mucosal surface. However, in her IgA knockout mice she was able to detect IgG at this surface. This makes you wonder whether or not these knockout mice had developed some compensatory mechanism to allow for the secretion of IgG onto the intestinal surface.

Greenberg: That is the point of what I was saying. In the IgA knockout mouse, those IgG B cells become α4β7 positive because the mouse compensates and allows its IgG cells to express high levels of the gut homing receptor α2β7.

Offit: It is still a polymeric immunoglobulin receptor at the basolateral surface.

Greenberg: I would rather have IgA and homing.

Offit: What gets IgG to the intestinal surface when it is a monomeric molecule? That is what is interesting.

Estes: We all know that knockout mice often have compensatory components, so we do have to interpret data from them with caution. Since you have raised the issue about IgG, we shouldn't forget its importance at the mucosal surface. It is clear from most of the natural studies looking at live rotavirus infection in animals or children, that the primary response that is measured is IgA. This doesn't exclude the fact that there is some IgG there, which is also a component of protection. If we are thinking about future vaccines, IgG at the mucosal surface could also be important.

Offit: I disagree. I am still not convinced that IgG plays an important role in protection against reinfection in the gut. I think it is true in the lower respiratory tract.

Greenberg: The critical question was what can play an important role. In natural rotavirus infection there is no doubt that in all the model systems tested to date, IgA appears to be a more important effector mechanism than IgG. This doesn't mean that IgG is not capable of being a fully powerful effector mechanism, depending on how one immunizes.

Offit: It still has to get to the intestinal mucosal surface.

Estes: It does. There is now evidence from a group at Harvard that there is a receptor in the intestine that will take IgG to the surface.

Matson: We evaluated children hospitalized for diarrhoea, but who did not have rotavirus diarrhoea at presentation (O'Ryan et al 1995). All were monitored and upon subsequent monitoring some developed nosocomial rotavirus diarrhoea and others did not. These children, whose mean age was 4 months, didn't have any IgA antibody, but they did have IgG. This IgG antibody was transplacental and they were not breastfeeding.

Offit: Did they have IgA antibodies in their blood?

Matson: No.

Offit: The question is, was the blood predictive of events that occurred in the intestinal mucosal surface?

Matson: They did not have serum IgA, but serum IgG titres predicted protection. This tells me that in natural infections transplacental IgG has some sort of a role in protection in the absence of IgA.

Saif: We have seen IgG antibody-secreting cells in the intestinal lamina propria which, in agreement with Paul Offit's comment, doesn't necessarily equate with IgG antibodies being secreted onto the luminal surface of the intestine. Just looking at the IgA literature on the secretory immune system, I would agree with the view that high levels of IgG antibodies on the surface of the mucosa is not highly desirable in resolving most natural infections, because IgG antibodies have the ability to fix complement and create inflammatory conditions there. I am not sure that this is the ideal situation. IgG antibodies can come in to play in situations where they act as a second line of defence but I think it is not desirable to have them in there in a long-term situation such as we see in the serum after infection to provide sterilizing immunity.

Estes: That is the classical interpretation of IgG being present in the intestine, but my feeling from all the experiments that Dr Conner has done in rabbits, where IgG is present at the mucosal surface, there is no evidence of any inflammatory reaction taking place there (Conner et al 1993, Ciarlet et al 1998, O'Neal et al 1998). There may be other regulatory mechanisms that, particularly in rotavirus infections, may be different from what has been seen in the past in other models.

Bishop: We may be confusing ourselves here with species differences, and perhaps with age differences. Grimwood et al (1988) looked at children with rotavirus infection, and compared duodenal mucosal antibody and serum antibody responses. With very few exceptions there was no detectable IgG response in gut contents at any level. However, circumstantial evidence implicates anti-rotavirus IgG in protection of newborn babies (R. F. Bishop & G. L. Barnes, unpublished results).

Estes: Let me clarify: in rabbits the primary response to live infection is an IgA response, but if you give inactivated virus or VLP it is an IgG response.

Greenberg: There are two critical questions. First, what happens in a natural infection. This is very important because as Paul Offit has said, natural infections do lead to protection. As you all know, however, many immunizations are not exactly the same as natural infection. Inactivated polio vaccination is not the same as wild-type polio infection, and it works just as well in terms of protection. It is wrong to assume that every strategy of vaccination has to recapitulate the exact form of immunity that occurs in natural infection. If we mix up these two concepts, we will be talking at cross-purposes. A virus-like particle administered systemically may or may not protect, but if it does protect it sure as heck is not going to protect by the same mechanism as a natural intestinal infection. We need to understand what the mechanism is. We will hear more about intussusception later in this meeting. It is not clear how big a problem this actually is, but to the degree that it is a problem, we need to think about what might be an alternative immunization strategy if this problem persists with all orally given replicating vaccine candidates.

Saif: However, the polio vaccine story may not be the best example for enteric viral vaccines (Saif 1990). With polio vaccines, one can either block viral infection locally at the primary site of infection in the intestine by induction of local immunity, or one can use inactivated vaccines parenterally to induce systemic immunity which blocks the systemic spread the virus to the secondary site of infection, the nervous system. Induction of local intestinal immunity appears essential to prevent the infection of enterocytes by enteric viruses such as rotavirus which do not induce secondary systemic infections outside the intestine.

Kapikian: Paul Offit, do we need a vaccine that protects better than natural infection? The elegant longitudinal studies of Velázquez and others of rotavirus infections in a cohort of 200 children studied from birth to 2 years of age show that after two natural rotavirus infections, symptomatic or asymptomatic, no child developed moderate-to-severe diarrhoea (Velázquez et al 1996). We also know from the rhesus rotavirus-based vaccine studies that it is possible to achieve 100% protection against hospitalization and severe diarrhoea in certain settings. If a controlled vaccine infection mimics the wild-type infection and thereby induces protection, why do we need to achieve better protection than occurs under natural conditions?

Offit: I agree. I would say that the goal of the rotavirus vaccine is to prevent the moderate-to-severe disease that is associated with hospitalization and death. The point I was trying to make was that in that second year after immunization, when children are still getting severe disease, it may be of value to give a booster dose to keep up that level of IgA antibody.

Kapikian: If you vaccinate a child three times, at 2, 4 and 6 months of age, the memory should be maintained.

Offit: Memory only offers you so much. But I agree: the goal of the vaccine is to keep the children out of the hospital and keep them from dying, and this is a consequence of natural infection.

Kapikian: Dr Chiba and his colleagues deserve credit for elucidating a mechanism of protection against rotavirus illness. They showed in an infant home in Japan that a serum neutralizing antibody level of 1:128 was protective against illness caused by a homotypic virus. I believe that this was the first study to demonstrate a clear-cut effect of serotype-specific protection in a naturally occurring rotavirus outbreak in humans (Chiba et al 1986).

Vesikari: He showed that serotype-specific neutralizing antibody protects against reinfection, but the great mystery of all rotavirus vaccine studies is why is it that these vaccines protect regardless of the serotype of the surface antigen? I think some light was starting to be shed on this question when Harry Greenberg discovered this intracellular-working IgA. Then the question is, what is the mechanism of the IgA that acts intracellularly against VP6? I was very impressed by Dr Prasad's talk last year in Amherst when he showed the VP6 antibody effect to be through blocking the channels of nucleic acid release. It is an extremely important question as to how a non-neutralizing antibody can actually block rotavirus infection.

Prasad: We have also done the structure of VLPs bound with IgA. The IgA binding to VP6 causes a conformational change down below. It is affecting the transcription, and particularly the translocation of the transcripts through the type I channel.

Greenberg: I want to remind all of you of the old literature, some from Ruth Bishop and Barbara Coulson, some by Ian Holmes, some by me, and some from Koki Tanaguchi, all of which showed that of the monoclonal antibodies to VP4 and VP7, some of the molecules were serotype specific, but in all groups there were antibodies that were not serotype specific and had varying degrees of heterotypic reactivity. While VP6 is a very interesting target, the fact is that both VP4 and VP7 also represent targets that are capable of generating both type-specific and cross-reactive antibodies. There are molecular mechanisms to account for heterotypic immunity at the level of VP4, VP7 and VP6 on a humoral basis. We keep forgetting this.

Saif: In regard to VP6, there may be some mechanism whereby it is moderating the infection, but apparently in the neonatal gnotobiotic pig model it is not enough to control the disease. We did see some degree of reduced virus shedding, although it wasn't significantly different from controls with the 2/6 VLPs alone (Yuan et al 2000). In terms of the adult mouse backpack model in John Burns' and Harry Greenberg's work, the problem there is that you had a physiologically unusually large amount of antibody to get to those sites that you would never be able to reproduce under normal conditions. In addition, in subsequent studies by Ruggeri et al (1998), IgA and IgG hybridomas to rotavirus VP6 implanted as backpack tumours in neonatal BALB/c mice failed to protect mice against rhesus rotavirus-induced diarrhoea, whereas hybridomas secreting IgA monoclonal antibodies to rotavirus VP8* protected the neonatal mice.

Greenberg: The most convincing part of the VP6 data is not the backpack but the 2/6 VLPs that have also all been shown to protect.

Saif: This is in an adult model of virus shedding, not in the neonatal model of rotavirus diarrhoea.

Greenberg: Absolutely correct; that is why I said there is a basis for heterotypic immmunity at the level of VP4 and VP7.

Glass: Paul Offit, in your presentation, you didn't distinguish that one key feature of the epidemiology of rotavirus is the fact that newborns get asymptomatic infections. I would guess this might be mediated by maternal antibody and raises another mechanism of immunization. I am intrigued that the vaccine developed by Drs Ward and Bernstein, strain 89-12, which is a serotype 1 human strain, has caused diarrhoea in volunteers and is only partially attenuated. By giving the vaccine to infants under 3 months old, it may be maternal antibody that prevents any diarrhoea. What does this say about the role of IgG and maternal antibodies?

Offit: You are trying to distinguish, then, the maternal antibody that is passively transferred placentally from the maternal antibody which is passively transferred in milk. I think this is not a practical strategy for immunization in the USA, because disease occurs commonly in the 6–24 month old, a group not commonly breast-fed.

Glass: The strategy there is to give the natural Wa infection to children who are protected by maternal antibody transplacentally.

Offit: It would surprise me if that immunization strategy could induce the kind of protective response that would be important up to two years of age.

References

Burns JW, Siadat-Pajouh M, Krishnaney AA, Greenberg HB 1996 Protective effect of rotavirus VP6-specific IgA monoclonal antibodies that lack neutralizing activity. Science 272:104–107

Chen SC, Fynan EF, Robinson HL et al 1997 Protective immunity induced by rotavirus DNA vaccines. Vaccine 15:899–902

Chiba S, Yokoyama T, Nakata S et al 1986 Protective effect of naturally acquired homotypic and heterotypic rotavirus antibodies. Lancet 2:417–421

Ciarlet M, Crawford SE, Barone C et al 1998 Subunit rotavirus vaccine administered parenterally to rabbits induces active protective immunity. J Virol 72:9233–9246

Conner ME Crawford SE, Barone C, Estes MK 1993 Rotavirus vaccine administered parenterally induces protective immunity. J Virol 67:6633–6641

Coulson BS, Masendycz PJ 1990 Measurement of rotavirus neutralizing coproantibody in children by fluorescent focus reduction assay. J Clin Microbiol 28:1652–1654

Desselberger U 1998 Prospects of vaccines against rotaviruses. Rev Med Virol 8:43–52

Grimwood K, Lund JSC, Coulson BS, Hudson IL, Bishop RF, Barnes GL 1988 Comparison of serum and mucosal antibody responses following severe acute rotavirus gastroenteritis in young children. J Clin Microbiol 26:732–738

Herremans MPT, van Loon AM, Reimerink JHJ et al 1997 Presence of poliovirus-specific IgA in persons vaccinated with inactivated (IPV) poliovirus in The Netherlands. Clin Lab Diagn Immunol 4:499–503

Herremans T, Reimerink J, Buisman A, Kimman T, Koopmans M 1999 Induction of mucosal immunity by inactivated poliovirus vaccine (IPV) is dependent on previous mucosal contact with live virus. J Immunol 162:5011–5018.

Herrmann JE, Chen SC, Fynan EF et al 1996 Protection against rotavirus infections by DNA vaccination. J Infect Dis 174:S93–S97

Johansen K, Granqvist L, Karlen K, Stintzing G, Uhnoo I, Svensson L 1994 Serum IgA immune responses to individual rotavirus polypeptides in young children with rotavirus infection. Arch Virol 138:247–259

Mazanec MB, Kaetzel CS, Lamm ME, Fletcher D, Nedrud JG 1992 Intracellular neutralization of virus by immunoglobulin A antibodies. Proc Natl Acad Sci USA 89:6901–6905

O'Neal CM, Clements JD, Estes MK, Conner ME 1998 Rotavirus 2/6 viruslike particles administered intranasally with cholera toxin, *Escherichia coli* heat-labile toxin (LT), and LT-R192G induce protection from rotavirus challenge. J Virol 72:3390–3393

O'Neal CM, Harriman G, Conner ME 2000 Protection of the villus epithelial cells of the small intestine from rotavirus infection does not require immunoglobulin A. J Virol 74:4102–2109

O'Ryan M, Mamani N, Avendaño LF et al 1995 Serum anti-rotavirus isotype- and G type-specific antibodies and protection against infection in Chilean children. Poster presentation, 35th Interscience conference on Antimicrobial Agents and Chemotherapy, San Francsico, CA, October 1995

Richardson SC, Grimwood K, Bishop RF 1993 Analysis of homotypic and heterotypic serum immune responses to rotavirus proteins following primary rotavirus infection using the RIP technique. J Clin Microbiol 31:377–385

Ruggeri FM, Johansen K, Basile G, Kraehenbuhl J, Svensson L 1998 Antirotavirus immunoglobulin A neutralizes virus in vitro after transcytosis through epithelial cells and protects infant mice from diarrhea. J Virol 72:2708–2714

Saif LJ 1990 Comparative aspects of enteric viral infections. In: Saif LJ, Theil KW (eds) Viral diarrheas of man and animals. CRC Press, Boca Raton, FL p 9–31

Saif LJ, Ward LA, Rosen BI, To TL 1996 The gnotobiotic piglet as a model for studies of disease pathogenesis and immunity to human rotaviruses. Arch Virol Suppl 12:153–161

Velázquez FR, Matson DO, Calva JJ et al 1996 Rotavirus infection in infants as protection against subsequent infections. N Engl J Med 335:1022–1028

Ward LA, Yuan L, Rosen BI, To TL, Saif LJ 1996 Development of mucosal and systemic lymphoproliferative responses and protective immunity to human group A rotaviruses in a gnotobiotic pig model. Clin Diag Lab Immunol 3:342–350

Yuan L, Ward LA, To TL, Saif LJ 1996 Systemic and intestinal antibody-secreting cell responses and correlates of protective immunity to human rotavirus in a gnotobiotic pig model of disease. J Virol 70:3075–3083

Yuan L, Kang S-Y, Ward LA, To TL, Saif LJ 1998 Antibody-secreting cell responses and protective immunity assessed in gnotobiotic pigs inoculated orally or intramuscularly with inactivated human rotavirus. J Virol 72:330–338

Yuan L, Geyer A, Hodgins DC et al 2000 Intranasal administration of 2/6-rotavirus-like particles with mutant *Escherichia coli* heat-labile toxin (LT-R1 92G) induces antibody secreting cell responses but no protective immunity in gnotobiotic pigs. J Virol 74:8843–8853

Rotavirus epidemiology and surveillance

Ulrich Desselberger, Miren Iturriza-Gómara and Jim J. Gray

Clinical Microbiology and Public Health Laboratory, Addenbrooke's Hospital, Cambridge, CB2 2QW, UK

Abstract. There is extensive antigenic and genomic diversity among co-circulating human rotaviruses. They are differentiated into groups, subgroups and types. There are at least 7 groups (A–G) and 4 subgroups within group A. To distinguish types within group A, a dual classification system has been established with the glycoprotein VP7 defining G types, and the protease-sensitive protein VP4 defining P types. At least 14 G types and more than 20 P types have been distinguished, of which at least 10 G types and at least 11 P types have been found in humans. Using the typing system, the complex molecular epidemiology of rotaviruses was investigated. Rotaviruses of different G and P types co-circulate. The main types found are G1P1A[8], G2P1B[4], G3P1A[8], G4P1A[8]; their relative incidence rates change over time in any one location and are different at the same time between different locations. Viruses with G/P constellations such as G1P1B[4] and G2P1A[8] are mostly natural reassortants of the co-circulating main virus types emerging after double infection of hosts. Viruses carrying G and or P types not represented in the four most common types, e.g. G8P[8], G1P[6] or G9P[6], could be introduced into the population by reassortment with animal viruses, or directly from animals or exotic human sources. Naturally circulating rotaviruses constantly undergo point mutations which can be used to classify lineages and sublineages within types. The full significance of human infections with group B and C rotaviruses remains to be established. Surveillance of rotavirus types in different parts of the world is essential to monitor the emergence of new types or of new G/P constellations which may predominate over time. The efficacy and effectiveness of any future rotavirus vaccine may differ depending on the predominant natural strain types. Detailed epidemiological and molecular surveillance data should be utilized to study the transmission dynamics of rotaviruses.

2001 Gastroenteritis viruses. Wiley, Chichester (Novartis Foundation Symposium 238) p 125–152

Rotaviruses are the major aetiologic agent of acute gastroenteritis in infants and young children and in the young of many animals (Kapikian & Chanock 1996). In humans, rotavirus infections are associated with high morbidity across the world and high mortality in developing countries accounting for over 800 000 deaths per year, mostly in children under 5 years old (Bern et al 1992, Glass et al

1996). For this reason the epidemiology has been studied intensely (Haffejee 1995, Kapikian & Chanock 1996, Glass et al 1996, Gentsch et al 1996, Barnes et al 1998, Koopmans & Brown 1999, Iturriza-Gómara et al 2000a). The high disease burden by rotavirus infections in infants and children in many countries has also motivated major efforts to develop rotavirus vaccines (e.g. Rennels et al 1996, Pérez-Schael et al 1997, Joensuu et al 1997). In 1998 a rhesus rotavirus tetravalent (RRV-TV) human reassortant vaccine was licensed in the USA, but serious side effects discovered during the implementation of this vaccine (Anonymous 1999) have necessitated the withdrawal in October 1999 (see Kapikian 2001, this volume). Alternative rotavirus vaccine candidates are on the horizon, and therefore this temporary setback does not diminish the case for continuous surveillance of rotavirus strains in the community to prepare for future vaccine implementation.

Here we review epidemiological and surveillance studies of rotaviruses and aspects of their evolution on which the epidemiology is based.

Rotavirus classification

Genome structure, proteins, gene–protein assignments and replication have been reviewed (Estes 1996) and discussed in previous chapters (see this volume: Prasad et al 2001, Arias et al 2001, Patton 2001).

Several viral components have been used to classify and differentiate rotavirus isolates:

- The 11 segments of double-stranded RNA constituting the viral genome can be easily separated by PAGE, and the RNA migration patterns or profiles thus obtained have been used to differentiate strains.
- Epitopes on VP6, the middle layer (inner capsid) trimeric protein of rotavirus, encoded by RNA segment 6, determine group and subgroup specificity.
- The two proteins constituting the outer capsid layer, VP7 and VP4, encoded by RNA segments 9, 7 or 8 (depending on strain) and 4, respectively, carry epitopes which specify neutralizing antibody responses and thus determine serotypes: VP7-specific serotypes are also termed G types (G standing for *g*lycoprotein), and VP4-specific serotypes are termed P types (P standing for *p*rotease sensitive protein). This dual classification system (Estes 1996) is now firmly established.
- The genes coding for VP4 and VP7 have also been used for genotypic classification of strains. For G types, genotypes and serotypes have been fully reconciled whereas many P genotypes have not been assigned to a serotype. Thus, a rotavirus strain designation is as follows: A/human/Wa (G1P1A[8]) indicating a human isolate of group A designated Wa of G genotype/serotype 1, P serotype 1A and P genotype 8, etc.

These classification criteria have revealed an enormous diversity of rotavirus strains:

(a) By PAGE so-called 'long', 'short', 'ultrashort' and 'abnormal' RNA profiles have been found, designating the relative migration of RNA segments 10 and 11.

(b) Rotavirus groups A–E have been firmly differentiated (Pedley et al 1986), and groups F and G are likely to be additional groups (Bridger 1987). Within group A there are at least four subgroups (I, II, I+II, nonI–nonII; Greenberg et al 1983).

(c) There are at least 14 different VP7-specific G types and at least 20 different VP4-specific P types of which at least 10 G types and at least 11 P types have been found among human rotavirus isolates (Estes 1996, Hoshino & Kapikian 1996).

Epidemiology

In temperate climates rotavirus infections occur in strict seasonal peaks during late autumn/winter/spring (Brandt et al 1983, Haffejee 1995, Bishop 1996) whereas in subtropical and tropical regions rotavirus infections are more evenly spread (Cook et al 1990, Ahmed et al 1991). The winter/spring outbreaks in infants and young children are based on a strong endemicity of the virus. Spread from West to East during a season has been observed in the USA (Anonymous 1997) and in Europe (Koopmans & Brown 1999). Rotavirus infections of the most common types (see below) are most frequently seen in children under 2 years of age, are relatively rare in children above the age of 5 years and in adults, but can again cause outbreaks of diarrhoeal disease in the elderly (Kapikian & Chanock 1996). The fact that G and P specificity are encoded by different RNA segments (see above) and the observation that viruses of the same group are able to reassort readily in doubly infected cells has resulted in a large variety of different G/P combinations observed in natural isolates (Desselberger 1998).

Here we review the main epidemiological observations of recent years. These are mainly derived from RT-PCR-based typing as the most reliable differentiating procedure (Gouvea et al 1990, Gentsch et al 1992, 1996, Iturriza-Gómara et al 1999, 2000a). RNA PAGE and serotyping based on ELISA techniques were mainly used before 1994, and cogent observations will also be reported.

The degree of diversity of co-circulating rotavirus strains is remarkable in most areas where investigations have been made. Most of the human rotaviruses are of group A. However, group B rotaviruses have caused outbreaks of diarrhoea among adults (the ADRV [Adult Diarrhoea Rotavirus] being the type strain; Hung 1988, Krishnan et al 1999), and group C rotaviruses have been found to cause small diarrhoea outbreaks in families and to occur sporadically in children (Caul et al 1990, Jiang et al 1995).

Among the group A rotaviruses there is co-circulation of viruses of long and short electropherotypes, different subgroups and of various serotypes/genotypes. In the 1980s and early 1990s only four G types and no P types were distinguished (Table 1) leaving many rotaviruses partially typed or untyped. However, already large regional and temporal differences were seen (see references in Table 1).

With the ability to distinguish more G types and the P types, the situation became more complex but also clearer (Table 2 and references therein). In most temperate climates viruses of types G1P1A[8], G2P1B[4], G3P1A[8] and G4P1A[8] were found to constitute over 90% of the co-circulating strains, isolates of G1P1A[8] usually, but not always, being of the highest incidence. G2P[4] viruses are usually of subgroup I and 'short' electropherotype whereas G1P[8], G3P[8] and G4P[8] viruses are subgroup II and 'long' electropherotype viruses. Subgroup I viruses of long electropherotype are infrequently found in humans but frequently in animals (see below). However, in other regions of the world (Asia, Africa, South America) viruses of other G types in combination with various P types have been found, e.g. G5P[8] (Brazil), G8P[6] (Malawi), G9P[6] (Bangladesh, India), G9P[8] (USA, Europe) and G9P[11] (India). Alternatively, viruses with common G types and less common P types were also found to prevail, e.g. G1P[4] (Argentina), G1P[6] (India), G2P[6] (Guinea-Bissau), G3P[6] (Malawi) and G4P[6] (South Africa) (Table 2). Various more recent studies worldwide on human rotavirus genotypes allow us to detect a wide diversity of G/P combinations involving G1–G6 and G8–G10 and P[1] to P[4], P[6], P[8]-P[12] and P[14] (Table 3).

Thus, in many areas of the world the type composition of co-circulating rotavirus strains is extremely variable; changes occur quickly over time in the same site, and vast differences are recorded between sites at the same time.

Rotavirus evolution

What are the explanations for this enormous diversity? Rotaviruses evolve, in principle, by three different mechanisms: point mutations, reassortment and intramolecular recombination (rearrangement).

The point mutation rate of rotaviruses was measured *in vitro* and found to be approximately 5×10^{-5} per nucleotide site (Blackhall et al 1996), i.e. per replication of one genome (of approximately 18.55 kbp size) on average one mutation occurs. This mutation rate is in close agreement with that of other RNA viruses (Smith & Inglis 1987) and approximately 1000 times higher than point mutation rates in DNA viruses. Point mutations in particular positions can be spontaneous events (i.e. only being found once or twice in isolates), but can also

TABLE 1a Rotavirus G types detected in epidemiological surveys: Europe/Mediterranean

Country (city)	Time period	n^a	Rotavirus types detected (percentage)						Reference
			G1	G2	G3	G4	Mixed	Non-typable	
Italy (Pavia)	1981–88	468	68	0	0	12	1	19	Gerna et al, Scand J Infect Dis 1988; **22**: 5–10
Italy	1981–88	450	76	3	<1	10	1	9	Gerna et al, Scand J Infect Dis 1988; **22**: 5–10
'Europe'	1981–88	831	65	3	1	19	1	12	Gerna et al, Scand J Infect Dis 1988; **22**: 5–10
UK (Birmingham)	1983–88	353	54	20	16	9		2	Beards et al, J Clin Microbiol 1989; **27**: 2827–2833
UK (London, Birmingham)	1984–90	781	52	9	3	21	1	14	Noël et al, J Clin Microbiol 1991; **29**: 2213–2219
Finland	1986–87	106	87	4	4	3		3	Vesikari in: Farthing (ed.), Viruses and the Gut 1988; pp121–122, London
Estonia	1989–92	314	36	5	4	6		50	Ginevskaja et al, Arch Virol 1994; **137**: 199–207
Israel	1987	97	54	10	0	19		16	Woods et al, J Clin Microbiol 1992; **30**: 781–785
Hungary	1984–92	1215	81	4	1	5		8	Szücs et al, Arch Virol 1995; **140**: 1693–1703
France	1997–98	170	29	7	2	60		2	Gault et al, J Clin Microbiol 1999; **37**: 2373–2375
Spain (Madrid, Barcelona)	1996–97	322	68	0	2	29	1		Wilhelmi et al, Enferm Infecc Microbiol Clin 1999; **17**: 509–514

a Number of rotavirus-positive faeces investigated.

TABLE 1b Rotavirus G types detected in epidemiological surveys: North and Central America

Country (city)	Time period	n^a	Rotavirus types detected (percentage)						Reference
			G1	G2	G3	G4	Mixed	Non-typable	
USA (diverse cities)	1987–89	232	78	2	19	0			Gouvea et al, J Infect Dis 1990; **162**: 362–367
USA (Houston, Daycare)	1986–88	134	45	0	30	0		25	O'Ryan et al, J Infect Dis 1990; **162**: 810–816
USA (Houston, Hospital)	1979–89	517	44	4	36	10	3	2	Matson et al, J Infect Dis 1990; **162**: 605–614
USA (Ohio)	1981–89	420	82	3	8	4	2	1	Matson et al, J Infect Dis 1990; **162**: 605–614
USA (diverse cities)	1981–88	478	73	3	17	1		6	Woods et al, J Clin Microbiol 1992; **30**: 781–785
Mexico	1984–87	132	29	11	10	17		33	Padilla–Noriega et al, J Clin Microbiol 1990; **28**: 1114–1119
Mexico	1986–89	166	24	16	31	6		23	Woods et al, J Clin Microbiol 1992; **30**: 781–785

[a] Number of rotavirus-positive faeces investigated.

TABLE 1c   Rotavirus G types detected in epidemiological surveys: South America

Country (city)	Time period	n^a	Rotavirus types detected in percent					Non-typable	Reference
			G1	G2	G3	G4	Mixed		
Venezuela	1981–83	134	39	13	18	11		19	Flores et al, J Clin Microbiol 1988; **26**: 2092–2095
Brazil (São Paulo)	1982–94	94	24	7	28	7		32	Timenetsky et al, J Clin Microbiol 1994; **32**: 2622–2624

[a]Number of rotavirus-positive faeces investigated.

TABLE 1d   Rotavirus types detected in epidemiological surveys: Australia

Country (city)	Time period	n^a	Rotavirus types detected in percent					Non-typable	Reference
			G1	G2	G3	G4	Mixed		
Australia (Melbourne)	1973–89	943	53	5	2	11	2	27	Bishop et al, J Clin Microbiol 1991; **29**: 862–868

[a]Number of rotavirus-positive faeces investigated.

TABLE 1e Rotavirus types detected in epidemiological surveys: Africa

Country (city)	Time period	n[a]	Rotavirus types detected in percent						Reference
			G1	G2	G3	G4	Mixed	Non-typable	
Central African Republic	1983–85	178	57	12	11	ND[b]		20	Georges-Courbot et al, J Clin Microbiol 1988; **26**: 668–671

[a]Number of rotavirus-positive faeces investigated.
[b]Not done

TABLE 1f Rotavirus types detected in epidemiological surveys: Asia

Country (city)	Time Period	n[a]	Rotavirus types detected in percent						Reference
			G1	G2	G3	G4	Mixed	Non-typable	
Thailand	1987–88	211	27	43	0	1		28	Sethabutr et al, J Infect Dis 1990; **162**: 368–372
Bangladesh	1987–88	718	20	27	5	15		33	Bern et al, J Clin Microbiol 1992; **30**: 3234–3238
China	1982–86	80	47	29	14	0		10	Woods et al, J Clin Microbiol 1992; **30**: 781–785
Korea	1988	138	38	4	1	0		43	Woods et al, J Clin Microbiol 1992; **30**: 781–785
India (Bangalore)	1988–94	200	19	11	33	4		35	Aijaz et al, Arch Virol 1996; **141**: 715–726
Bangladesh	1987–92	2199	12	16	4	19		49	Unicomb et al, J Clin Microbiol 1999; **37**: 1885–1891

[a]Number of rotavirus-positive faeces investigated.

TABLE 2a Rotavirus G/P constellations detected in epidemiological surveys: Europe/Mediterranean

Country (city)	Time period	n^a	Rotavirus types detected in percent							Reference
			G1P[8]	G2P[4]	G3P[8]	G4P[8]	Others	Mixed	Non-typable	
Israel	1991–94	355[b]	52	6	1	28	G1P[9] 1		13	Silberstein et al, J Clin Microbiol 1995; **33**: 1421–1422
		432[c]	44	6	1	20	G3P[9] 3		26	
Italy (Palermo)	1990–94	108	38	2	1	52	G9P[8] 3 G1P[4] 2 G1P[6] 1 G4P[6] 1		1	Arista et al, Arch Virol 1997; **42**: 2065–2071
Ireland (diverse cities)	1996–98	158	65	18	<1	12			4	O'Mahoney et al, J Clin Microbiol 1999; **37**: 1699–1703
UK (diverse cities)	1995–98	3303	65	10	3	5	G1P[4] 1 G9P[6] 1 G9P[8] 2 G2P[8] <1 G3P[6] <1 G4P[4] <1	2	10	Iturriza-Gómara et al, J Clin Microbiol 2000; **38**: 4394–4401

[a] Number of rotavirus-positive faeces investigated.
[b] From children admitted to hospital.
[c] From children attending outpatient departments.

TABLE 2b   Rotavirus G/P constellations detected in epidemiological surveys: North & Central America

Country (city)	Time period	n[a]	G1P[8]	G2P[4]	G3P[8]	G4P[8]	Others	Mixed	Non-typable	Reference
			— Rotavirus types detected in percent							
USA	1990–92	171	71	2	20	2	G1P[6] 1 G2P[6] 1	3	0	Santos et al, J Clin Microbiol 1994; **32**: 205–208
USA	1996–97	348	66	8	7	1	G9P[6] 6 G9P[8] 2 G1P[6] 1		8	Ramachandran et al, J Clin Microbiol 1988; **36**: 3223–3229

[a] Number of rotavirus-positive faeces investigated.

TABLE 2c   Rotavirus G/P constellations detected in epidemiological surveys: South America

Country (city)	Time period	n[a]	G1P[8]	G2P[4]	G3P[8]	G4P[8]	Others	Mixed	Non-typable	Reference
			— Rotavirus types detected in percent							
Brazil (diverse cities)	1982–94	130	43	12	6	6	G5P[8] 9 G2P[8] 1 G4P[6] 1 G3P[9] 2		21	Leite et al, Arch Virol 1996; **141**: 2365–2374
Argentina (Buenos Aires)	1996–98	310	12	43	0	4	G1P[4] 14	10	17	Arguëlles et al, J Clin Microbiol 2000; **38**: 252–259

[a] Number of rotavirus-positive faeces investigated.

TABLE 2d   Rotavirus G/P constellations detected in epidemiological surveys: Africa

Country (city)	Time period	n^a	G1P[8]	G2P[4]	G3P[4]	G3P[8]	G4P[8]	Others	Mixed	Non-typable	Reference
South Africa (diverse cities)	1988–89	377	57	22		<1	11	G4P[6] 10 G3P[9] 1 G1P[6] <1			Steele et al, J Clin Microbiol 1995; **33**: 1516–1519
Kenya	1991–94	317	24[b]	17[b]		1	42[b]	G8P[4] 2		15	Nakata et al, J Med Virol 1999; **58**: 291–303
Malawi (Blantyre)	1997–98	100	0	0		20	2	G8P[6] 42 G8P[4] 9 G3P[6] 10 G9P[6] 3 G4P[6] 2 G3P[4] 1	1	9	Cunliffe et al, J Med Virol 1999; **37**: 308–312
Guinea-Bissau	1996–98	167	8	11			4	G2P[6] 24 G1P[6] 2 G8P[2] 1 G3P[6] 1 G3P[9] 1 G4P[9] 1	4	48[c]	Kolsen–Fischer et al, J Clin Microbiol 2000; **38**: 264–267

[a]Number of rotavirus-positive faeces investigated.
[b]P types not determined in many cases.
[c]Of those 67 percent were partially typable (G or P).

TABLE 2e Rotavirus G/P constellations detected in epidemiological surveys: Asia

Country (city)	Time period	n^a	Rotavirus types detected in percent					Mixed	Non-typable	Reference
			G1P[8]	G2P[4]	G3P[8]	G4P[8]	Others			
India (New Delhi)	1986–88 1992–93	75	0	1	0	0	G9P[11]70 G9P[6]13 G3P[11]3	2	11	Das et al, J Clin Microbiol 1994; **32**: 1820–1822
India	1993	63	1	21	8	3	G9P[6]24 G1P[6]10 G2P[6]2 G3P[6]3 G4P[6]5	11	11	Ramachandran et al, J Clin Microbiol 1996; **34**: 436–439
China	1994–95	289	41	18	8	0	G1P[4]1 G3P[4]	7	23	Wu et al, J Med Virol 1998; **55**: 168–176
Bangladesh	1993–97	333	11	11	0	26	G1P[4,6, other] G2P[6,8, other] G3P[4,6, other] G9P[6,8, other]	6 10 11 17	8	Unicomb et al, J Clin Microbiol 1999; **37**: 1885–1891

^{a} Number of rotavirus-positive faeces investigated.

TABLE 3 G/P combinations of human rotaviruses

P Type	G Type													
	G1	G2	G3	G4	G5	G6	G7	G8	G9	G10	G11	G12	G13	G14
P1	+													
P2								+						
P3			+											
P4	+[g]	**+**	+	+				+				+		
P5														
P6	+[c]	+[b]	+	+[i]				+[a]	+[d,f]					
P7														
P8	**+**	+	**+**	**+**	+[h]				+[f]					
P9	+		+	+										
P10			+	+				+						
P11			+						+[c]	+				
P12		+												
P13														
P14						+		+		+				

From data of Table 2 of this paper, Estes (1996; Tables 2 and 3) and Hoshino & Kapikian (1996, Table 3).
The generally highest incidences are in bold.

[a] High incidence in Malawi.
[b] High incidence in Guinea Bissau.
[c] High incidence in India.
[d] High incidence in India.
[e] High incidence in India.
[f] High incidence in Bangladesh.
[g] High incidence in Argentina.
[h] High incidence in Brazil.

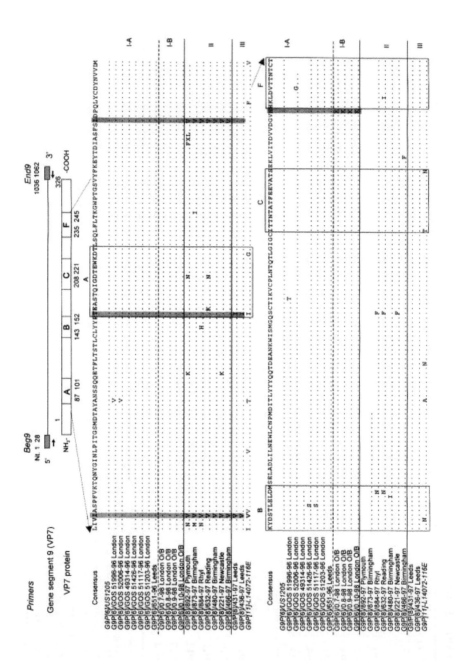

be 'fixed' and be accumulated over time, then serving to differentiate lineages and sublineages within types (Maunula & von Bonsdorff 1998, Iturriza-Gómara et al 2000b; Fig. 1).

Genome reassortment, occurring readily *in vitro* after double infection of cells with different strains of group A rotaviruses, has been widely used for gene–protein assignments and also gene function assignments (for review see Ramig 1997, Desselberger 2001). The comparison of natural isolates has provided ample evidence that reassortment occurs *in vivo* (Browning et al 1992, Cunliffe et al 1999, Santos et al 1999, Zao et al 1999, Unicomb et al 1999).

Intramolecular recombination (rearrangement) has been shown to occur both *in vivo* and *in vitro* and to contribute to genomic and also protein variation (for review see Desselberger 1996, Ramig 1997).

In our collection of over 3000 fully genotyped rotavirus isolates obtained in the UK between 1995/96 and 1997/98, the four most common genotypes constituted 94.7% (Table 4; Iturriza-Gómara et al 2000a). Among the uncommon genotypes there were 47 (1.5%) of types G1P[4] ($n=33$), G2P[8] ($n=9$), and G4P[4] ($n=5$); for some of those (the G1P[4] strains) there is now evidence that they are natural reassortants emerging as progeny from the most frequent co-circulating strains (Fig. 2; Iturriza-Gómara et al 2001). Similar possible intra-human strain reassortment events are likely to have occurred elsewhere (Table 2; Arista et al 1997, Wu et al 1998, Unicomb et al 1999, Argüelles et al 2000). In addition, there were 18 isolates carrying the human VP7 protein G1, G3 or G4, but the unusual VP4 proteins P[6] and P[9], the origin of which is still under investigation.

G9 rotaviruses

Human G9 rotavirus strains were first detected in the USA in 1983 and then a decade later in the USA and Bangladesh as epidemic strains (Ramachandran et al 1998, Unicomb et al 1999). They were first detected in the UK in 1995/96, carrying a P[6] VP4 (Table 4; Iturriza-Gómara et al 2000c, Cubitt et al 2000). Those strains decreased in incidence towards 1997/98 but seemed to be replaced by G9P[8] strains. It is likely that the P[8] gene has been picked up by natural reassortment with the co-circulating G1P[8], G3P[8] and G4P[8] strains (Unicomb et al 1999, Iturriza-Gómara et al 2000a,c, 2001).

FIG. 1. Schematic representation of the VP7 gene and protein (indicating sequencing primer positions and antigenic sites), and alignment of the deduced amino acid sequences from position 40–245. Substitutions differing from the consensus are indicated, lineage and sub-lineage defining amino acid substitutions are highlighted. Antigenic regions A, B, C and F are boxed. (From Iturriza-Gómara et al 2000c, with permission).

TABLE 4   G/P genotype combinations of rotavirus strains collected in the UK, 1995–98

Type by RT-PCR	Number	Percentage[a]
Common:		
G1P[8]	2156	74.0
G2P[4]	326	11.2
G3P[8]	95	3.3
G4P[8]	181	6.2
Subtotal	2758	94.7
Uncommon:		
G1P[4]	33	1.1
G2P[8]	9	0.3
G4P[4]	5	0.2
Others[b]	20	0.7
Subtotal	67	2.3
G9P[6]	26	0.9
G9P[8]	61	2.1
Subtotal	87	3.0

[a]Of those typed.
[b]G1P[6], 2; G1P[9], 3; G3P[6], 11; G3P[9], 1; G4P[6], 1; G8P[8], 2.
Data from Iturriza-Gómara et al (2000a).

Animal rotaviruses

The diversity of co-circulating rotaviruses in any one region is mainly driven by a constant sequence of point mutations and reassortment events (see above). A further mechanism to explain the great variability of human isolates is the possible transmission to humans of animal rotaviruses, either as whole viruses (Das et al 1993) or by contributing individual genes in a reassortant event

---

FIG. 2.   Phylogenetic tree constructed from nt sequences of the VP7 gene (nt 417–784) of the rotavirus strains G1P[8] and possible reassortants G1P[4] using *Clustal* and Neighbour Joining methods. Laboratory number, rotavirus season, G/P combination and geographical origin of the strains are indicated. Prototype strains KU and Wa were included (GenBank accession numbers D16343 and K02033, respectively). VP7 sequences derived from G1P[4] strains are underlined. Bootstrap values are indicated in the dendrogram (from Iturriza-Gómara et al 2001, with permission).

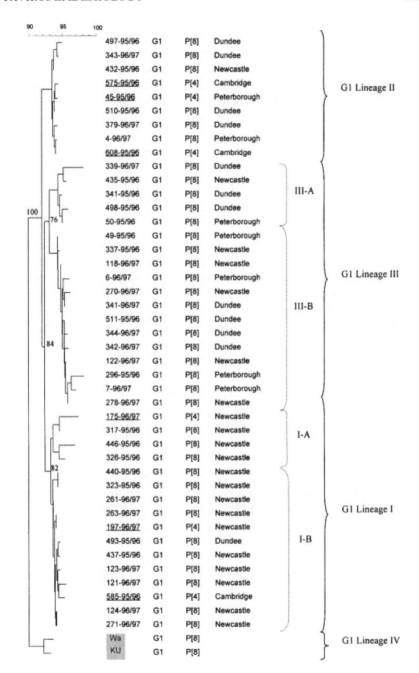

90	95	100				
			497-95/96	G1	P[8]	Dundee
			343-96/97	G1	P[8]	Dundee
			432-95/96	G1	P[8]	Newcastle
			575-95/96	G1	P[4]	Cambridge
			45-95/96	G1	P[4]	Peterborough
			510-95/96	G1	P[8]	Dundee
			379-96/97	G1	P[8]	Dundee
			4-96/97	G1	P[8]	Peterborough
			608-95/96	G1	P[4]	Cambridge
			339-96/97	G1	P[8]	Dundee
			435-95/96	G1	P[8]	Newcastle
			341-95/96	G1	P[8]	Dundee
			498-95/96	G1	P[8]	Dundee
			50-95/96	G1	P[8]	Peterborough
			49-95/96	G1	P[8]	Peterborough
			337-95/96	G1	P[8]	Newcastle
			118-96/97	G1	P[8]	Newcastle
			6-96/97	G1	P[8]	Peterborough
			270-96/97	G1	P[8]	Newcastle
			341-96/97	G1	P[8]	Dundee
			511-95/96	G1	P[8]	Dundee
			344-96/97	G1	P[8]	Dundee
			342-96/97	G1	P[8]	Dundee
			122-96/97	G1	P[8]	Newcastle
			296-95/96	G1	P[8]	Peterborough
			7-96/97	G1	P[8]	Peterborough
			278-96/97	G1	P[8]	Newcastle
			175-96/97	G1	P[4]	Newcastle
			317-95/96	G1	P[8]	Newcastle
			446-95/96	G1	P[8]	Newcastle
			326-95/96	G1	P[8]	Newcastle
			440-95/96	G1	P[8]	Newcastle
			323-95/96	G1	P[8]	Newcastle
			261-96/97	G1	P[8]	Newcastle
			263-96/97	G1	P[8]	Newcastle
			197-96/97	G1	P[4]	Newcastle
			493-95/96	G1	P[8]	Dundee
			437-95/96	G1	P[8]	Newcastle
			123-96/97	G1	P[8]	Newcastle
			121-96/97	G1	P[8]	Newcastle
			585-95/96	G1	P[4]	Cambridge
			124-96/97	G1	P[8]	Newcastle
			271-96/97	G1	P[8]	Newcastle
			Wa	G1	P[8]	
			KU	G1	P[8]	

G1 Lineage II

III-A

III-B

G1 Lineage III

I-A

I-B

G1 Lineage I

G1 Lineage IV

(Gentsch et al 1993). Rotaviruses are ubiquitous, with many more G and P types found in animals than in humans. This is reminiscent of the situation encountered with influenza viruses, where only three out of the 15 haemagglutinin subtypes and two of the nine neuraminidase subtypes known cause the vast majority of human infections (Murphy & Webster 1996). Table 5 lists rotavirus G and P types that are found in humans but also commonly in animals. In some cases the genetic relatedness determined through nucleotide sequencing has made the origin of human isolates from an animal source very likely (Browning et al 1992, Gentsch et al 1993, Santos et al 1999). We are still very much at the beginning of exploring this area as the surveillance and characterization of animal rotaviruses is not of the same scale as that of human rotaviruses.

Surveillance

On the basis of the observation that co-circulating rotaviruses show a great degree of diversity and that apparently animal strains can contribute to the gene pool of strains circulating in man, a continuous surveillance of human but also animal rotaviruses including genotyping seems to be vital at various stages of testing of rotavirus candidate vaccines and of implementation of licensed vaccines (Kapikian 2001, this volume). The vaccine candidates in the past, among them the RRV-TV human reassortant vaccine, were tailored to elicit immune responses of relevance with regard to the most frequently co-circulating human strains. Although there is evidence both from natural infections (Velasquez et al 1996) and vaccine studies (e.g. Rennels et al 1996) that infection/vaccination with single strains can elicit cross-reactive immune responses sufficient to prevent severe disease after infection with heterologous rotavirus strains, the true correlates of protection and cross-protection are far from being fully identified (see Offit 2001, this volume).

The epidemiological characteristics of the recent introduction of G9 strains in various populations may suggest that pre-existing rotavirus immunity was insufficient to prevent infection and spreading of these strains (Cubitt et al 2000, Koopmans 2000, Iturriza-Gómara et al 2000a,c). Therefore, as in influenza vaccinology, rotavirus vaccines used in widely different areas of the world may need constant tailoring to adapt their composition to that of locally or regionally most prevalent and co-circulating type strains. Again, like in influenza surveillance, it now seems to be of paramount importance to include the characterization of animal rotaviruses, particularly of domestic animals and pets.

Transmission dynamics

Although some of the genetic mechanisms underlying rotavirus diversity are known, the transmission dynamics of rotaviruses effecting this diversity in

TABLE 5   G and P types of human rotavirus strains commonly found in animal rotavirus strains

Type	Animal Source	References
G3	Cats, dogs, monkeys	Nakagomi et al 1989; *Arch. Virol.* **106**: 145–150 Mochizuki et al 1997; *J. Clin. Microbiol.* **35**: 1272–1275
G5	Pigs, horses	Gouvea & Santos 1999; *Vaccine* **17**: 1291–1292 Santos et al 1999; *J. Clin. Microbiol.* **37**: 2734–2736
G6	Calves	Snodgrass et al 1990; *J. Clin. Microbiol.* **28**: 504–507 Gerna et al 1992; *J. Clin. Microbiol.* **30**: 9–16 Palombo & Bishop 1995; *J. Med. Virol.* **47**: 348–354 Gulati et al 1999; *J. Clin. Microbiol.* **37**: 2074–2076
G8	Calves	Adah et al 1997; *Arch Virol.* **142**: 1881–1887 Santos et al 1998; *J. Clin. Microbiol.* **36**: 2727–2729 Cunliffe et al 1999; *J. Med. Virol.* **57**: 308–318 Steele et al 1999; *J. Gen. Virol.* **80**: 3029–3034 Palombo et al 2000; *J. Med. Virol.* **60**: 56–62
G9	Lambs, pigs	Das et al 1993; *Virology* **197**: 99–107 Fitzgerald et al 1995; *Arch. Virol.* **140**: 1541–1548 Ramachandran et al 1996; *J. Clin. Microbiol.* **34**: 436–439 Ramachandran et al 1998; *J. Clin. Microbiol.* **36**: 3223–3229 Santos et al 1999; *J. Clin. Microbiol.* **37**: 2734–2736
G10	Calves	Snodgrass et al 1990; *J. Clin. Microbiol.* **28**: 504–507 Beards et al 1992; *J. Clin. Microbiol.* **30**: 1432–1435 Santos et al 1998; *J. Clin. Microbiol.* **36**: 2727–2729 Gulati et al 1999; *J. Clin. Microbiol.* **37**: 2074–2076
P[6]	Pigs	Leite et al 1996; *Arch. Virol.* **141**: 2365–2374 Ramachandran et al 1996; *J. Clin. Microbiol.* **34**: 436–439 Arista et al 1997; *Arch. Virol.* **142**: 2065–2071 Ramachandran et al 1998; *J. Clin. Microbiol.* **36**: 3223–3229 Cunliffe et al 1999; *J. Med. Virol.* **57**: 308–312 Cubitt et al 2000; *J. Med. Virol.* **61**: 150–154 Fischer et al 2000; *J. Clin. Microbiol.* **38**: 264–267 Racz et al 2000; *J. Clin. Microbiol.* **38**: 2443–2446
P[9]	Cats	Mochizuki et al 1997; *J. Clin. Microbiol.* **35**: 1272–1275
P[11]	Calves, horses	Gentsch et al 1993; *Virology* **194**: 424–430 Gulati et al 1999; *J. Clin. Microbiol.* **37**: 2074–2076
P[14]	Pigs, rabbits	Huang et al 1993; *Virology* **196**: 319–327 Ciarlet et al 1997; *Arch. Virol.* **142**: 1059–1069 Arista et al 1999; *J. Clin. Microbiol.* **37**: 2706–2708
P[19]	Pigs	Okada et al 2000; *J. Med. Virol.* **60**: 63–69

populations are much less so. Their description will require knowledge of a number of parameters: annual human birthrate in area of study; duration of presence of maternal antibodies after birth; age-related susceptibility and prevalence of specific antibodies, specified by G and P type; age-related incidence of rotavirus infections; transmission effectiveness; reduction of susceptibility in non-primary infections; and significance of animal reservoirs (Desselberger & Estes 2000). On the other hand, modern techniques of phylogenetic analysis of cognate sequences of an appropriate sample will allow characterization of some of the factors determining the spread of rotaviruses (Page & Holmes 1998, E. Holmes, personal communication). Much more work will have to be done to be able to establish an accurate model of the epidemiology and transmission dynamics of rotaviruses.

Conclusion

The detailed analysis of rotavirus isolates obtained throughout the world has on the one hand revealed the enormous diversity of co-circulating rotavirus strains and also taught us about some of the driving forces behind their diversity (point mutations, reassortment and animal reservoirs). On the other hand, the strain characterization has demonstrated that the complexity of rotavirus epidemiology is far from being understood. Rotavirus surveillance comprising human and animal strains will be necessary to evaluate the efficacy of rotavirus candidate vaccines in different settings.

Acknowledgements

The authors gratefully acknowledge the support by Mrs Lynne Bastow in typing of the manuscript. Relevant work from authors' laboratory was supported by a grant of the Public Health Laboratory Service, London.

References

[References cited only in the tables are not in this list.]

Ahmed MU, Urasawa S, Taniguchi K et al 1991 Analysis of human rotavirus strains prevailing in Bangladesh in relation to nationwide floods brought by the 1988 monsoon. J Clin Microbiol 29:2273–2279

Anonymous 1997 Laboratory-based surveillance for rotavirus — United States, July 1996–June 1997. Morb Mort Wkly Rep 46:1092–1094

Anonymous 1999 Intussusception among recipients of rotavirus vaccine — United States, 1998–1999. Morb Mort Wkly Rep 48:577–581

Arguëlles MH, Villegas GA, Castello A et al 2000 VP7 and VP4 genotyping of human group A rotavirus in Buenos Aires, Argentina. J Clin Microbiol 38:252–259

Arias CF, Guerrero CA, Méndez E et al 2001 Early events of rotavirus infection: the search for the receptor(s). In: Gastroenteritis viruses. Wiley, Chichester (Novartis Found Symp 238) p 47–63

Arista S, Vizzi E, Ferraro D, Cascio A, Di Stefano R 1997 Distribution of VP7 serotypes and VP4 genotypes among rotavirus strains recovered from Italian children with diarrhea. Arch Virol 142:2065–2071

Barnes GL, Uren E, Stevens KB, Bishop RF 1998 Etiology of acute gastroenteritis in hospitalized children in Melbourne, Australia, from April 1980 to March 1993. J Clin Microbiol 36:133–138

Bern C, Martines J, de Zoysa I, Glass RI 1992 The magnitude of the global problem of diarrhoeal disease: a ten-year update. Bull World Health Organ 70:705–714

Bishop RF 1996 Natural history of human rotavirus infection. Arch Virol Suppl 12:119–128

Blackhall J, Fuentes A, Magnesson G 1996 Genetic stability of a porcine rotavirus RNA segment during repeated plaque isolation. Virology 225:181–190

Brandt CD, Kim HW, Rodriquez WJ et al 1983 Pediatric viral gastroenteritis during eight years of study. J Clin Microbiol 18:71–78

Bridger JC 1987 Novel rotaviruses in animals and man. In: Novel diarrhoea viruses. Wiley, Chichester (Ciba Found Symp 128) p 5–23

Browning GF, Snodgrass DR, Nakagomi O, Kaga E, Sarasini A, Gerna G 1992 Human and bovine serotype G8 rotaviruses may be derived by reassortment. Arch Virol 125:121–128

Caul EO, Ashley CR, Danville JM, Bridger JC 1990 Group C rotavirus associated with fatal enteritis in a family outbreak. J Med Virol 30:201–205

Cook SM, Glass RI, LeBaron CW, Ho MS 1990 Global seasonality of rotavirus infections. Bull World Health Organ 68:171–177

Cubitt WD, Steele AD, Iturriza-Gómara M 2000 Characterisation of rotaviruses from children treated at a London hospital during 1996. Emergence of strains G9P2A[6] and G3P2A[6]. J Med Virol 61:150–154

Cunliffe NA, Gondwe JS, Broadhead RL et al 1999 Rotavirus G and P types in children with acute diarrhea in Blantyre, Malawi, from 1997 to 1998: predominance of novel P[6]G8 strains. J Med Virol 57:308–312

Das BK, Gentsch JR, Hoshino Y et al 1993 Characterization of the G serotype and genogroup of New Delhi newborn rotavirus 116E. Virology 197:99–107

Desselberger U 1996 Genome rearrangements of rotaviruses. Adv Virus Res 46:69–95

Desselberger U 1998 Reoviruses. In: Mahy BWJ, Collier L (eds) Topley and Wilson's microbiology and microbial infections, 9th edn, vol 1: Virology. Arnold, London, p 537–550

Desselberger U 2001 Rotaviruses: Génétique et virulence. In: Pothier P, Garbarg-Chenon A, Cohen J (eds). Gastroentérétis virales. Elsevier Science Publishers, Amsterdam

Desselberger U, Estes MK 2000 Future rotavirus research. In: Gray JJ, Desselberger U (eds), Rotaviruses: methods and protocols. Humana Press, Totowa, NJ, p 239–258

Estes M 1996 Rotaviruses and their replication. In: Fields BN, Knipe DM, Howley PM et al (eds), Fields Virology, 3rd edn. Lippincott-Raven, Philadelphia, PA, p 1625–1655

Gentsch JR, Glass RI, Woods P et al 1992 Identification of group A rotavirus gene 4 types by polymerase chain reaction. J Clin Microbiol 30:1365–1373

Gentsch JR, Das BK, Jiang B, Bhan MK, Glass RI 1993 Similarity of the VP4 protein of human rotavirus strain 116E to that of the bovine B223 strain. Virology 194:424–430

Gentsch JR, Woods PA, Ramachandran M et al 1996 Review of G and P typing results from a global collection of rotavirus strains: implications for vaccine development. J Infect Dis 174:S30–S36

Glass RI, Kilgore PE, Holman RC et al 1996 The epidemiology of rotavirus diarrhea in the United States: surveillance and estimates of disease burden. J Infect Dis 174:S5–S11

Gouvea V, Glass RI, Woods P et al 1990 Polymerase chain reaction amplification and typing of rotavirus nucleic acid from stool specimens. J Clin Microbiol 28:276–282

Greenberg HB, McAuliffe V, Valdesuso J et al 1983 Serological analysis of the subgroup protein of rotavirus, using monoclonal antibodies. Infect Immun 39:91–99

Haffejee IE 1995 The epidemiology of rotavirus infections: a global perspective. J Pediatr Gastroenterol Nutr 20:275–286

Hoshino Y, Kapikian AZ 1996 Classification of rotavirus VP4 and VP7 serotypes. Arch Virol Suppl 12:99–111

Hung T 1988 Rotavirus and adult diarrhoea. Adv Virus Res 35:193–218

Iturriza-Gómara M, Green J, Brown DW, Desselberger U, Gray JJ 1999 Comparison of specific and random priming in the reverse transcriptase polymerase chain reaction of genotyping group A rotaviruses. J Virol Methods 78:93–103

Iturriza-Gómara M, Green J, Brown DWG, Ramsay M, Desselberger U, Gray JJ 2000a Molecular epidemiology of human group A rotavirus infections in the United Kingdom between 1995 and 1998. J Clin Microbiol 38:4394–4401

Iturriza-Gómara M, Green J, Brown DWG, Desselberger U, Gray JJ 2000b Diversity within the VP4 gene of rotavirus P[8] strains: implications for reverse transcription-PCR genotyping. J Clin Microbiol 38:898–901

Iturriza-Gómara M, Cubitt D, Steele D et al 2000c Characterization of rotavirus G9 strains isolated in the UK between 1995 and 1998. J Med Virol 61:510–517

Iturriza-Gómara M, Isherwood B, Desselberger U, Gray JJ 2001 Reassortment in vivo: a driving force for diversity of human rotavirus strains isolated in the UK between 1995 and 1999. J Virol, in press

Jiang B, Dennehy PH, Spangenberger S, Gentsch JR, Glass RI 1995 First detection of group C rotavirus in fecal specimens of children with diarrhea in the United States. J Infect Dis 172: 45–50

Joensuu J, Koskenniemi E, Pang XL, Vesikari T 1997 Randomised, placebo-controlled trial of rhesus-human reassortant rotavirus vaccine for prevention of severe rotavirus gastroenteritis. Lancet 350:1205–1209

Kapikian AZ, Chanock RM 1996 Rotaviruses. In: Fields BN, Knipe DM, Howley PM et al (eds) Fields virology, 3rd edn. Lippincott-Raven, Philadelphia, PA, p 1657–1708

Kapikian AZ 2001 A rotavirus vaccine for prevention of severe diarrhoeal of infants and young children: development, utilization and withdrawal. In: Gastroenteritis viruses. Wiley, Chichester (Novartis Found Symp 238) p 153–179

Koopmans M 2000 Rotavirus G9P[6] in the Netherlands: Eurosurveillance Weekly, ProMED 200000107124931.

Koopmans M, Brown D 1999 The seasonality and diversity of group A rotaviruses in Europe. Acta Paediatr Suppl 88:14–19

Krishnan T, Sen A, Choudhury JS, Das S, Naik TN, Bhattacharya SK 1999 Emergence of adult diarrhoea rotavirus in Calcutta, India. Lancet 353:380–381

Maunula L, von Bonsdorff CH 1998 Short sequences define genetic lineages: phylogenetic analysis of group A rotaviruses based on partial sequences of genome segments 4 and 9. J Gen Virol 79:321–332

Murphy BR, Webster RG 1996 Orthomyxoviruses. In: Fields BN, Knipe DM, Howley PM et al (eds) Fields virology, 3rd edn. Lippincott Raven, Philadelphia, PA, p 1397–1445

Offit PA 2001 Correlates of protection against rotavirus infection and disease. In: Gastroenteritis viruses. Wiley, Chichester (Novartis Found Symp 238) p 106–124

Page RDM, Holmes EC 1998 Molecular evolution. A phylogenetic approach. Blackwell Science, Oxford

Patton JT 2001 Rotavirus RNA replication and gene expression. In: Gastroenteritis viruses. Wiley, Chichester (Novartis Found Symp 238) p 64–81

Pedley S, Bridger JC, Chasey D, McCrae MA 1986 Definition of two new groups of atypical rotaviruses. J Gen Virol 67:131–137

Pérez-Schael I, Guntiñas MJ, Pérez M et al 1997 Efficacy of the rhesus rotavirus-based quadrivalent vaccine in infants and young children in Venezuela. N Engl J Med 337:1181–1187 (erratum: 1998 N Engl J Med 338:1002)

Prasad BVV, Crawford S, Lawton JA, Pesavento J, Hardy M, Estes MK 2001 Structural studies on gastroenteritis viruses. In: Gastroenteritis viruses. Wiley, Chichester (Novartis Found Symp 238) p 26–46

Ramachandran M, Gentsch JR, Parashar UD et al 1998 Detection and characterization of novel rotavirus strains in the United States. J Clin Microbiol 36:3223–3229 (erratum: 1999 J Clin Microbiol 37:2392)

Ramig RF 1997 Genetics of the rotaviruses. Annu Rev Microbiol 51:225–255

Rennels MB, Glass RI, Dennehy PH et al 1996 Safety and efficacy of high dose rhesus-human reassortant rotavirus vaccines — report of the national multicenter trial. United States rotavirus vaccine efficacy group. Pediatrics 97:7–13

Santos N, Lima R, Nozawa C, Linhares R, Gouvea V 1999 Detection of porcine rotavirus type G9 and a mixture of types G1 and G5 associated with Wa-like VP4 specificity: evidence for natural human-porcine genetic reassortment. J Clin Microbiol 37:2734–2736

Smith DB, Inglis SC 1987 The mutation rate and variability of eukaryotic viruses: an analytical review. J Gen Virol 68:2729–2740

Unicomb LE, Podder G, Gentsch JR et al 1999 Evidence of high frequency genomic reassortment of group A rotavirus strains in Bangladesh: emergence of G9 strains in 1995. J Clin Microbiol 37:1885–1891

Velazquez FR, Matson DO, Calva JJ et al 1996 Rotavirus infections in infants as protection against subsequent infections. N Engl J Med 335:1022–1028

Wu H, Taniguchi K, Urasawa T, Urasawa S 1998 Serological and genomic characterization of human rotaviruses detected in China. J Med Virol 55:168–176

Zao CL, Yu WN, Kao CL, Taniguchi K, Lee CY, Lee CN 1999 Sequence analysis of VP1 and VP7 genes suggest occurrence of a reassortant G2 rotavirus responsible for an epidemic of gastroenteritis. J Gen Virol 80:1407–1415

DISCUSSION

Estes: Could you clarify what you mean by lineages?

Desselberger: The term 'lineage' is an arbitrary one. People sequence a number of G types, for example, and then try to place them in phylogenetic trees. Some of the amino acid residues are conserved in certain subsections of such a tree, and viruses of that tree are said to form a lineage. Only a few amino acids may determine a lineage. I think lineages have meaning when you look at these strains in a close-up epidemiological context. Certain lineages or, for that matter sublineages thereof, identify strains that may be taken from an outbreak, but also some unconnected strains. These genetic relationships may teach us how these strains have possibly migrated and how long this has taken.

Bishop: Lineages can have antigenic respectability, since G1 lineages can be correlated with reactivities using anti-VP7 G1 neutralizing monoclonal antibodies (Diwakala & Palombo 1999).

Desselberger: Not always. In some of the lineages I showed here, most of the lineage-determining amino acids were outside the antigenically relevant domains.

Glass: It is interesting to see how all this diversity has come into this field in the last couple of years, especially with the G9 strains. When we started with our studies in India, it was unusual to find G9 strains. In fact, in India, G9 strains now represent about 40% of rotavirus strains. G9 has to be considered one of the world's most common strains: among the top four. In the USA, we started with the G9P[6] strains, then as we looked further we found both lineages. When we compared the sequences of the US G9 strains to other strains, the US lineage by sequence is much closer to Malawian strains that we have examined and less closely related to Indian strains. When G9 strains appeared, we worried that this new serotype might cause disease of increased severity in older children who were not previously exposed or immune to this serotype. We found no such evidence, but we will be going back to revisit this issue. You started out showing the PAGE difference in the subgroups. As you have looked at this diversity, have you found evidence for other reassortment combinations? Unicomb et al (1999) found that in the G9 strains from Bangladesh that she had all different subgroups and electropherotypes as well as P types. These G9s are particularly promiscuous, just like the P[6] strains, and they mix with many other genes.

Desselberger: P[6] genes are found frequently in animal strains. I have taken on board what was said yesterday: better proof that animal strains contribute to human infection and disease has to be obtained. There are many data, but they are not systematic in the epidemiological context. You mentioned the situation in Bangladesh. This is an ideal situation to study, because you find almost every G/P combination. There is a paper from Bangladesh by Ahmed et al (1991) in which they reported high numbers of mixed electropherotypes over a monsoon season. In the peak month of the monsoon season, 30% of their isolates were mixed infections. In the UK, we found mixed infections very infrequently; in Bangladesh they are much more common.

Glass: In your unusual strains, do you have any that come from immigrants from places such as India, or people with animals who might have animal strains, or recent travellers?

Desselberger: We haven't looked at this yet in detail.

Greenberg: You just have to walk around in London to realize that there is a tremendous degree of communication and interaction between India and England. At the same time, the G types in England are pretty much what we have seen in the USA for the last 30 years. Except for in India, these still represent relatively infrequent strains. Why have G9 strains not replaced G1–G4 strains in England?

Desselberger: There are also many Indian subpopulations in the USA. They tend to form a relatively discrete subpopulation.

Greenberg: Could anyone clarify the biological meaning of all of this? We all know that in influenza, every 10–30 years a new pandemic occurs and some novel haemagglutinin or neuraminidase genes get into the human population. Are you warning us that this is what will happen with rotavirus? Does the pool of animal genes represent a new group of serotypes that could move through the human population?

Desselberger: In influenza, it is clear that the H2 and H3 genes of human strains have been introduced from animal strains via reassortment events; there is good molecular evidence for this. Recently, we have seen H5 and H9 strains being introduced into humans in Hong Kong: H5 strains only caused a small epidemic and H9 strains were only found in two or three cases because the genomes of these strains are completely animal, i.e. they are not reassortants. From various data it seems that they don't have the ability to circulate widely in the human population. In terms of our knowledge of the natural history of rotavirus diversity, I think we are at the stage where the flu people were a few decades ago.

Clarke: I think it is wrong to draw parallels with influenza, because the mode of transmission changes from faecal–oral to airborne as the virus goes through different animal hosts. The expectation that we will see a new pandemic with G9 is not something that one might expect because there is no history of pandemics of viral gastroenteritis.

Estes: The key point here is, what is the biological significance of all this diversity, and is it telling us that there will be some shift in a phenotypic property that will be biologically relevant in terms of children suddenly getting much more severe disease because there is no antibody in the population? Do we have any evidence that directly addresses this?

Koopmans: I don't have direct evidence, but I do have some suggestive indirect observations. In a recent WHO meeting on rotavirus in Europe, it was striking that in three of the countries present, there seems to be a recent increase in the detection of non-common rotavirus serotypes. We have looked at some more G9s, which have translated into severe hospital outbreaks (Widdowson et al 2000), and Dr Svensson presented data about something happening between the 1997 and 1998 rotavirus season, where he has a sudden increase in the number of non-typeable rotaviruses and a concomitant shift in the ages of people infected (L. Svensson, personal communication). This suggests that there is also something going on. From my perspective, looking at RNA viruses, these are events waiting to happen. They may not be frequent, but I think you have to always think about RNA viruses as being genetically flexible enough to undergo sudden changes. What we describe in molecular epidemiology is the current situation, but what we need to think about is what happens if you introduce a genetic bottleneck by starting vaccinating against predominant strains. If you give them a disadvantage, you would probably open up the population for more infections with these uncommon genotypes.

Desselberger: There is a lot of conjecture about the vaccine issue. We have heard from Paul Offit that it is possible to get heterotypic protection with a monotypic vaccine. If there is a vaccine when G9 strains are circulating, we don't know whether this situation will be covered by the vaccine or not.

Saif: The bovine rotavirus vaccine has been out since 1973 in the USA. Granted it is not highly efficacious, but the predominant G type is G6, which is the same as the vaccine, although the predominant P type in the field (P[5]) is different from the P[1] type in the vaccine (Parwani et al 1993, Chang et al 1996). The other major type that we see in the USA is G10P[11]. There should be ways to study this with the more recent introduction of the bovine rotavirus vaccine in Europe, and then in Argentina where the G6P[5] vaccine is used in cattle.

Koopmans: The problem is that it is not clear how high the vaccine coverage is. Before you can conclude that the serotypes are not changing, you need to know this.

Kapikian: I think Harry Greenberg's question is highly relevant. These new serotypes that are emerging are really outliers as far as the developed countries of the world are concerned. Ulrich Desselberger showed that 94% of serotypes in the UK were G1–G4. If someone said that we could make a magic vaccine that could protect against only one rotavirus type, we would select the G1 serotype and this would be a major achievement, because overall the G1 serotype still predominates. I don't think that a vaccine is going to facilitate the emergence of other strains, because the live rotavirus vaccines don't induce 'sterilizing immunity'; reinfections occur frequently. Even adults undergo reinfections but characteristically they are asymptomatic. From my perspective, the four serotypes (G1, G2, G3 and G4) are the epidemiologically important ones and we should develop vaccines to cover them. Roger Glass, what have you found recently about the distribution of the G9 serotype in the USA?

Glass: From the point of view of immunity and vaccination, these things could well be irrelevant. In the USA, 98% of the population is naturally immune to rotavirus by exposure in the first few years of life. We have never had a huge epidemic of a new strain coming in an infecting people of all ages. These are interesting for the epidemiology of the virus, but are much less relevant for the protection by vaccines. We have the same pattern in the USA: G9 has been much more prevalent over the last several years than serotypes three and four. The question we haven't addressed is, if there is this entire population of Americans who are completely immune to G1, why is G1 the most common strain? We have all these variants, but none of them really take over.

Desselberger: In my opinion this statement is not tenable on a global scale. If you look at some of the African and Asian countries, other strains are more prevalent than the G1–G4 strains: there are unusual G/P constellations that are most prevalent. You say that there are not many of the other strains in the USA, but perhaps there is a sampling problem.

Matson: There is G1 subtype replacement in the same population. This was shown in Dimitrov's study in Houston (Dimitrov et al 1984). He did the initial characterization by electropherotype, but when we went back and typed those samples with different electopherotypes, they were different G1s that were replacing the previously predominant G1 subtype (Matson et al 1990).

Brown: I remain to be convinced that there is a biological significance to the diversity of group A rotavirus strains. Epidemiologically, we have not seen a shift in the age distribution of cases of group A rotavirus infections. Perhaps it would be worth turning our attention to some of the non-group A rotavirus infections, for example, group B, which showed a very distinct epidemiological pattern when they emerged in the early 1980s with a high proportion of adult cases (Hung et al 1984). We need to look for non-group A rotaviruses, which may be more of a pandemic threat to human population.

Matson: In addition to these viruses having a tremendous diversity of P and G type combinations within communities, within a type there is extraordinary diversity. We have published a study from Argentina where we looked at 68 different G1s recovered from one city with a panel of monoclonal antibodies (Espul et al 2000). We saw 28 different monotype patterns for neutralizing epitopes of G1. This is an amazing diversity. If there is subtype replacement and there is this type of diversity, there can be pressure for shifting of predominating subtypes.

Green: How do you explain the epidemics beginning in the southernmost parts of the USA and Europe and then spreading up to the North? Is this a climate issue?

Estes: It is important that we understand that although there are patterns of temporal spread of disease, it is not spread of one strain but of multiple strains. It is very different from the influenza situation where you can follow a strain moving around the world.

Bishop: This also occurs in Australia, where the peak rotavirus season in Perth on the west coast always precedes the peaks in the eastern states which are 2000 miles distant (Carlin et al 1998).

Matson: The same occurs in South America. We tried to look at this wave phenomenon in the USA, and received data from the US National Weather Service on mean temperature, maximum temperature, minimum temperature, rainfall, humidity and so on and could find no correlates.

Bishop: Perhaps we ignore the physiological effect of weather on the host. There is animal research showing that if pigs are infected with transmissible gastroenteritis virus and exposed to alternating temperatures in 24 h, they are much more susceptible to disease than pigs that are kept at a sustained level temperature (Shimizu et al 1978).

References

Ahmed MV, Urasawa S, Taniguchi K et al 1991 Analysis of human rotavirus strains prevailing in Bangladesh in relation to nationwide floods brought by the 1988 monsoon. J Clin Microbiol 29:2273–2279

Carlin JB, Chondros P, Masendycz P, Bugg H, Bishop RF, Barnes GL 1998 Rotavirus infection and rates of hospitalisation for acute gastroenteritis in young children, Australia 1993–1996. Med J Aust 169:252–256

Chang KO, Parwani AV, Saif LJ 1996 The characterization of VP7 (G type) and VP4 (P type) genes of bovine group A rotaviruses from field samples using RT-PCR and RFLP analysis. Arch Virol 141:1727–1739

Dimitrov DH, Graham DY, López J et al 1984 RNA electropherotypes of rotaviruses from North and South America. Bull WHO 62:321–329

Diwakala CS, Palombo EA 1999 Genetic and antigenic variation of capsid protein VP7 of serotype G1 human rotavirus isolates. J Gen Virol 80:341–344

Espul C, Cuello H, Martinez N et al 2000 Genomic and antigenic variation among rotavirus strains circulating in a large city of Argentina. J Med Virol 61:504–509

Huang T, Wang C, Fang Z et al 1984 Waterborne outbreak of rotavirus diarrhoea in adults in China caused by a novel rotavirus. Lancet i:1139–1142

Matson DO, Estes MK, Burns JW, Greenberg HB, Taniguchi K, Urasawa S 1990 Serotype variation of human group A rotaviruses in two regions of the United States. J Infect Dis 162:605–614

Parwani AV, Hussein HA, Rosen BI, Lucchelli A, Navarro L, Saif LJ 1993 Characterization of field strains of group A bovine rotaviruses using polymerase chain reaction-generated G and P type-specific cDNA probes. J Clin Microbiol 31:2010–2015

Shimizu M, Shimizu Y, Kodama Y 1978 Effects of ambient temperatures on induction of transmissible gastroenteritis in feeder pigs. Infect Immun 21:747–752

Unicomb LE, Podder G, Gentsch JR et al 1999 Evidence of a high frequency genomic reassortment of group A rotavirus strains in Bangladesh: emergence of G9 strains in 1995. J Clin Microbiol 37:1885–1891

Widdowson MA, Doornum GJ, van der Poel WHM, de Boer AS, Mahdi U, Koopmans M 2000 Emerging group-A rotavirus and a nosocomial outbreak of diarrhoea. Lancet 356:1161–1162

Novartis 238: Gastroenteritis Viruses.
Copyright © 2001 John Wiley & Sons Ltd
Print ISBN 0-471-49663-4   eISBN 0-470-84653-4

A rotavirus vaccine for prevention of severe diarrhoea of infants and young children: development, utilization and withdrawal

Albert Z. Kapikian

Epidemiology Section, Laboratory of Infectious Diseases, National Institute of Allergy and Infectious Diseases, National Institutes of Health, Bethesda, MD 20852, USA

Abstract. The importance of rotaviruses (RVs) as the single most important cause of severe diarrhoea of infants and young children is well recognized. At NIH, we developed a quadrivalent (tetravalent [TV]) vaccine to protect against the four epidemiologically important RV serotypes. It is comprised of live attenuated rhesus RV (RRV), a VP7 serotype G3 strain (the 'Jennerian' approach), and three reassortant RVs, each containing 10 RRV genes and one human RV gene that codes for the major outer protein, VP7, that determines serotype G1, G2 or G4 specificity (the 'modified Jennerian' approach). The vaccine was safe and effective against severe diarrhoea in a major pre-licensure collaborative effort of phase III trials. In February 1998 and again in June 1998, the Advisory Committee on Immunization Practices (ACIP) recommended routine immunization with three oral doses at 2, 4 and 6 months of age. The tetravalent vaccine (RotaShield) was licensed in the USA by the FDA in August 1998. In July 1999, after about 1.5 million doses had been given, the CDC recommended suspending administration of the vaccine because post-licensure surveillance of adverse events had suggested an association with intussusception. After further investigation by CDC, in October 1999, the ACIP withdrew its recommendation concluding that '... intussusception occurs with significantly increased frequency in the first 1–2 weeks after vaccination with RRV-TV, particularly following the first dose'. The implications of these developments from a practical, epidemiological, analytical and ethical perspective are discussed.

2001 Gastroenteritis viruses. Wiley, Chichester (Novartis Foundation Symposium 238) p 153–179

It is clear from this Symposium that rotaviruses are the single most important etiological agents of severe diarrhoea in infants and young children in both developed and developing countries. These viruses are responsible for 35–50% of severe diarrhoeal diseases in infants and young children less than two years of age. Rotaviruses have the unique characteristic of being quite egalitarian as they infect nearly every child in the first few years of life in both developed and developing countries regardless of hygienic conditions. But the consequences of such infections are strikingly different: in the USA they are responsible for over 500 000 visits to physicians, 50 000 hospitalizations and 20 deaths, whereas in the developing countries 600 000–873 000 children under 5 years of age die from rotavirus disease each year, which translates to about 2000–2400 deaths per day or 100 deaths each hour for this age group (Kapikian & Chanock 1996, Bresee et al 1999).

The need for a rotavirus vaccine

Since the golden age of viral gastroenteritis commenced in the early 1970s, many viruses have been implicated as etiological agents of diarrhoeal illnesses. However, rotaviruses reign as the number one cause of severe diarrhoeal disease worldwide, surpassing the enteric adenoviruses, astroviruses, caliciviruses and bacterial agents. Thus, the need for a rotavirus vaccine is clear and compelling, with the goal being the prevention of severe rotavirus diarrhoea during the first two years of life when the consequences of such illnesses are most serious.

Rotavirus features relevant to vaccine development

Rotaviruses are 70 nm in diameter, non-enveloped and possess a distinctive double-shelled outer capsid. Within the inner shell is a third layer, the core, which contains the viral genome comprised of 11 segments of double-stranded (ds)RNA. During coinfection with different rotavirus strains, the segmented genomes readily undergo genetic reassortment. With regard to vaccine development, the two outer capsid proteins, VP4 and VP7, deserve special attention (Kapikian & Chanock 1996).

VP7, a glycoprotein, comprises one of two major neutralization antigens located on the outer capsid and is encoded by RNA segment 7, 8 or 9 (depending on strain). The other outer capsid protein, VP4, is encoded by RNA segment 4; it protrudes from the outer capsid in the form of 60 spikes. Antibodies to both VP7 and VP4 are independently associated with protection against illness in various animal models. Serotypes are characteristically determined by VP7, but a VP4 serotyping scheme has also been developed recently. Although there are 14 VP7 (or G for glycoprotein) serotypes, 10 in humans, 13 in animals and 9 shared between humans and animals, the antigenic variation is not a formidable problem in vaccine development because only four serotypes, numbered 1, 2, 3 and 4, are of major epidemiological importance; therefore efforts have been focused on developing a vaccine to protect against each of these four serotypes (Hoshino & Kapikian 2000). Although the mechanism of protection is still not certain, early studies in animals suggested that antibodies in the lumen of the small intestine are a major determinant of resistance to rotavirus illness (Offit 1994, Kapikian & Chanock 1996, Matson 1996). In addition, we sought the development of an oral, live, attenuated vaccine which would mimic natural infection, thus inducing local intestinal immunity.

The Jennerian approach

Our initial approach was to adopt the strategy pioneered by Edward Jenner in 1796 for human smallpox vaccination in which a related, live, attenuated agent from a non-human host is used as the immunogen. Early serological and animal studies were instrumental in suggesting the feasibility of the Jennerian approach to rotavirus vaccination (Kapikian et al 1996). We pursued this approach with a rhesus rotavirus strain, designated MMU18006, which belongs to serotype VP7:3 (=G3), and which grew efficiently in a semi-continuous simian diploid cell strain FRhL2. This vaccine was administered orally in a single 10^4 or 10^5 pfu dose to over 1500 infants and young children 1–20 months of age in field trials in the USA and overseas. Vaccine efficacy ranged from 0–85% against moderate-to-severe diarrhoea. It appeared from these studies that serotype specific immunity was an important factor in determining vaccine efficacy (Kapikian et al 1996).

The modified Jennerian approach

The likelihood that serotype-specific immunity was important in protection became the impetus for our modification of the Jennerian strategy. The objective was to evaluate a quadrivalent rotavirus vaccine that incorporates the VP7 specificity of each of the four epidemiologically important serotypes as well as the attenuation phenotype of RRV in order to achieve protection against each of these four human rotavirus serotypes.

This was achieved by generating reassortants which possessed a single VP7 gene from human rotavirus serotypes G1, G2 or G4, and 10 genes from RRV, and combining these three reassortants with the RRV strain, the latter providing coverage for serotype G3 (Midthun et al 1985, 1986) (Fig. 1). This quadrivalent (tetravalent) rotavirus vaccine (RRV-TV) was evaluated in major field trials in the US and overseas. When used at a dose of 4×10^5 pfu, it characteristically induced about 50% protection against any rotavirus diarrhoea, whereas against severe diarrhoea its protective efficacy reached as high as 100% (Table 1). For example, in Finland, the quadrivalent vaccine induced 68% protection against any rotavirus diarrhoea, 91–100% against severe and very severe rotavirus diarrhoea, respectively, and 100% against hospital admission due to rotavirus (Joensuu et al 1997).

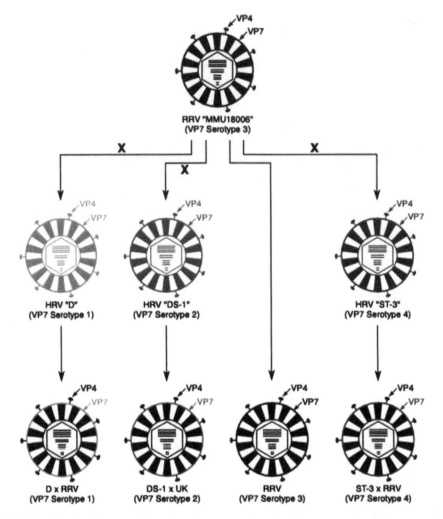

FIG. 1.   The development of a quadrivalent (tetravalent) rotavirus vaccine (RRV-TV) in order to achieve protection against each of the four human rotavirus serotypes. Reassortants were generated which possessed a single VP7 gene from human rotaviruses G1, G2 or G4, and 10 genes from RRV, and these three reassortants were combined with the RRV strain, the latter providing coverage for serotype G3. (Reproduced from Kapikian et al 1996, with permission).

Regulatory issues

Because of the data regarding the safety and efficacy of this quadrivalent vaccine, on 11 February 1998 and again on 25 June 1998 the Advisory Committee on Immunization Practices (ACIP) recommended routine immunization with three

TABLE 1   Protective efficacy of quadrivalent rotavirus (RV) vaccine (4×10^5 PFU) on the occurrence of RV diarrhoea of varying severity in infants and young children

	No. of individuals		Protective efficacy vs.		
Trial	Vaccine	Placebo	All RV diarrhoea	Severe RV diarrhoea	Dehydration
US National Mulitcenter[a]	398	385	49%	80%	100%
Finland[b]	1128	1145	68%	91–100%	75%
Venezuela[c]	112	1095	48%	88%	75%
US Native American[d]	347	348	50%	69%	—*

*Only a few cases (aggressive use of oral rehydration therapy). Note: the efficacy figures were all statistically significant. [a]Rennels et al (1996); [b]Joensuu et al (1997); [c]Perez-Schael et al (1997); [d]Santosham et al (1997), Mack (personal communication).

oral doses of this vaccine at 2, 4 and 6 months of age (CDC 1999a). Later on August 31, 1998 the FDA granted a biologics license to Wyeth Laboratories for manufacture and distribution of the rotavirus vaccine known commercially as RotaShield.

Rotavirus Vaccine and intussusception

Postponement of administration

After over 9 months of apparently successful use of the vaccine in the USA, on 16 July 1999 the CDC reported that between 1 Sept 1998 and 7 July 1999, according to the Vaccine Adverse Event Reporting System (VAERS), a passive system operated by FDA and CDC, 15 cases of intussusception had occurred following vaccination with RRV-TV (CDC 1999b). It was estimated that 1.8 million doses of RRV-TV had been distributed and that 1.5 million doses had been given. Although the number of intussusception cases reported was within the expected value (considering a New York State background rate of 51 per 100 000 infants < 12 months of age in the period 1991–1997 [prior to RRV-TV licensure]), it was of concern that 11 of the 15 cases had occurred within 1 week of administration of the first dose of vaccine. Thus, the CDC recommended suspending further vaccination until additional data could be obtained.

Withdrawal of ACIP recommendation

In a follow-up CDC–ACIP meeting on 22 October 1999, CDC estimated that approximately one million infants had received RRV-TV and that a total of 102 confirmed or presumptive cases of intussusception had been reported to VAERS

(ACIP 1999). Moreover, 57 of the cases had onset within 7 days of vaccination and 46 (81%) of the 57 cases had onset within 7 days of the first dose. Case-series and case-control studies supported the observation of highest risk during the first week (3–7 days) after the first dose of vaccine. Therefore, the ACIP on 22 October 1999 concluded that, '... intussusception occurs with significantly increased frequency in the first one-to-two weeks following vaccination with RRV-TV, particularly following the first dose' (CDC 1999c). Thus, the ACIP withdrew its recommendation for RRV-TV and no longer recommended its use in the USA.

Pre-licensure studies

It is noteworthy that in pre-licensure studies, five of 10 054 infants who received rotavirus vaccine (in three dosage levels, two vaccine formulations and two buffering methods) and one of 4633 never-vaccinated infants developed intussusception, $(P = 0.45)$ (Rennels et al 1998). None of the five cases occurred after the first dose; one case each had onset on day 6, 15 or 51 after the 2nd dose, and two cases on day 7 after the third dose. Further analyses of these data indicated that 8240 of the 10 054 infants who received rotavirus vaccine had received the vaccine at the dosage that had been proposed for licensure: two of these 8240 children developed intussusception, one on day 51 after the second dose, and one on day 7 after the third dose. It was concluded that the pre-licensure studies failed to demonstrate an aetiological association between the rotavirus vaccine and intussusception. It should be noted, however, that the rate of intussusception in the 10 054 vaccinees and 4633 placebo recipients was described in the package insert of RotaShield.

Wild-type rotavirus and intussusception

Because of the association of the vaccine with intussusception and its withdrawal from use, earlier studies that had examined the relationship between naturally occurring rotavirus infection and intussusception have taken on special importance. In 1978, in Japan, rotavirus was detected in stools of 11 (37%) of 30 children (6–49 months old) with intussusception; a serologic response was observed in five of seven rotavirus-positive children (Konno et al, 1978). It was concluded that human rotavirus '... may be an infectious agent causing intus-susception in infants and young children'. In addition, in 1981, in an extension of this study, evidence of rotavirus infection was reported in 20 (33%) of 61 cases, including the 30 patients above (Katsushima 1981). In 1982 in Australia, no virological or serological evidence of rotavirus infection was found in 22 of 24 children during a 6 month prospective study which included the winter peak of gastroenteritis (Mulcahy et al 1982). In a retrospective study, a negative correlation was found between the occurrence of rotavirus gastroenteritis and the occurrence of intussusception. It was concluded that there was 'no evidence... of an etiological role of rotavirus in intussusception.' In 1982 in France, in a 1 year prospective study of 64 infants and young children with intussusception, it was concluded that, '... rotavirus does not seem to be a good candidate for having a role in the aetiology of intussusception ...' (Nicolas et al 1982). In 1998 in a 10 year German study of 155 cases of intussusception in children (49.6% < 1 year of age), rotavirus was not found to be a significant cause of this condition (Staatz et al 1998).

Because of the reported rotavirus vaccine–intussusception link, in 2000 in the USA, the distribution of infectious enteritis and intussusception was evaluated retrospectively over a 5 year period. It was postulated that if wild-type rotavirus infection was linked to more cases of intussusception than the vaccine, then it would not be necessary to limit use of the vaccine (Hellems et al 2000). It was found that, 'intussusception occurs in a monthly distribution similar to that of infectious enteritis with peak incidence during rotavirus season. Since rotavirus is responsible for most wintertime enteritis, rotavirus may be an important aetiologic factor in intussusception.'

Unresolved issues regarding rotavirus vaccine and intussusception

The CDC data regarding the clustering of cases particularly during the first week after the first dose of vaccine are significant and important, and this needs to be studied further. However, the key question that has even greater public health importance and which has not been answered satisfactorily relates to the attributable risk, if any, of RRV-TV among the one million infants who were vaccinated. How many cases of intussusception did the RRV-TV vaccine cause in excess of the background baseline incidence of 51 cases per 100 000 (or 1 per 1961 infants) during the first year of life? Surprisingly, it is still not known whether an 'epidemic' of intussusception occurred in the USA following the administration of RRV-TV to one quarter of the US birth cohort, or whether there was a decrease in the number of cases. This is a major, as yet unanswered, question for both developed and developing countries where in the former (for example the USA), over 500 000 infants and young children seek medical attention for rotavirus diarrhoea annually, but especially in the latter where approximately 1 in 160 infants and young children less than 5 years of age die of rotavirus disease annually (Glass et al 1994). The attributable risk question will be discussed in further detail later in this presentation.

Other important questions include:

(1) Did the rotavirus vaccine 'trigger' the onset of intussusception in high-risk susceptible individuals who may have developed it later under natural conditions?

(2) Does naturally occurring rotavirus infection cause intussusception? If it does, did the rotavirus vaccine prevent intussusception later in the year in high-risk infants who did not experience the putative early 'triggering' effect, and prevent it in non high-risk infants as well?

(3) During pre-licensure studies, why were no cases of intussusception observed in the more than 8000 children who received RRV-TV following administration of the first dose (Rennels et al 1998), especially since CDC has reported odds ratios of 25 during the first week after vaccination (ACIP 1999)? Did the routine administration of other childhood vaccines along with RRV-TV post-licensure play any role in this inconsistency, or was the inconsistency due to an overall very rare occurrence of intussusception following administration of RRV-TV?

Ethical considerations for developing countries

A meeting at the WHO in Geneva, 9–11 February 2000, considered the future directions for rotavirus vaccine research in developing countries (World Health Organization 2000). Ethical considerations were a feature of this meeting. Some of the issues that were addressed in this regard included whether a vaccine withdrawn from the US market could be used in developing countries. Should testing a vaccine with known adverse risks that can be fatal be supported? What safeguards would be necessary? Was it ethical not to use a vaccine that could prevent a large burden of fatal disease? How should new candidate vaccines be tested: simultaneously in developed and developing countries, or in sequence? These were noted to be difficult ethical issues for consideration for a vaccine aimed at a disease that is commonly fatal in developing countries but rarely fatal in the developed world (World Health Organization 2000).

The WHO Ethical Issues Working Group deliberations were summarized by Dr Charles Weijer who noted that: (1) failure to proceed with further trials of RRV-TV would further any existing inequities in health between developed and developing countries; (2) data developed for RRV-TV far exceed the data available on other rotavirus vaccines; (3) inaction, waiting for comparable data on other vaccines is not morally neutral, since the disease burden cannot be ignored in the interim; and (4) it would be immoral not to proceed with RRV-TV in developing countries (World Health Organization 2000).

The deliberations of this WHO meeting recommended that ' . . . further studies of the current rotavirus vaccine (RRV-TV) in developing countries were ethical, given the higher disease burden and potential higher benefit:risk ratio in a developing country. The group was careful, however, in insisting that further testing of RRV-TV not occur without the assurance that the vaccine would be available for general use should the results of the trial prove to be positive'. This latter comment was addressing the question of whether Wyeth Laboratories, the producer of the vaccine, would continue to make vaccine if it were not used in the USA.

Evolution and impact of the attributable risk issue

Despite the WHO recommendation, overall the developing country representatives had no desire to evaluate RRV-TV because of the reported magnified risk of RRV-TV that led to its withdrawal. The future of this vaccine and of other rotavirus vaccines under development rests on an accurate determination of its overall attributable risk, if any, for intussusception. The CDC has presented various estimates of the attributable risk with a continuing downward trend from the figures that were presented at the CDC-ACIP meeting on 22 October 1999, when the vaccine was withdrawn (Fig. 2).

At this meeting, CDC presented data indicating that the excess risk of intussusception attributable to RRV-TV was 1.8, 1.7 or 1.6 as determined from the case-control, single managed care cohort and case-series studies, respectively (ACIP 1999). Thus, CDC presented data indicating that the overall risk of intussusception was increased 80%, 70% or 60% (over the expected baseline value of 51 cases per 100 000 infants < 12 months of age) after RRV-TV vaccination, and thus, they projected that there would be 1600, 1400 or 1200 excess cases of intussusception in the entire birth cohort annually if RRV-TV was used universally in the USA (i.e. 40 per 100 000 [or 1 per 2500 vaccinees]; 35 per 100 000, or 30 per 100 000, respectively, in addition to the background rate of 51 per 100 000 noted earlier) (Fig. 2). These projections were made using the New York State baseline rate of 51 cases of intussusception per 100 000 children (or 1 per ~ 2000 children) during the first year of life cited earlier (e.g. 80%×2000 background rate=1600 excess annual cases; 70%×2000=1400 excess annual cases; 60%×2000=1200 excess annual cases due to RRV-TV) (Fig. 2).

At this meeting, the CDC emphasized the increased risk during the first week after RRV-TV administration reporting that the risk of developing intussusception during days 3–7 post vaccination was increased 25-fold, 19-fold and 13-fold from analysis of the case-control, case-series and expanded cohort studies, respectively (ACIP 1999).

The CDC also presented figures at this meeting from this expanded cohort study of six managed care organizations (MCOs) which included approximately 50 000 children who received at least one dose of RRV-TV. They reported that nine children developed intussusception within the first 3 weeks after vaccination (and

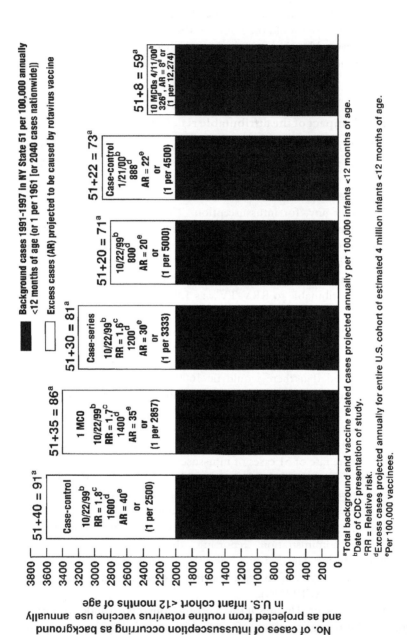

FIG. 2. Number of projected cases of intussusception (attributable risk [AR]) caused by rotavirus vaccine according to CDC in various analyses and times.

53 developed intussusception in a larger never-vaccinated group of children observed over a longer period of time but whose absolute number was not available) (ACIP 1999). It was noted in this expanded cohort study that RRV-TV had an attributable risk of 1 case of intussusception per > 12 000 doses (ACIP 1999). In another estimate at this meeting, they also noted that the RRV-TV was causally related with one case of intussusception per 5000 vaccinees or 800 excess cases.

Three months later, in January 2000, CDC reported the attributable risk from the case-control study, to be 1 case of intussusception per 4500 vaccinees (or 22.2 per 100 000 infants, or 888 excess cases) (Fig. 2) (NIH/NVPO Workshop 1/21/2000).

Moreover, on 11 April 2000, at the CDC EIS Conference, the CDC reported that from a further expanded cohort study, which now included 10 MCOs, the risk of developing intussusception after vaccination was 1 case per 12 274 infants—an almost fivefold reduction from a figure presented to the ACIP in October 1999 when the vaccine was withdrawn (Fig. 2). In this further expanded cohort study, six cases of intussusception were detected in 61 371 RRV-TV-vaccinated infants in the first 3 weeks after vaccination (or one case per 20 100 doses of vaccine). The 10 MCOs cohort study provided the most reliable data available up to that time regarding attributable risk because it included the largest number of vaccinated children and, in addition, the rate of intussusception in relation to the absolute number of vaccinees was available rather than only person-year calculations.

We have consistently had a problem with the odds ratios and attributable risk figures presented by CDC. The attributable risk of 1 case per 12 274 (or 8.1 cases/100 000) vaccinated infants) (CDC-EIS Conference 4/11/00) is in sharp contrast to the reported relative risk of 1.8 from the case-control study (i.e. 40 excess cases per 100 000) and the odds ratios which had ranged from 13–25 for rotavirus vaccine recipients during the first week after vaccination in the case-control, case-series and cohort studies (Fig. 2) (ACIP 1999). These magnified odds ratios observed during the first week after the first dose received special emphasis and attention by the ACIP and public health community, whereas the overall attributable risk figure of ~ 1:12 000 which has not been available until recently, has not been placed in proper perspective.

Was there an 'epidemic' of intussusception because of vaccine use?

Our initial doubts about the overall risk of this vaccine arose from evaluation of published data from CDC which failed to reveal a striking increase in the overall number of cases of intussusception that would have been anticipated from the extremely high odds ratios, noted above, that were presented for the first week following vaccination. For example, CDC reported the occurrence of three cases of intussusception in 9802 vaccinees in a California managed care study, which translated to an overall incidence of 30 cases per 100 000 over an unspecified period of time. However, because one of the three cases occurred during the first week after vaccination, CDC reported that the incidence of intussusception was 314 per 100 000 individuals during that period (CDC 1999b). However, the overall risk of the vaccine in this large cohort of children was not presented.

Similarly, in a Minnesota study, five cases were reported in recipients of 53 479 doses, an incidence of ~9 per 100 000 doses over an unspecified period of time; however because three of the infants developed intussusception within 1 week of vaccination, the rate of intussusception was calculated to be 292 per 100 000 infant years (CDC 1999b).

In addition, the CDC reported that 102 cases of intussusception were detected by the VAERS in the ~1 million vaccinated infants (ACIP 1999). This translates to an incidence of ~10 cases per 100 000 vaccinees over an unspecified period of time. Although VAERS is a passive reporting system, even assuming a 50% sensitivity of detection, the maximum incidence from these data would translate to ~20 cases per 100 000 vaccinees, a figure well below the background rate of 51 cases per 100 000 infants during the first year of life. Because of the low number of cases overall, we considered that there was a 'disconnect' between the extremely high odds ratios calculated from case/control, case series, and cohort studies, and the relative risks of 1.8, 1.6 and 1.7, noted earlier, with the actual number of cases observed.

The results of the 10 MCOs study are of particular interest (CDC-EIS Conference 2000). Of the 61 371 infants who received at least a single dose of the RRV-TV vaccine, six infants developed intussusception during the 3 week period after vaccination, which yields an incidence of 9.8 cases per 100 000 vaccinees (i.e. 1 per 10 229 infants) over an overall unspecified period of time, a figure well below the predicted 1 per ~2000 infants during the first year of life as baseline from the NY State study. It is clear to us from the further expanded cohort study and from the figures cited above, that an 'epidemic' of intussusception did not occur following administration of the rotavirus vaccine in the USA, confirming our conclusion that there was a 'disconnect' or major inconsistency between the odds ratios during the first week after vaccination and the attributable risk figure of 1 case per 12 274 vaccinees derived from the 10 MCOs cohort study.

Magnification of relative risk by comparing unequal groups

A greatly magnified rate of intussusception for the vaccinated group was created by the 'window analysis' because CDC compared vastly unequal person-year values which artificially inflate the time denominator for the non-vaccinated group. In this way, the initial clustering of cases during the first week after vaccination is assumed to persist at the same elevated rate even though such data are not available, and were, in fact clearly ruled out.

For example, in data presented by CDC at the CDC-ACIP meeting on 22 October 1999, an elevated risk of intussusception of 13 among rotavirus vaccinees vs. non-vaccinees was reported in the six MCOs cohort study, which included seven cases of intussusception days 3–7 post-vaccination in ∼50 000 vaccinees and 53 cases in an unspecified but larger group of non-vaccinated individuals over an extended period of time. The elevated risk figure of 13 was derived by fragmenting the person-years of exposure into windows of varying periods. In comparing the 5 day period embracing days 3–7 for the vaccinees (i.e. 1001 person-years) with a considerably longer period for the non-vaccinated group (i.e. 135 067 person-years), the assumption is that the increased rate of intussusception on days 3–7 for the vaccinees will persist at the same elevated rate over the longer period used for the non-vaccinated group, and thus the incidence risk ratio is derived using the unexposed group as the referent with a value of 1.00. However, by stating that the incidence risk ratio (IRR) was 13, the implication for those not familiar with the limits (i.e. days 3–7) of this IRR was that the acknowledged background level of intussusception of 51 cases per 100 000 infants during the first year of life would (because of the vaccine) be 13×51 or 663 cases of intussusception per 100 000 infants, or 6630 cases per million vaccinees, or 26 520 excess cases if the entire newborn population of ∼4 million infants had been vaccinated.

Of course, we know this was not the case, but the perception was that a great excess occurred and it was this type of information that was widely disseminated. The same type of analysis was carried out when the data for the expanded cohort study of 10 MCOs was reported at the April 2000 CDC meeting in which the attributable risk figure of 1 case per 12 274 vaccinees was presented. Despite the rarefied attributable risk figure with six cases of intussusception among of 61 371 vaccinees within the first 3 weeks after the first dose, the window analysis yielded an incidence risk ratio of 15 for days 3–7 for the vaccinated group. The disparity between the attributable risk of 1 case per 12 274 vaccinees and the relative risk of 15 was once again very difficult to place in practical perspective.

The issue of the attributable risk of the vaccine can only be settled if the incidence of intussusception in the vaccinated and non-vaccinated groups is compared over the same periods and for the same length of time, rather than extrapolating a rate by person-years for the vaccinated group for a fragmented early segment of time, because of the disproportionate clustering of cases in days 3–7 post vaccination.

An analogy for this statistical anomaly

By way of illustration of this statistical anomaly of increased initial risk versus overall attributable risk, a baseball analogy regarding a pitcher's earned run average (ERA) provides an excellent example. The ERA is probably the most critical statistic in determining a pitcher's performance. It is calculated by dividing the number of earned runs allowed by the number of innings pitched and multiplying by nine to determine the number of earned runs yielded per normal nine-inning game.

In this illustration, let's assume that pitcher 'A' gives up two earned runs in the first inning of a game and then leaves the game. His ERA is calculated as 18.00 (i.e. 2 runs divided by 1 inning=2; 2 × 9 innings=18.00). However, pitcher 'B' plays the entire game and yields 2 in the 9th inning. His ERA is calculated as 2.00 (i.e. 2 runs divided by 9 innings × 9 innings=2.00 ERA). As the season progresses, 'A' and 'B' each pitch 100 total innings and each gives up a total of 20 earned runs. The ERA of each pitcher is now 1.80 (i.e. 20 runs divided by 100 innings=0.20; 0.20 × 9 innings=1.80 ERA). The initial high ERA of pitcher 'A' is stabilized as the season progresses.

CDC has presented an odds ratio of 24.8 on days 3–7 post vaccination in their case-control study (ACIP 1999), and an incidence rate ratio of 15.05 during days 3–7 post vaccination in the 10 MCOs cohort study (CDC-EIS conference April 2000). However, we still do not know the risk of developing intussusception following RRV-TV vaccination. The attributable risk has ranged from one case per 2500 vaccinees to the current value of one case per 12 274 vaccinees.

We also do not know the risk of intussusception in vaccinated and never-vaccinated infants when they are studied for the same length of time (e.g. 12 months) or whether there was an 'epidemic' of intussusception following vaccination. Although the odds ratio during the first week predicts that an 'epidemic' should have occurred, the population-based cohort data do not support this position.

The future of RRV-TV

It is clear that the developing countries of the world will not use the rotavirus vaccine as long as the ACIP recommendation for its withdrawal remains in force. How can this barrier be removed? There are three possible options that need consideration: (i) a recommendation for routine use of the vaccine would remove the barrier, but the prospect of this option being selected is highly unlikely and appears not possible at present, based on the currently available data; (ii) a 'permissive recommendation' would remove the barrier but the likelihood of this option being selected is unlikely, but possible at this time because of the recent

TABLE 2 Candidate oral rotavirus (RV) vaccines evaluated in efficacy trials in infants and young children

Venue	Vaccine	Serotype [Genotype]	Composition	Status
Jennerian approach				
Tampere, Finland	Bovine RV (BRV) NCDV (RIT 4237)	G6; P6[1]	Monovalent	Discontinued
Philadelphia, USA	BRV-WC3	G6; P[5]	Monovalent	Discontinued
Bethesda, USA	Rhesus RV (RRV)-MMU 18006	G3; P5B[3]	Monovalent	Discontinued
Modified Jennerian approach				
Bethesda, USA	Human RV (HRV) × RRV, Reassortants+RRV*	G1, 2, 3, 4; P5B[3]	Quadrivalent	Licensed by FDA; use suspended
Philadelphia, USA	HRV × BRV (WC3), Reassortants*	G1, 2, 3; P1A[8]; P[5]	Quadrivalent	Active
Bethesda, USA	HRV × BRV (UK), Reassortants	G1, 2, 3, 4; P7[5]	Quadrivalent	Active
Non-Jennerian approach				
Bethesda, USA	HRV-M37	G1; P2A[6]	Monovalent	Discontinued
Cincinnati, USA	HRV-89–12	G1; P[8]	Monovalent	Active

*Selected individual components evaluated for efficacy also.

References: Midthun, & Kapikian (1996); Kapikian & Chanock (1996); Clark et al (1996); Vesikari (1996); Offit et al (1997); Bresee et al (1999); Clements et al (1999); Hoshino & Kapikian (2000); World Health Organization (2000).

revised attributable risk data; and (iii) a statement indicating that on the basis of new information, the risk of intussusception following vaccination is considerably less than originally projected, is likely to be selected but would be totally ineffective in removing the barrier. Thus, the only realistic way to remove the barrier to evaluation of this vaccine in the developing countries under the present circumstances would be for the ACIP to approve a 'permissive recommendation', thus validating the concept that children in the developing countries are on an equal footing to their counterparts in the USA. With a permissive recommendation the rotavirus vaccine could be evaluated in double-blind placebo-controlled trials in both the USA and the developing countries, and we could finally have an answer regarding the true risk, if any, of this vaccine.

Other rotavirus vaccines

A presentation on rotavirus vaccines would not be complete if it did not consider the prospects for other rotavirus vaccines that may fill the void left by the withdrawal of the rhesus rotavirus-based vaccine. Table 2 summarizes the status of the various rotavirus vaccines that have been evaluated in efficacy trials in infants and young children. Evaluation of monovalent bovine or rhesus rotavirus vaccine has been discontinued because of the variable efficacy of these immunogens. The quadrivalent WC3 bovine rotavirus-based reassortant vaccine with G1, G2, G3 and P1A[8] specificity is undergoing active field testing. A quadrivalent UK bovine rotavirus-based reassortant vaccine with G1, G2, G3 and G4 specificity is 'on hold' pending developments with its counterpart rhesus rotavirus tetravalent vaccine. A monovalent attenuated human rotavirus G1 vaccine is under active clinical evaluation. As shown in Table 3, various other vaccine candidates have been evaluated in phase 1 safety and immunogenicity studies. Some of these vaccine candidates are no longer under development, others are in active development or 'on hold'.

Conclusion

Although the list of vaccines under evaluation includes several promising candidates, there is no certainty that any of them will be immune to the difficulties encountered by the rhesus rotavirus-based reassortant vaccine. It is estimated that it will take 4–7 years before a new rotavirus vaccine could be licensed, even if shown to be safe and effective. Tragically and lamentably, during this interval about 4 million infants and young children will die from rotavirus diarrhoea. For this reason, it is imperative that risk/benefit decisions relating to the currently licensed rotavirus vaccine be made as soon as possible, so that public health authorities can make informed decisions regarding its use.

TABLE 3 Candidate oral rotavirus (RV) vaccines in phase I–II safety and immunogenicity trials in infants and young children

Venue	Vaccine	Serotype [Genotype] Composition		Status
Jennerian approach				
Lanzhou, China	Lamb Rotavirus (LLR)	G10, P[12]	Monovalent	Active
Modified Jennerian approach				
Bethesda, USA	HRV (Wa) × BRV, (UK) Reassortant	P1A; G6	Monovalent	Active
Bethesda, USA	HRV (Wa × DS-1) × BRV (UK), Reassortant	P1A, G2	Monovalent	Active
Philadelphia, USA	HRV (WI 79 4+9) × BRV (WC3), Reassortant	P1A; G1	Monovalent	Discontinued
Non-Jennerian approach				
Philadelphia, USA	HRV-WI78	G3; P[8]	Monovalent	Discontinued
Philadelphia, USA	HRV-30° cold-adapted WI78	G3; P[8]	Monovalent	Discontinued
Philadelphia, USA	HRV-WI61	G9; P1A[8]	Monovalent	Discontinued
Philadelphia, USA	HRV-30° cold-adapted WI61	G9; P1A[8]	Monovalent	Discontinued
Bethesda, USA	HRV-30° cold-adapted D	G1; P1A[8]	Monovalent	Active
Parkville, Australia	HRV-neonatal RV3	G3; P[6]	Monovalent	Active

Other approaches not in human trials include: synthetic viral proteins; viral proteins expressed by cloned rotavirus DNA; empty capsids expressed by a baculovirus recombinant; synthetic peptides; DNA vaccines; and an inactivated G1 P[4] strain (AU64) for parenteral administration.
References: Clark et al (1996); Offit et al (1997); Bresee et al (1999); Hoshino & Kapikian (2000); World Health Organization (2000).

References

ACIP 1999 Transcript of Advisory Committee on Immunization Practices (ACIP) Meeting at CDC, October 22, 1999. N. Lee and Associates, Certified Court Reporters, Atlanta GA, vol 3, p 1–174

Bresee JS, Glass RI, Ivanoff B, Gentsch JR 1999 Current status and future priorities for rotavirus vaccine development, evaluation and implementation in developing countries. Vaccine 17:2207–2222

CDC 1999a Rotavirus vaccine for the prevention of rotavirus gastroenteritis among children. Recommendations of the Advisory Committee on Immunization Practices (ACIP). Morb Mortal Wkly Rep 48:1–23

CDC 1999b Intussusception among recipients of rotavirus vaccine—United States, 1998–1999. Morb Mortal Wkly Rep 48:577–581

CDC 1999c Withdrawal of rotavirus vaccine recommendation. Morb Mortal Wkly Rep 48:1007

Clark HF, Offit PA, Ellis RW et al 1996 WC3 reassortant vaccines in children. Arch Virol Suppl 12:187–198

Clements ML, Makhene MK, Mrukowicz et al 1999 Safety and immunogenicity of live attenuated human-bovine (UK) reassortant rotavirus vaccines with VP7—specificity for serotypes 1, 2, 3 or 4 in adults, children and infants. Vaccine 17:2715–2725

Glass RI, Gentsch J, Smith JC 1994 Rotavirus Vaccines: success by reassortment? Science 265:1389–1391

Hellems MA, Waggoner-Fountain L, Borowitz SM 2000 Association between intussusception and rotavirus gastroenteritis. Pediatric Res Program Issue 2000:1562 (abstr)

Hoshino Y, Kapikian AZ 2000 Rotavirus serotypes: classification and importance in epidemiology, immunity and vaccine development J Health Popul Nutr 18:5–14

Joensuu J, Koskenniemi E, Pang XL, Vesikari T 1997 Randomised placebo-controlled trial of rhesus-human reassortant rotavirus vaccine for prevention of severe rotavirus gastroenteritis. Lancet 350:1205–1209

Kapikian AZ, Chanock RM 1996 Rotaviruses. In: Fields BN, Knipe DM, Howley PM et al (eds) Fields Virology, 3rd edn. Lippincott-Raven, Philadelphia, PA, p1657–1708

Kapikian AZ, Hoshino Y, Chanock RM, Pérez-Schael I 1996 Efficacy of a quadrivalent rhesus rotavirus-based human rotavirus vaccine aimed at preventing severe rotavirus diarrhea in infants and young children. J Infect Dis 174:S65–S72

Katsushima N 1981 Epidemiology, clinical features and diagnosis of intussusception (in Japanese). Jap J Pediatr Surg 13:563–570

Konno T, Suzuki H, Kutsuzawa T et al 1978 Human rotavirus infection in infants and young children with intussusception. J Med Virol 2:265–269

Matson 1996 Protective immunity against group A rotavirus infection and illness in infants. Arch Virol Suppl 12:129–139

Midthun K, Kapikian AZ 1996 Rotavirus vaccines: an overview. Clin Microbiol Rev J 9: 423–434

Midthun K, Greenberg HB, Hoshino Y, Kapikian AZ, Wyatt RG, Chanock RM 1985 Reassortant rotaviruses as potential live rotavirus vaccine candidates. J Virol 53:949–954

Midthun K, Hoshino Y, Kapikian AZ, Chanock RM 1986 Single gene substitution rotavirus reassortants containing the major neutralization protein (VP7) of human rotavirus serotype 4. J Clin Microbiol 24:822–826

Mulcahy DL, Kamath KR, de Silva LM, Hodges S, Carter IW, Cloonan MJ 1982 A two-part study of the aetiological role in intussusception. J Med Virol 9:51–55

Nicolas JC, Ingrand D, Fortier B, Bricout F 1982 A one-year virological survey of acute intussusception in childhood. J Med Virol 9:267–271

Offit PA 1994 Immunologic determinants of protection against rotavirus disease. Curr Top Microbiol Immunol 185:229–254

Offit PA, Clark HF, Kapikian AZ 1997 Vaccines against rotavirus. In: Levine MM, Woodrow GC, Kaper JB, Cobon GS (eds) New Generation Vaccines, 2nd edn. Marcel Dekker, New York, p 659–671

Pérez-Schael I, Guntiñas MJ, Pérez M et al 1997 Efficacy of the rhesus rotavirus-based quadrivalent vaccine in infants and young children in Venezuela. N Engl J Med 337: 1181–1187 (erratum: 1998 N Engl J Med 2:1002)

Rennels MB, Glass RI, Dennehy PH et al 1996 Safety and efficacy of high-dose rhesus-human reassortant rotavirus vaccines—report of the National Multicenter trial. United States Rotavirus Vaccine Efficacy Group. Pediatrics 97:7–13

Rennels MB, Parashar UD, Holman RC, Le CT, Chang HG, Glass RI 1998 Lack of an apparent association between intussusception and wild or vaccine rotavirus infection. Pediatr Infect Dis J 17:924–925

Santosham M, Moulton LH, Reid R et al 1997 Efficacy and safety of high-dose rhesus-human reassortant rotavirus vaccine in Native American populations. J Pediatr 131:632–638

Staatz G, Alzen G, Heimann G 1998 Intestinal infection, the most frequent cause of invagination in childhood: results of a 10-year clinical study (in German). Klin Paediatr 210:61–64

Vesikari T 1996 Trials of oral bovine rhesus rotavirus vaccines in Finland: a historical account and present status. Arch Virol Suppl 12:177–186

World Health Organization 2000 Report of the meeting on future directions for rotavirus vaccine research in developing countries, Geneva 9–11 February 2000 p 1–62

DISCUSSION

Vesikari: I wanted to share some data on the viral aetiology of diarrhoea, which are relevant to the question of whether the rotavirus vaccine is needed. We have data from a cohort of 1200 children that we are following to the age of 2 years (Fig. 1 [*Vesikari*]). 764 episodes of gastroenteritis were detected during this follow-up and were searched for all gastroenteritis viruses by PCR. We scored the episodes using the traditional 20 point score (Pang et al 2000). Approximately 60% of the episodes were mild. In this group, we have a miscellaneous collection of viruses but most of the episodes remain aetiologically unresolved. On the other hand, we may not really need to resolve them, because these are not significant illnesses; the children will not see a doctor. Also, because the threshold for detection of a case was low, we were probably also detecting other childhood diseases which are associated with either diarrhoea or some vomiting. The picture changes completely when we go to a score of 8 or higher, which is moderately severe to severe gastroenteritis. About 40% of the episodes fell into this category. This is the same score that was used in the US rotavirus vaccine studies as a definition of moderately severe disease. Here rotavirus is responsible for 42% of episodes, and a little bit more where it is associated with co-infection with other viruses. There are two points here. First, human caliciviruses are an important group of aetiological agents in the moderately severe category. These children may or may not see a doctor. Second, only 20% of the episodes in this category remain unresolved.

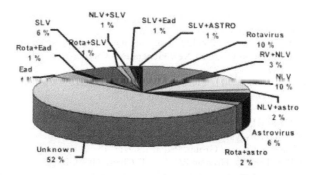

Mild episodes (Score <7, *n* = 481)

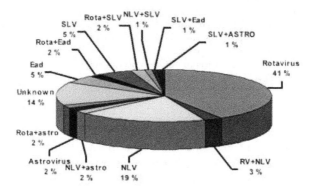

Moderately severe and severe episodes (Score ≥ 8, *n* = 335)

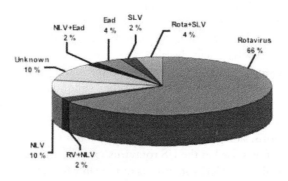

Very severe episodes (Score 1 4, *n* = 56)

FIG. 1.   *(Vesikari)* Distribution of viral findings according to severity score of gastroenteritis episodes.

Finally, I would like to show the really severe episodes, which represent the top 10% of all gastroenteritis cases we saw. These are children who are likely to end up in hospital; if they don't, they should. In this category we can find a virus in virtually all of the cases. Rotavirus is responsible for 72%. We still have some caliciviruses and enteric adenoviruses.

Is there anything that we could do to improve the detection rate still beyond this into the unknown category? I don't think we have to presume totally unknown viruses. The causative agents are probably among those that we already looked for. I suspect that one of the culprits is enteric adenoviruses: we are not detecting them all and we have some evidence that by using a combination of primers we can detect more. There is a hope that we can narrow the aetiological void still further, and that there won't be much room left for novel gastroenteritis viruses as aetiological agents in human gastroenteritis.

Greenberg: Is the attributable risk from the managed care facilities of about 1 in 12 000 excess cases per year after being vaccinated?

Kapikian: Yes, this is the most recent figure that the CDC has calculated from an expanded cohort study of participants enrolled in 10 managed care organizations.

Offit: As a member of the ACIP, I would love to be able to go back to them and convince them to use this vaccine. Here is what I need from this group to help me convince them. Let us say that we use your lowest attributable risk of 1 in 12 274, with a birth cohort of roughly 4 million this would mean potentially at least 320 excess cases of intussusception per year with a universal recommendation. In the USA, roughly 55 000 children are hospitalized with severe gastroenteritis. So we are comparing 55 000 versus 320 hospitalizations, 20–40 deaths versus say 4 deaths. There are some assumptions here that are probably false: we assume that all deaths would be preventable by vaccination, and ignore the fact that now we are aware of intussusception, deaths are less likely to occur from this. The best way to compel people to still give this vaccine — and I think that it is going to have to be given in the USA if it is going to be given in developing countries — is to convince people that it is safe, with safety being defined as the benefits clearly outweighing the risks. The most compelling way to do this is not going to be with these data. Any upper middle class parent is not going to want their child to take this vaccine because of intussusception. I don't think the members of the ACIP are going to give a permissive recommendation if they are not going to give it to their own children. Rotashield was withdrawn from the market in July of 1999. We have a year's worth of information. If you can show that there is a decrease in the rate of intussusception because the child was vaccinated, which I think is a decent formal way of proving that natural infection does cause intussusception, and therefore vaccination prevents it, this would be the most compelling set of data to convince people that the benefit outweighs the risk. I would argue very strongly before June 20th that we should do whatever we can do to make that information available. The way it looks now, this is not going to happen.

Kapikian: The increased risk during the first week after the first dose appears to be significant and deserves further evaluation. Is it possible that the vaccine had a triggering effect in an infant who would have developed intussusception later if they had not been vaccinated? It should also be noted that the package insert notes intussusception as a possible adverse reaction. Is it possible that some of those early cases resulted from recall or reporting bias? For example, a mother calls the paediatrician and says that her child is having abdominal complaints, the paediatrician says that since the child had rotavirus vaccine three days ago, she should bring the child in for further evaluation. An X-ray suggests to the paediatrician that it is intussusception. Another mother calls her paediatrician with the same complaint. Because the paediatrician didn't vaccinate this child, he suggests watchful waiting to see if the condition will improve. These are scenarios we can only speculate about at this time. The only way to answer this issue would be in a double-blind placebo-controlled study, which may no longer be possible.

Offit: If we can get those data before June that is helpful, or if anyone can provide me with some other piece of information that convinces this group that makes decisions about vaccines in our country that the benefits of Rotashield clearly outweigh its risks, I would love to hear it.

Matson: I think that the June meeting is too soon. That date is simply asking people to crush data that need to be cleaned up. The October meeting might be the better time. With regard to the issue about the upper- and middle-class mother who says that her child doesn't die from intussusception, that child also won't die from diarrhoea. The risk factors for mortality occur in a different population than the risk factors for intussusception in the USA.

Glass: One thing that has come from all of these studies, whether they are biased or not, is that there is an excess risk in the week after immunization with the first dose of Rotashield. Regardless of what the attributable risk is, the relationship is present.

Greenberg: There is a spectrum of 'informedness' about this issue. Our colleagues from Europe are probably as not yet fully on top of the issue. I simply want to say that as you try to think this through, the USA, like any country, is complicated. There is the FDA that has the legal power to licence and unlicence; there is the ACIP which is an advisory committee that consists of a group of experts in the area of vaccines; and there is the CDC that is doing the epidemiological analysis. Paul asked a question for the ACIP group of experts, what should we do? Everyone listens to what they say. I am an FDA advisor, but I am not on the ACIP committee. My feeling is that you can only deal with the data provided, but the ACIP did not, in its initial discussion, present to the public a process of how to weigh the problem in terms of risk and benefit. They simply said that there was a risk and that the risk seemed unacceptable. They didn't discuss in detail the potential benefit also. If we can't figure out the benefit, we can't make an informed decision. The US public may decide that if there is a risk, they do not care about the benefit. This is a public decision. But they have to be presented with the data about the potential benefits as well as the risks, and how one goes about weighing these two factors.

Offit: Your point is excellent, in that we lost an opportunity in the ACIP in discussing issues of risk–benefit. For this or any vaccine, that is the point: do the benefits clearly outweigh any potential risk? In defence of the ACIP, two things happened. One is that the vaccine was withdrawn by the company two days before we met, so to some extent it was a *fait accompli*. Secondly, the antivaccine groups sit in that meeting and are very vociferous. People are scared to have the discussion that they should have. I agree with you, we should have this vaccine if it is what is best for children in our country.

Desselberger: We saw that various calculations lead to different results in assessing the risks. But you pointed out clearly that the clustering of cases after the first dose of the vaccine is significant and has to be looked at in respect of all the other factors. What has been done further with these 56 intussusception cases in terms of trying to analyse what is going on? There is an epidemiological suspicion of association with the vaccine. About 20% of the cases have been operated on. What do the surgical resection specimens look like? Have they been investigated by ELISA, RT-PCR or immunofluorescence?

Kapikian: This is in progress, and can be answered better by Roger Glass, since the CDC is coordinating this activity.

Glass: The epidemiological investigation is being handled by the National Immunization Program at CDC. This has been one of the largest adverse event investigations they have ever conducted, covering 19 states with lots of analyses. We are in the process of trying to get the pathology tissue from some of those patients who had surgery. This has been very slow, because we have had to go back and get informed consent.

Desselberger: Paul Offit made some interesting comments at the WHO meeting in February 2000 that there might be some link between this event early after the first infection and viral replication. It is certainly worth looking at this.

Offit: I'd like to add to the comments that I made at the WHO meeting. Three to seven days is certainly when one sees replication, but it is not clear that natural infection causes intussusception — it may, but if it does, it doesn't do it at a high and obvious rate. Yet in natural infection of children with human rotavirus, the virus replicates very well. When you look at the simian viruses — the rhesus × human reassortants — these viruses replicate much less well, and clearly cause intussusception at a low but reproducible rate. There was a case of intussusception in the WC3 × human reassortant in Finland. This was in a 7 month old child who got a vaccine. Stools at days 3 and 5 and biopsy material at the time of surgery didn't show any evidence for virus. Initially this was somewhat surprising, but there is a very compelling animal model of transient intussusception in mice that are parenterally inoculated with lipopolysaccharide. What is compelling about this is that one can see this transient intussusception occurring in the absence in inflammation and a clear lead point. It is also an intussusception that can be modified by giving agents that decrease the effects of cytokines. One could argue, then, that there is something about immunization — whether it is with polio virus, simian × human rotavirus reassortants or with bovine × human rotavirus reassortants — where one gives a lot of virus at one time and it is taken up in a site or processed by an antigen-presenting cell (APC) type that is different from that which occurs after natural infection. It is associated with a profile of cytokines that causes this increase in motility and the subsequent intussusception event. One could even argue that there would be a preventive strategy where one could give an anticytokine-specific agent and prevent this. If it is true that any oral bolus of a lot of virus causes intussusception and is prohibited for use as a vaccine, this doesn't bode well for rotavirus vaccines. It is hard to prime the intestine by a non-mucosal route. I hope we can get around this.

Vesikari: I want to comment on the cases of intussusception that we have seen in Finland. The first one was associated with the Rotashield vaccine, and the question in retrospect is could the subsequent events in the USA have been predicted from our experience? I always have an uneasy feeling when I look at the table compiled by Rennels and others, because it puts together cases from very different studies (Rennels et al 1998). In our series we had one case in 1191 children in the vaccine group, and one case in 1207 children in the placebo group. Thus the two populations were very comparable. The one case in the vaccine group had intussusception six days after the third dose, given at the age of 5 months, and the placebo case was 44 days after the second dose. We reported that this was possibly associated, but because there was the other case in the placebo group, the external safety monitor group said it was all right.

Intussusception can happen with other vaccines. We have had one case of intussusception in a child who received a WC3-based reassortant vaccine. It was a 7 month old child, 8 days after the first dose, out of about 1600 who received the vaccine in Finland. We had another case in a UK-based bovine reassortant vaccine recipient, which was a five month old child six days after administration. In these more recent studies, we are giving the vaccine to children at this age, because the rhesus-based rotavirus vaccine cannot be given to such children due to a high febrile reaction rate. We thought that with the use of the bovine vaccine strains we could extend rotavirus vaccination to older children. However, it turns out that this approach may also run into problems, because 6–9 months is the peak age of naturally occurring intussusception. The children are susceptible to developing intussusception, whether this is due to another virus or the rotavirus vaccine — the two can even coincide, and it is difficult to rule out one or the other. The response to this situation has been that anyone who is contemplating a new candidate vaccine has moved down with the age of vaccination. In the future vaccine studies, the first dose is about to be given at the age of six weeks. One reason might be that this age fits with the EPI schedule, but the real reason is to avoid intussusception. Probably the safest way would be to give rotavirus vaccine to neonates. The reason why such studies are not being conducted is because neonatal immunization is not part of the US immunization schedule.

Arias: Are there any data about the rate of intussusception in developing countries?

Kapikian: The incidence of intussusception in developing countries was discussed at the WHO meeting on rotavirus vaccines in Geneva in February 2000. Although the rates seemed to be characteristically lower in developing countries than in developed countries, it appeared that the issue needed to be studied further to exclude the possibility of incomplete reporting of cases.

Glass: We have tried to look at the intussusception rates in developing countries, and we don't have population-based data. We have two experiences which are quite contrasting. One is that in Dehli, where Dr M. K. Bhan at PIIMs looked at the largest hospitals in the city. In the last five years, they have had very few cases of intussusception, so it is rare. In Ho Chi Min City in Vietnam, Dr Ngoun takes care of two cases per day, which is several hundred a year from a huge area. The rates seem to differ greatly. This could all be irrelevant: one of the great discoveries that Al Kapikian's vaccine has made is that the approach of using a live oral vaccine really works well and can protect children from subsequent severe disease. Even with a low rate of intussusception, it could be a life-saver in these other countries.

Kapikian: Unfortunately, a recommendation for evaluation of the rotavirus vaccine in developing countries may turn out to be merely a Pyrrhic victory because the vaccine will not be used in developing countries as long as it is not recommended in the USA. It is a tragedy that every day about 2000 infants and young children die from rotavirus diarrhoea in the developing countries. It will be another 4–7 years before another rotavirus vaccine becomes available for licensure, and there is no guarantee that this vaccine will not have a similar problem. In the meantime, about 4 million children will have died. Wyeth-Lederle, the producers of the rotavirus vaccine have indicated that they would consider staying in the business of making the vaccine if three conditions were met: (1) WHO recommends use of the vaccine; (2) the attributable risk becomes rarefied; and (3) the ACIP would at a minimum grant a permissive licence for its use. If a permissive licence is not granted in the USA, I do not believe that developing countries will use the vaccine.

Pollok: Is there pathological evidence that rotavirus infection is associated with Peyer's patch hypertrophy? This is critical: is it an association or is there a causal link?

Greenberg: There are not enough data. It is anecdotal.

Koopmans: Laying aside the issue of the risk of intussusception, in the USA there may be a consensus that it is useful to vaccinate every child for rotavirus, but this discussion is still being held in Europe. In The Netherlands the issue is not so much one of informing the public: rather, the paediatricians are not all convinced that we need to vaccinate against rotavirus.

Estes: I have one other point I would like to raise about intussusception. One of the things that is most interesting to me about this story is the fact that a virus that is clearly associated with intussusception is respiratory adenovirus, and not the enteric adenovirus. Why does the enteric virus not seem to be associated? Barbara Coulson's papers describe integrins as the rotavirus receptor, and the receptor that is clearly identified for the respiratory adenovirus is an integrin (Coulson et al 1997, Hewish et al 2000). There has been some discussion that perhaps these integrins are found in the intestine in the region of the ileal–caecal junction. I don't know whether there is any connection here, but it is interesting to think about this.

Greenberg: I think the receptor for the respiratory adenovirus is also the receptor for some of the enteroviruses. This receptor is more broadly used in the enteric environment than just for those adenoviruses.

Prasad: It is also the receptor for foot-and-mouth disease virus.

Glass: One of the other differences with the adenoviruses is that pathologists tell us that the adenovirus inclusions in the mesenteric lymph nodes are longer and more well defined. This provides a nice leading edge from which intussusception can occur. This is the only one that is well defined besides polyps.

Estes: Intussusception is a very important clinical problem for children. Paediatric surgeons say that this is the most important problem that they deal with. How people resolve it is very different in different countries and even in different cities in the USA. In some cities it is resolved by the radiologists; in other cities, particularly in today's litigious environment, the children always go to surgery. This is one area where we as virologists might consider interacting with the physicians in our institutions to see whether we can help resolve this difficulty in children, regardless of its association or not with the rotavirus vaccine.

References

Coulson BS, Londrigan SL, Lee DJ 1997 Rotavirus contains integrin ligand sequences and a disintegrin-like domain that are implicated in virus entry into cells. Proc Natl Acad Sci USA 94:5389–5394
Hewish MJ, Takada Y, Coulson BS 2000 Integrins $\alpha2\beta1$ and $\alpha4\beta1$ can mediate SA11 rotavirus attachment and entry into cells. J Virol 74:228–236

Pang X-L, Honma S, Nakata S, Vesikari T 2000 Human caliciviruses in acute gastroenteritis of young children in the community. J Infect Dis 181:S288–S294

Rennels MB, Parashar UD, Holman RC, Le CT, Chang HG, Glass RI 1998 Lack of an apparent association between intussusception and wild or vaccine rotavirus infection. Pediatr Infect Dis J 17:924–925

Novartis 238: Gastroenteritis Viruses.
Copyright © 2001 John Wiley & Sons Ltd
Print ISBN 0-471-49663-4 eISBN 0-470-84653-4

The molecular biology of human caliciviruses

Ian N. Clarke and Paul R. Lambden

Virus Group, Mailpoint 814, Division of Cell and Molecular Medicine, University of Southampton Medical School, Southampton SO16 6YD, UK

Abstract. Within the last decade molecular analyses of the genome of Norwalk-like viruses (NLVs) have confirmed that this important group of infectious agents belongs to the *Caliciviridae* family. NLVs have a positive-sense, single-stranded RNA genome of approximately 7700 nucleotides excluding the polyadenylated tail. The genome encodes three open reading frames: ORF 1 is the largest (~ 1700 amino acids) and is expressed as a polyprotein precursor that is cleaved by the viral 3C-like protease; ORF 2 encodes the viral capsid (550 amino acids); and ORF 3 encodes a small basic protein of unknown function. Comparative sequencing studies of human caliciviruses have revealed a second distinct group of viruses known as Sapporo-like viruses (SLVs). SLVs also have a single-stranded, positive-sense RNA genome of approximately 7400 nucleotides and the small 3′ terminal ORF (NLV-ORF3 equivalent) is retained. Phylogenetic analyses of NLV and SLV genomic sequences have assigned these viruses to two different genera with each genus comprised of two distinct genogroups. The fundamental difference in genome organization between NLVs and SLVs is that the polyprotein and capsid ORFs are contiguous and fused in SLVs. Progress in understanding the molecular biology of human caliciviruses is hampered by the lack of a cell culture system for virus propagation. Studies on viral replication and virion structure have therefore relied on the expression of recombinant virus proteins in heterologous systems. Norwalk virus capsid expressed in insect cells assembles to form virus-like particles (VLPs). Structural studies have shown that Norwalk virus VLPs are comprised of 90 dimers of the capsid protein.

2001 Gastroenteritis viruses. Wiley, Chichester (Novartis Foundation Symposium 238) p 180–196

Caliciviruses

The application of electron microscopy to the examination of stool samples from patients with diarrhoeal disease resulted in the discovery of the viruses associated with gastroenteritis. Whilst rotaviruses and enteric adenoviruses have obvious and distinguishable morphological features there was considerable confusion about the role of 'small round viruses' found in stool samples from patients with non-bacterial gastroenteritis. An interim classification scheme described in 1982

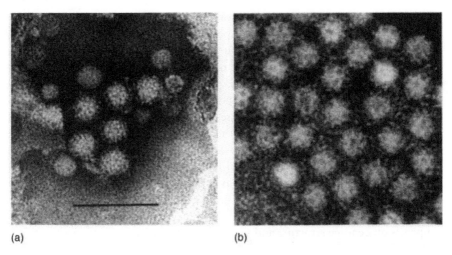

(a)   (b)

FIG. 1.   Electron microscopic appearance of (a) NLVs and (b) SLVs. NLVs have a ragged edge
and amorphous structure whereas SLVs display the classic cup-shaped morphology from which
caliciviruses derive their name. Scale bar = 100 nm. (Fig. 1a courtesy of Mr P. Pead, Fig. 1b
reproduced courtesy of Mrs B. Cosgrove and Prof R. Madeley.)

allowed the clear differentiation of these viruses (Caul & Appleton 1982). In this
scheme two distinctive morphological groups of human viruses (now known to be
caliciviruses), both approximately 30–35 nm in diameter were recognized. The
small round structured viruses (currently known as 'Norwalk-like viruses' or
NLVs) have an amorphous structure with a ragged outer edge (Fig. 1a) and the
'classic' caliciviruses ('Sapporo-like viruses' or SLVs) display the true cup-shaped
structures from which the calicivirus family derives its name (Fig. 1b). SLV
infections are rarely diagnosed and are usually found in symptomatic young
children whereas NLV infections are common in all age groups.

Caliciviruses possess a single-stranded, positive-sense RNA genome
approximately 7400–7800 nucleotides in length (excluding the polyadenylate
tail). Calicivirus genomes have a characteristic arrangement of their open reading
frames (ORFs) that clearly distinguishes them from the genomes of picornaviruses
(Clarke & Lambden 1997). The 5′ region of the genome encodes a large non-
structural polyprotein that precedes a single viral capsid protein ORF. At the 3′
terminus of the genome there is a small ORF that encodes a basic protein.
Calicivirus replication can be distinguished from picornavirus replication by the
production of a subgenomic RNA species that serves as the main template for the
synthesis of the capsid protein.

Phylogenetic analysis of genome sequences has divided the calicivirus family
into four distinct genera (Green et al 2000). These genera map with some of the

biological properties of the viruses: for example, caliciviruses have long been associated with veterinary diseases especially involving marine mammals and respiratory infections of cats (*Vesivirus* genus) and more recently with hepatic diseases in lagomorphs (*Lagovirus* genus). However, viruses naturally infecting humans are found only in two of the genera: the NLVs and the SLVs. These generic names are themselves only temporary until more suitable and appropriate terms can be derived. Very little progress was made in the study of the human viruses until the early 1990s because they cannot be grown in cell culture and there is no reliable animal model. The application of modern molecular techniques to study virus genome structure and organisation has led to the production of new reagents that have provided further insights into the molecular biology of these viruses. Our aim is to review the most important advances in the molecular biology of the human caliciviruses with particular emphasis on genome structure and virus gene expression.

Norwalk-like viruses

The prototype virus for this genus is the Norwalk virus (NV), the first human virus to be described with an aetiological association with non-bacterial gastroenteritis (Kapikian et al 1972). The NV was the cause of an outbreak of gastroenteritis amongst adults and children in an elementary school in Norwalk, Ohio, USA. NV was visualized in human stool samples by immune electron microscopy using convalescent serum from a volunteer who had been experimentally infected with a faecal filtrate from the original outbreak. Subsequently other morphologically indistinguishable viruses have been described from similar outbreaks. The low numbers of virus particles shed during infection and the lack of a cell culture system has made it very difficult to characterize the Norwalk and related viruses. Early studies relied on the use of volunteers to produce enough virus for biochemical analysis. The NV has a buoyant density of 1.38–1.41 g/cm^3 and a single capsid protein of 60 kDa (Greenberg et al 1981). Major advances came with the description of the NV genome (Jiang et al 1990) and the sequence of some small genome fragments (Jiang et al 1993, Matsui et al 1991). This work showed that the NV genome is comprised of positive-sense, single-stranded RNA approximately 7.5 kb in length with a 3′ polyadenylated tail. Complete genome sequences of NV and another related virus, Southampton virus (SV) soon followed (Jiang et al 1993, Lambden et al 1993). The genome organisation of these viruses (5′ region encoding a large non-structural polyprotein, preceding a single viral capsid protein ORF and a small ORF encoding a basic protein at the 3′ terminus of the genome) confirmed that the NLVs should be classified within the *Caliciviridae*. The availability of these genome sequences made it possible to develop primer sets for the further investigation of the nature and extent of sequence diversity amongst the NLVs. Sequence comparisons showed that the viruses could be divided further into two genetic groupings or genogroups (Lew et al 1994) with SV and NV belonging to genogroup 1. Complete genome sequences are available for the following genogroup 2 viruses, Lordsdale (LV; Dingle et al 1995), Camberwell (CV; Seah et al 1999) and Hawaii virus (K. Green, personal communication). A generalized genome map for the NLVs is shown in Fig. 2.

ORF1/polyprotein processing

Alignment of the nucleotide sequences from the 5′ region of ORF1 showed significant divergence between viruses from the two genogroups (Dingle et al 1995). Whilst the initiation codon for ORF1 has not been defined in the NLVs, comparison of the 'N-terminal' 150 amino acids also showed little amino acid sequence identity. Beginning at the first in frame AUG, ORF1 encodes a polyprotein of approximately 200 kDa containing motifs for 2C-like NTPase, 3C-like protease and 3D-like RNA-dependent RNA polymerase (Lambden & Clarke 1995). Because NLVs cannot be grown in cell culture, studies of polyprotein processing have been based on transcription/translation of RNA generated from cDNA clones, expression of the polyprotein in *Escherichia coli* and transfection of mammalian cells with cDNA. In these systems genogroup 1 (SV) and genogroup 2 (CV and LV) polyproteins undergo similar proteolytic cleavages (Liu et al 1996, 1999a, Seah et al 1999). Cleavage by the 3C-like protease occurs in *cis* at five specific sites liberating six defined polypeptides. The kinetics and order of cleavage have yet to be determined although preliminary work also suggests that the SV 3C-like protease has activity in *trans*. By analogy with animal caliciviruses further assignment of the biological functions of the cleavage products has been possible: the 3B fragment is thought to be the viral genome linked protein (VPg).

Capsid

Immunoprecipitation of radiolabelled gradient-purified NV with acute and convalescent sera indicated that these viruses were comprised of a single major capsid protein with a molecular weight of 59 kDa (Greenberg et al 1981). Later studies with the Snow Mountain agent confirmed this observation (Madore et al 1986). A major breakthrough in studying the NLVs came with the discovery that expression of NV ORF2 in insect cells using a recombinant baculovirus led to the export of the capsid protein to the cell culture supernatant where it self-assembles to form virus-like particles (VLPs) (Jiang et al 1995). The VLPs appeared as 'empty' virions when viewed by negative-stain electron microscopy but were

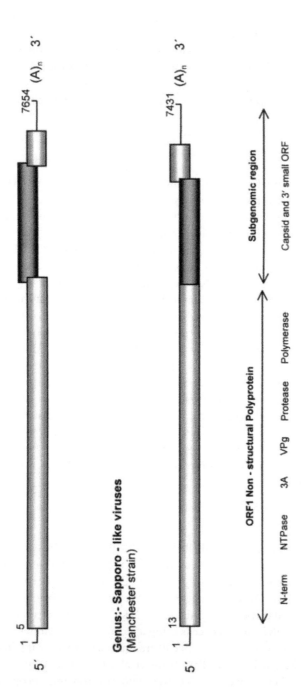

FIG. 2. Diagrammatic representation of the organization of ORFs in the two genera of human enteric caliciviruses. The 5' region of the genome encodes the viral non-structural proteins as part of a larger polyprotein precursor. The 3' region (subgenomic region) of the genome encodes the viral capsid structural protein and a 3'-terminal small basic protein of unknown function.

otherwise antigenically indistinguishable from NV particles (Green et al 1993). Subsequently ORF2 has been expressed in insect cells as VLPs from a number of different NLVs (both genogroup 1 and genogroup 2). NV VLPs also occur when ORF2 is expressed in transgenic potatoes and tobacco — these products could have the potential to form the basis of a new oral vaccine (Mason et al 1996). By contrast expression of the capsid protein in mammalian cells does not result in the formation of VLPs (Pletneva et al 1998). VLPs are now available as an abundant source of antigen which has been used to study the seroprevalence of NLV infections (Gray et al 1993) as well as used to generate specific antisera for use in antigen detection ELISAs (Graham et al 1994).

3′ terminal ORF

All caliciviruses possess a short ORF located towards the 3′ terminus of their genome. In the NLVs this ORF is termed ORF3 and the predicted protein product is basic in structure but has no significant homologies to other proteins within the sequence databases. ORF3 is variable in size amongst the NLVs ranging from 211–268 amino acids. In genogroup 2 viruses the ORF is some 50 amino acids longer than its counterpart in genogroup 1 viruses. The conservation of this ORF in all NLVs strongly suggests that it has a functional biological role. Studies with the rabbit haemorrhagic disease virus (RHDV) have suggested that the 3′ terminal ORF may be a minor structural component of the virion (Wirblich et al 1996), however this protein is not seen to be associated with feline calicivirus (FCV) particles (Tohya et al 1999). In addition X-ray crystallographic studies with NV VLPs have not identified the ORF3 product as a structural entity in NV VLPs (Prasad et al 1999). The basic nature of the ORF3 product has also led to a suggestion that it may have a role in RNA binding (Neill et al 1991). However, in our laboratory we have been unable to detect the ORF3 product from faecal specimens positive for SV or LV.

Sapporo-like viruses

It is now clearly established that human enteric caliciviruses which display the classic surface structure have a fundamentally different genome organization to the NLVs (Liu et al 1995). They are also phylogenetically distinct from NLVs and have been assigned to a separate genus (Berke et al 1997, Noel et al 1997). The classic caliciviruses were first described in the UK (Madeley & Cosgrove 1976), but it was not until some years later that the prototype Sapporo virus was identified (Terashima et al 1983). The 'interim' classification system allowed differentiation of these viruses by their distinctive morphology but there are also important epidemiological differences (Caul & Appleton 1982). Infections are mainly found in children under 4 years of age suggesting that immunity develops early and is life-long. In contrast to the NLVs, infections caused by the SLVs are seldom associated with large outbreaks, diagnosis is by electron microscopy and positive specimens usually occur as single sporadic cases of gastroenteritis.

The first complete SLV sequence was determined for 'Manchester virus' (Liu et al 1995) with a genome length of 7431 nucleotides. The first open reading frame of Manchester virus starts at nucleotide 12 and contains the characteristic motifs of the 2C-like NTPase, 3C-like protease and RNA polymerase seen in the NLVs. However, the major difference between the genome of Manchester virus and the NLV genomes (Fig. 2) is that the capsid structural protein gene is in the same frame as ORF1 and is contiguous with the RNA-dependent RNA polymerase, giving rise to a single large polyprotein that covers most of the genome. This type of genomic organization is also found in the caliciviruses that infect lagomorphs (Clarke & Lambden 1997). Like all other caliciviruses the SLVs have repeated nucleotide sequence motifs located at the genome 5' terminus and at the start of the capsid open reading frame. Whilst SLVs cannot be grown in cell culture it is assumed that expression of the capsid protein can occur through two routes, either by cleavage from the polyprotein or by direct expression from a separate subgenomic RNA. Preliminary work using a full-length genomic clone of Manchester virus in an *in vitro* transcription/translation system has shown that the polyprotein undergoes proteolytic cleavage liberating the capsid protein.

Although no volunteer studies have been performed to regenerate SLVs for detailed biochemical studies, it has been possible to purify virions directly from stool samples for further characterization. These studies have shown that the Sapporo virions are comprised of a single major capsid protein of 62 kDa (Terashima et al 1983). Attempts to produce the capsid protein in heterologous expression systems have met with mixed fortunes. The Sapporo virus capsid protein is exported to the cell culture supernatant when expressed in insect cells using recombinant baculoviruses but formation of VLPs appears to be dependent on the length and nature of 5' leader sequences (Jiang et al 1999). In our hands expression of the Manchester virus capsid protein from a recombinant baculovirus produces abundant capsid protein in the cell culture supernatant but we have not been able to obtain VLPs.

Computer analysis of the Manchester virus genome sequence predicts a typical calicivirus short 3' terminal ORF of 165 amino acids. This is frame shifted -1 relative to main ORF (ORF1) and encodes a 17.8 kDa basic protein, hydrophilic in nature. A second short ORF (encoding 161 amino acids) is also predicted to overlap the capsid region of the genome but is in a different reading frame. This overlapping ORF is found in several SLV isolates but its significance remains unknown.

The availability of the genome sequence has led to the development of oligonucleotide primers for further amplification of related SLV sequences and

Norwalk like Viruses | **Sapporo like Viruses**

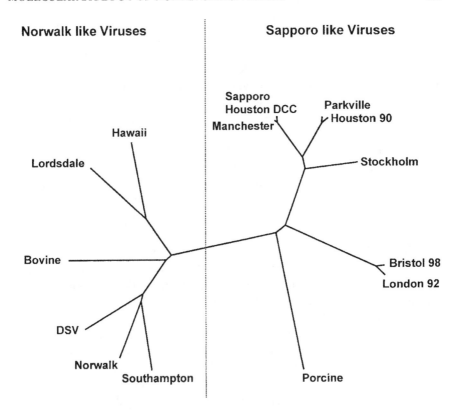

FIG. 3. An unrooted phylogenetic tree comparing the amino acid sequences of calicivirus structural capsid proteins. The tree shows the relationship of the 'Norwalk-like' calicivirus genus with the 'Sapporo-like' virus genus. Accession numbers (in parentheses) for caliciviruses are as follows: Manchester SLV (X86560), Houston DCC SLV (U95643), Parkville SLV (U73124), Houston 90 SLV (U95644), Stockholm (AF194182), Bristol 98 SLV (AJ249939), London/92 SLV (U95645), Porcine enteric calicivirus (AF182760), Southampton NLV (L07418), Norwalk virus (M87661), Desert Shield NLV (U04469), Bovine Jena virus (AJ011099), Lordsdale NLV (X86557), Hawaii NLV (U07611).

there are now a number of partial sequences available. Immune electron microscopical studies suggested that there are a number of SLV 'serotypes'. This observation has been supported by phylogenetic analysis of the accumulating SLV sequences (Berke et al 1997, Noel et al 1997). It is now clear that the human SLVs can also be divided into two discreet genogroups based on sequence comparison of both RNA polymerase and capsid regions of the genome (Fig. 3). Within these two genogroupings there are distinctive but clearly related 'types' of virus (e.g. Parkville, Houston/90).

Recent advances in virion and genome structure

A great deal of progress has been made in the molecular characterization of the human caliciviruses over the past decade. The aetiological role of NLVs as the primary cause of adult viral gastroenteritis is established, furthermore NLVs are now recognized as the major cause of food-borne viral gastroenteritis. One of the major obstacles to research is the lack of a cell culture system, which has driven researchers to investigate other caliciviruses to study as model systems. In particular feline calcivirus (FCV) has been the focus of much research because this virus grows well in CRFK cells. An infectious cDNA clone of FCV has been constructed (Sosnovtsev & Green 1995) and this has been used to investigate structure/function relationships in the FCV capsid (Neill et al 2000). Whilst FCV is a useful model for calicivirus replication this virus belongs to a different genus to the enteric viruses. Caliciviruses causing enteric disease in domestic animals have been known for a long time. However, the economic importance of enteric disease in animals caused by caliciviruses is not established. Recently genome sequences have become available for both bovine (Jena virus, JV) and porcine enteric caliciviruses (PEC). Interestingly these viruses are phylogenetically related to the human caliciviruses (Fig. 3).

The bovine enteric calicivirus genome (7338 nucleotides) has a similar organization to the NLVs with 3 separate open reading frames encoding polyprotein, capsid and ORF 3 (Liu et al 1999b). Sequence comparisons using both the RNA polymerase and capsid sequences have shown that the JV is most closely related to the genogroup 1 NLVs. In Japan, a study designed to survey for caliciviruses in swine using primers based on NLV sequences identified four unique amplicons (Sugieda et al 1998). Phylogenetic analysis showed these sequences to be most closely related to the NLV genogroup 2 viruses. These observations suggest that the animal and human 'NLVs' share a recent common ancestor and whilst there is currently no evidence for cross species infection by 'NLVs' there exists the possibility that there might be an animal reservoir for human infection.

The genome sequence of a PEC, PEC/Cowden (7320 nucleotides), associated with diarrhoea in pigs, has also recently been completed (Guo et al 1999). The PEC virus genome has two ORFs similar to the SLVs and lagoviruses. Incorporation of the intestinal contents of uninfected gnotobiotic piglets into the culture medium was necessary to adapt this virus to grow and it remains the only enteric calicivirus that has been adapted to growth in cell culture. It was thus possible to compare the nucleotide sequence differences between the cell culture-adapted virus and the wild-type virus. Only nine point mutations were observed and occurred across the coding regions of the genome with six mutations resulting in an amino acid change. Three of the substitutions were clustered within a seven amino acid region of the predicted hypervariable part of the capsid. The contribution of each of the mutations to adaptation of PEC to growth in cell culture has yet to be evaluated. Whilst phylogenetic analysis of the PEC genome places it with the SLVs it clearly belongs to a separate third genogroup (Vinjé et al 2000).

The structure of NV VLPs has been determined by cryoelectron microscopy and 3D image reconstruction. This study showed that the NV VLPs have T=3 icosahedral symmetry and that the virion is composed of 90 dimers of the capsid protein. Recently the detailed structure of NV VLPs has been determined at 3.2 Å resolution by X-ray crystallography (Prasad et al 1999). This elegant work combined with mutation analysis of the expressed capsid protein has provided new insights into the structure of the NV capsid. The capsid protein is comprised of a shell domain (S) joined by a flexible hinge to a protruding P domain. The P domain is further subdivided into two sub domains P1 and P2. Sub domain P2 has a fold like the domain 2 of the eukaryotic translation elongation factor EF-Tu and thus may have a role in regulating viral/cellular translation processes. Furthermore a monoclonal antibody to the P2 sub domain inhibits the binding of NV VLPs to cells suggesting this region may also have role in cell attachment.

Summary

Progress in the characterization of the human caliciviruses has been severely hampered by the lack of a cell culture system, the very low numbers of viruses shed during infection and the absence of a reliable animal model. Molecular characterization of the NV genome has opened a new era in our understanding of these fastidious viruses. The burgeoning number of sequences in the databases is providing a clearer picture of the nature and extent of diversity of these viruses. Application of recombinant DNA techniques has allowed a ready supply of capsid protein for developing immunoassays and expanding our understanding of the virion structure. The adaptation of animal viruses to growth in cell culture and the further development of infectious cDNA clones will serve as useful models for the development of culture systems for the human viruses.

References

Berke T, Golding B, Jiang X et al 1997 Phylogenetic analysis of the caliciviruses. J Med Virol 52:419–424
Caul EO, Appleton H 1982 The electron microscopical and physical characteristics of small round human fecal viruses: an interim scheme for classification. J Med Virol 9:257–265
Clarke IN, Lambden PR 1997 The molecular biology of caliciviruses. J Gen Virol 78:291–301
Dingle KE, Lambden PR, Caul EO, Clarke IN 1995 Human enteric *Caliciviridae*: the complete genome sequence and expression of virus-like particles from a genetic group II small round structured virus. J Gen Virol 76:2349–2355

Graham DY, Jiang X, Tanaka T, Opekun AR, Madore HP, Estes MK 1994 Norwalk virus infection of volunteers: new insights based on improved assays. J Infect Dis 170:34–43

Gray JJ, Jiang X, Morgan-Capner P, Desselberger U, Estes MK 1993 Prevalence of antibodies to Norwalk virus in England: detection by enzyme-linked immunosorbent assay using baculovirus-expressed Norwalk virus capsid antigen. J Clin Microbiol 31:1022–1025

Green KY, Lew JF, Jiang X, Kapikian AZ, Estes MK 1993 Comparison of the reactivities of baculovirus-expressed recombinant Norwalk virus capsid antigen with those of the native Norwalk virus antigen in serologic assays and some epidemiologic observations. J Clin Microbiol 31:2185–2191

Green KY, Ando T, Balayan MS et al 2000 Taxonomy of the caliciviruses. J Infect Dis 181: S322–S330

Greenberg HB, Valdesuso JR, Kalica AR et al 1981 Proteins of Norwalk virus. J Virol 37:994–999

Guo M, Chang KO, Hardy ME, Zhang O, Parwani AV, Saif LJ 1999 Molecular characterization of a porcine enteric calicivirus genetically related to Sapporo-like human caliciviruses. J Virol 73:9625–9631

Jiang X, Graham DY, Wang K, Estes MK 1990 Norwalk virus genome cloning and characterization. Science 250:1580–1583

Jiang X, Wang M, Wang K, Estes MK 1993 Sequence and genomic organization of Norwalk virus. Virology 195:51–61

Jiang X, Matson DO, Ruiz-Palacios GM, Hu J, Treanor J, Pickering LK 1995 Expression, self-assembly, and antigenicity of a Snow Mountain agent-like calicivirus capsid protein. J Clin Microbiol 33:1452–1455

Jiang X, Zhong WM, Kaplan M, Pickering LK, Matson DO 1999 Expression and characterization of Sapporo-like human calicivirus capsid proteins in baculovirus. J Virol Methods 78:81–91

Kapikian AZ, Wyatt RG, Dolin R, Thornhill TS, Kalica AR, Chanock RM 1972 Visualization by immune electron microscopy of a 27 nm particle associated with acute infectious nonbacterial gastroenteritis. J Virol 10:1075–1081

Lambden PR, Clarke IN 1995 Genome organization in the caliciviridae. Trends Microbiol 3:261–265

Lambden PR, Caul EO, Ashley CR, Clarke IN 1993 Sequence and genome organization of a human small round-structured (Norwalk-like) virus. Science 259:516–519

Lew JF, Kapikian AZ, Valdesuso J, Green KY 1994 Molecular characterization of Hawaii virus and other Norwalk-like viruses: evidence for genetic polymorphism among human caliciviruses. J Infect Dis 170:535–542

Liu BL, Clarke IN, Caul EO, Lambden PR 1995 Human enteric caliciviruses have a unique genome structure and are distinct from the Norwalk-like viruses. Arch Virol 140:1345–1356

Liu BL, Clarke IN, Lambden PR 1996 Polyprotein processing in Southampton virus: identification of 3C-like protease cleavage sites by in vitro mutagenesis. J Virol 70:2605–2610

Liu BL, Viljoen GJ, Clarke IN, Lambden PR 1999a Identification of further proteolytic cleavage sites in the Southampton calicivirus polyprotein by expression of the viral protease in E. coli. J Gen Virol 80:291–296

Liu BL, Lambden PR, Günther H, Otto P, Elschner M, Clarke IN 1999b Molecular characterization of a bovine enteric calicivirus: relationship to the Norwalk-like viruses. J Virol 73:819–825

Madeley CR, Cosgrove BP 1976 Caliciviruses in man. Lancet 1:199–200

Madore HP, Treanor JJ, Dolin R 1986 Characterization of the Snow Mountain agent of viral gastroenteritis. J Virol 58:487–492

Mason HS, Ball JM, Shi J-J, Jiang X, Estes MK, Arntzen CJ 1996 Expression of Norwalk virus capsid protein in transgenic tobacco and potato and its oral immunogenicity in mice. Proc Natl Acad Sci USA 93:5335–5340

Matsui SM, Kim JP, Greenberg HB et al 1991 The isolation and characterization of a Norwalk virus-specific cDNA. J Clin Invest 87:1456–1461

Neill JD, Reardon IM, Heinrikson RL 1991 Nucleotide sequence and expression of the capsid protein gene of feline calicivirus. J Virol 65:5440–5447

Neill JD, Sosnovtsev SV, Green KY 2000 Recovery and altered neutralization specificities of chimeric viruses containing capsid protein domain exchanges from antigenically distinct strains of feline calicivirus. J Virol 74:1079–1084

Noel JS, Liu BL, Humphrey CD et al 1997 Parkville virus: a novel genetic variant of human calicivirus in the Sapporo virus clade, associated with an outbreak of gastroenteritis in adults. J Med Virol 52:173–178

Pletneva MA, Sosnovtsev SV, Sosnovtseva SA, Green KY 1998 Characterization of a recombinant human calicivirus capsid protein expressed in mammalian cells. Virus Res 55:129–141

Prasad BVV, Hardy ME, Dokland T, Bella J, Rossmann MG, Estes MK 1999 X-ray crystallographic structure of the Norwalk virus capsid. Science 286:287–290

Seah EL, Marshall JA, Wright PJ 1999 Open reading frame 1 of the Norwalk-like virus Camberwell: completion of sequence and expression in mammalian cells. J Virol 73:10531–10535

Sosnovtsev S, Green KY 1995 RNA transcripts derived from a cloned full-length copy of the feline calicivirus genome do not require VpG for infectivity. Virology 210:383–390

Sugieda M, Nagaoka H, Kakishima Y, Ohshita T, Nakamura S, Nakajima S 1998 Detection of Norwalk-like virus genes in the caecum contents of pigs. Arch Virol 143:1215–1221

Terashima H, Chiba S, Sakuma Y et al 1983 The polypeptide of a human calicivirus. Arch Virol 78:1–7

Tohya Y, Shinchi H, Matsuura Y et al 1999 Analysis of the N-terminal polypeptide of the capsid precursor protein and the ORF3 product of feline calicivirus. J Vet Med Sci 61:1043–1047

Vinjé J, Deijl H, van der Heide R et al 2000 Molecular detection and epidemiology of Sapporo-like viruses. J Clin Microbiol 38:530–536

Wirblich C, Thiel HJ, Meyers G 1996 Genetic map of the calicivirus rabbit hemorrhagic disease virus as deduced from *in vitro* translation studies. J Virol 70:7974–7983

DISCUSSION

Patton: I am not clear on the structural differences between the genome of NLVs and SLVs. Is it true that SLVs do not produce a subgenomic RNA while NLVs do? How do SLVs make sufficient capsid protein if they do not produce subgenomic RNAs?

Clarke: That is a good question. Our knowledge of subgenomic RNAs comes from studying viruses of other genera. In the case of NLVs, because none of these viruses grow in cell culture there is only one report of a subgenomic RNA. I think this was in Jason Jiang's paper in which he blotted stool samples and saw a small subgenomic RNA (Jiang et al 1993). I suspect, therefore, that there is a subgenomic RNA for NLVs. In the case of the SLVs, their genome organization is much like that of the lagoviruses: the caliciviruses that infect rabbits and hares. In those cases, there is clearly a subgenomic RNA produced in rabbit livers. Again, these viruses don't grow in cell culture, but in a rabbit liver that has been infected by rabbit haemorrhagic disease virus (RHDV), there is clear subgenomic RNA. In fact, the virions have been purified and there is some evidence that the virions actually package (perhaps mistakenly) subgenomic RNA.

Monroe: Another piece of evidence in support of this is the finding of the conserved motif at the 5' end of the genome.

Offit: In what cell type does the virus principally replicate in human hosts?

Clarke: We don't really know. The only evidence that exists comes from taking biopsies from the human small intestine of volunteers that have been infected. From these studies viral replication appears to occur in the enterocytes.

Kapikian: Virus was not detected in the epithelial cells of the jejunal mucosa of volunteers challenged with the Norwalk or Hawaii viruses. However, there was broadening and blunting of villi (Agus et al 1973, Dolin et al 1975).

Clarke: So you saw stunting of the villi but no cell target was ever identified in these studies. This pathology was also true in the case of Newbury agent 1, a bovine 'NLV'. It was possible to look at infected bowel samples under the SEM that showed stunting of the villi in the proximal part of the small intestine. The actual target cell was not identified.

Estes: In more recent volunteer studies done in Houston, Dr Tomoyuki Tanaka did some antigen staining (Graham et al 1994). We saw the characteristic stunting of the villi in the upper small intestine. Using our new antibodies to the VLPs we could see an occasional enterocyte that was stained. There was actually much more staining in the lamina propria, but we couldn't identify what the cell types were.

Offit: Have people tried to grow these viruses in human intestinal epithelial cells?

Estes: Yes, but without success.

Saif: We have done a lot of pathogenesis studies with the NLV that we have from cattle (Chang et al 1999). We have seen moderate-to-severe villous atrophy in the proximal small intestine, but when we tried to do immunofluorescent staining with specific antibodies, we weren't able to see any evidence of immunofluorescent cells in the small intestine. However, with the porcine enteric calicivirus (PEC), it is very easy to identify the viral antigen: it is in the villus enterocytes in the proximal small intestine (Flynn et al 1988). This is something that is different between caliciviruses and rotaviruses. In our experience the major replication site of rotavirus is in the mid-to-distal small intestine (Theil et al 1978, Ward et al 1996), but for the caliciviruses it is mostly the proximal small intestine (Flynn et al 1988). We can identify the PEC, which is an SLV, in the enterocytes, but we can't find the NLV virus or antigen in infected calves. Hall et al (1984) reported a similar distribution of lesions in the proximal small intestine of calves infected with the NLV Newbury agent and also failed to identify viral particles in enterocytes of the infected calves.

Vesikari: I don't know what cells these viruses are multiplying in humans, but in children under two years of age, the clinical picture of NLV disease versus SLV is totally different. NLVs are predominantly associated with a vomiting disease; the SLV infection is characterized by mild diarrhoea with virtually no vomiting. SLV disease is clearly endemic in Finland. SLVs follow closely the rotavirus epidemiology: there is a winter peak, but it never goes away. NLV disease has a winter peak and we have not been able to detect NLVs all year round in children. I would presume that because the clinical picture is so different that the sites of multiplication of NLVs and SLVs are also different.

Monroe: We have seen a number of outbreaks where we have been able to detect the virus by PCR in vomitus. What mechanism of replication exists where replicating virus shows up in vomitus, and how does this relate to how the virus grows?

Greenberg: The most noxious experiment that I have ever done was to thaw several litres of vomitus that Dr Kapikian had stored from the early Norwalk studies. I am probably the only person who has ultracentrifuged several litres of vomitus! We didn't have the advantage of PCR, but we did see a few viral particles by IEM. What is amazing with the caliciviruses is how rapidly people get sick, even within 8–12 hours. In the early days, people talked about a toxin or a phage or some sort of rapid onset agent, because it hits them so fast.

Estes: My understanding was that the regulation of what controls vomiting is quite complex. There are some animals that never vomit; humans are quite good at it. The earlier volunteer studies showed that there were changes in the rate of stomach emptying which can affect vomiting. We have taken the idea that perhaps this virus is growing in the stomach. We tried to put the virus into AGS cells from the stomach, and it still didn't grow. There is still something missing.

Greenberg: People looked at this histologically in the early studies.

Estes: What is the current understanding of the pathophysiology of vomiting?

Farthing: Obviously, there are central mechanisms. If you go in a rollercoaster and your vestibular mechanisms are activated, you may vomit. This is due to activation of the central vomiting pathways. There are also peripheral pathways. Stimulation of vagal afferents is thought to be important. This can probably be achieved in a number of ways. It may be possible to stimulate the vagus directly or by the presence of inflammation or infection in the gut. In particular, proximal infections in the gut such as acute viral infections may act in this way. Another important mechanism is via serotonin. Perhaps the best model of acute vomiting is chemotherapy-induced vomiting. If a cancer patient is given intravenous cisplatin, they may vomit within minutes. This is thought to be due to acute, massive release of serotonin (5-HT) from enterochromaffin cells in the gut. This then activates 5-HT3 receptors on enteric nerves — vagal afferents — that terminate in the vomiting centre and promote vomiting. The dramatic clinical intervention in chemotherapy has been to give patients a 5-HT3 receptor antagonist which minimizes the vomiting. An area that we are particularly interested in is the importance of 5-HT release during intestinal infection. One of the enterotoxins that releases 5-HT is cholera toxin. I suspect that the vomiting seen early in cholera is related to 5-HT release. We believe that about 50% of the diarrhoea in cholera is due to cholera toxin-activated enterochromaffin cell release of 5-HT. This mechanism may be important in other infections, and is interesting, because it links vomiting and diarrhoea together with the same chemical mediator.

Estes: Has anyone done a study with these drugs to prevent acute vomiting with NLV disease?

Farthing: I do not think it has ever been looked at in any acute viral enteritis.

Holmes: I think it is fascinating that for two related viruses, one is likely to cause vomiting and the other is not.

Glass: There are a number of interesting issues here with relation to transmission and public health. First, we always think of these viruses as being spread by the faecal–oral route. Here we have enteric spread, but by vomitus and not faeces. Second, we have had a number of outbreak investigations where vomitus has been critical to virus spread. Third, over the last few years we have been just as successful in getting virus out of vomitus than out of stools in the same outbreak, which to me suggests that this is something we should think about in epidemiological investigations. We have never had a public health message about what to do for vomitus. In the outbreak I presented from the football team, these guys were vomiting. The risk as some sort of contact through vomitus is probably high.

Brown: We have been doing some studies of environmental contamination. We have been able to show the presence of NLVs by RT-PCR in places where it wouldn't get apart from being aerosolized. We have recently done some air sampling studies, and when people are changing sheets, virus can be found in the air (Cheesbrough et al 1999). A number of routes of transmission from environmental contamination are possible.

Desselberger: I have a question about the direct repeats you have described. In some studies we have found a co-circulation of two different genogroups in the same setting (Gray et al 1997). As direct repeats are known to be a signal of recombination, is there any evidence for inter-genogroup recombinants?

Clarke: Yes, recombination does appear to occur. There have been reports of PCR of the RNA polymerase fragment of the viral genome, and also fragments of the capsid. Even the RNA polymerase will give a genogroup 1 or 2 score. Others have found mixtures of genogroup 1 and 2. The break point for template shifting, which I guess must have happened in the same cell, presumably occurs between those two points which would be where the repeated sequence is.

Matson: We amplified a single clone that straddles the polymerase and capsid genes from a strain recovered in Argentina (Jiang et al 1999). It is a recombinant. The issue is that because there is so much sequence conservation right at the junction of the ORF1 and the beginning of the capsid gene, defining an exact recombination site was impossible on the basis of sequence alone.

Koopmans: We had exactly the same experience with the same virus, which we have named Rotterdam virus (Vinjé & Koopmans 2000).

Greenberg: Linda Saif, I was surprised about rotavirus. I have always thought of rotavirus, from the old literature, as replicating primarily in the proximal gut. I am thinking this mostly from Chuck Mebus' data in cattle and the early studies in mice. Were you talking about pigs, or is it your general impression that all rotaviruses grow mostly in the distal small intestine?

Saif: I was talking about our experience with pigs and cattle. There is a sequence of rotaviral replication. Early on after an infection of pigs with human rotavirus, we see only a few fluorescing cells in the duodenum, and this appears to progress laterally, so that peak numbers of immunofluorescing cells are then present in the jejeunum and ileum by 24–48 hours (Ward et al 1996). Similar findings were reported by Theil et al (1978) after infection of pigs with porcine rotaviruses.

Greenberg: The literature says that the jejunum is the major site. But you are saying that in pigs and cattle most replication is in the ileum.

Saif: It is time-related, but initially we see some immunofluorescing cells in the duodenum, but as the infection progresses in the peak and later stages of infection most of the antigen is seen in the jejunum and ileum.

Desselberger: There are data from Janice Bridger's group showing that in cattle differences in pathogenicity are correlated with the extent of the area of infection of the small intestine (Hall et al 1993). The highly pathogenic strain infected the duodenum and most of the small intestine, whereas the strain with less pathogenicity infected the proximal small intestine poorly, and although it infected enterocytes in the mid and distal small gut, it did not damage intestinal structure.

Monroe: One other comment about the junction between ORF1 and ORF2: not only is it conserved, but it also is predicted to have a high degree of secondary structure. Although it is conserved and one would think that is a great target for PCR, it is actually a very poor target for PCR primers, presumably because of that high secondary structure.

Matson: I wanted to point out that there are more than two genogroups ('subgenera') in each of the calicivirus genera. For SLVs there are at least four distinct clades ('subgenera').

References

Agus SG, Dolin R, Wyatt RG, Tousimis AJ, Northrup RS 1973 Acute infectious nonbacterial gastroenteritis: intestinal histopathology. Norwalk agent in man. Ann Int Med 79:18–25

Chang K-O, Parwani AV, Cho K-O, Guo M, Nielsen PR, Saif LJ 1999 Pathogenesis of a bovine enteric calicivirus in gnotobiotic calves. Conference of Research Workers in Animal Disease, Abstr #107, Chicago, IL, Nov 8–9, 1999

Cheesbrough J, Green J, Brown D, Wright P 1999 The detection of small round structured virus by nested reverse transcriptase polymerase chain reaction. International Workshop on Human Caliciviruses, Centers for Disease Control and Prevention, Altanta, Georgia, USA, March 1999

Dolin R, Levy AG, Wyatt RG, Thornhill TS, Gardner JD 1975 Viral gastroenteritis induced by the Hawaii agent: jejunal histopathology and serologic response. Am J Med 59:761–768

Flynn WT, Saif LJ, Moorhead PD 1988 Pathogenesis of a porcine enteric calicivirus in gnotobiotic pigs. Am J Vet Res 49:819–828

Graham DY, Jiang X, Tanaka T, Opekun AR, Madore HP, Estes MK 1994 Norwalk virus infection of volunteers: new insights based on improved assays. J Infect Dis 170:34–43

Gray JJ, Green J, Cunliffe C, Gallimore CI, Lee JV, Neal K, Brown DWG 1997 Mixed genogroup SRSV infections among a party of canoeists exposed to contaminated recreational water. J Med Virol 52:425–429

Hall GA, Bridger JC, Brooker BE, Parsons KR, Ormerod E 1984 Lesions of gnotobiotic calves experimentally infected with a calcivirus-like (Newbury) agent. Vet Pathol 21:208–215

Hall GA, Bridger JC, Parsons KR, Cook R 1993 Variation in rotavirus virulence: a comparison of pathogenesis in calves between two rotaviruses of different virulence. Vet Pathol 30:223–233

Jiang X, Wang M, Wang K, Estes MK 1993 Sequence and genomic organization of Norwalk virus. Virology 195:51–61

Jiang X, Espul C, Zhong WM, Cuello H, Matson DO 1999 Characterization of a novel human calicivirus that may be a naturally occurring recombinant. Arch Virol 144:2377–2387

Theil KW, Bohl EH, Cross RF, Kohler EM, Agnes AG 1978 Pathogenicity of porcine rotaviral infection in experimentally inoculated gnotobiotic pigs. Am Vet Med Assoc 39:213–220

Vinjé J, Koopmans M 2000 Simultaneous detection and genotyping of Norwalk-like viruses by oligonucleotide array in a reverse-line blot hybridisation format. J Clin Microbiol 38:2595–2601

Ward LA, Rosen BI, Yuan L, Saif LJ 1996 Pathogenesis of an attenuated and a virulent strain of group A human rotavirus in neonatal gnotobiotic pigs. J Gen Virol 77:1431–1441

Novartis 238: Gastroenteritis Viruses.
Copyright © 2001 John Wiley & Sons Ltd
Print ISBN 0-471-49663-4 eISBN 0-470-84653-4

Molecular epidemiology of human enteric caliciviruses in The Netherlands

Marion Koopmans, Jan Vinjé, Erwin Duizer, Matty de Wit and Yvonne van Duijnhoven

Research Laboratory for Infectious Diseases and Center for Infectious Diseases Epidemiology, National Institute of Public Health and the Environment, Bilthoven, The Netherlands

Abstract. Caliciviruses are among the most common causes of gastroenteritis in people of all age groups. These antigenetically and genetically diverse viruses have been grouped into two genera within the family *Caliciviridae*, designated Norwalk-like viruses (NLV) and Sapporo-like viruses (SLV). To gain more insight in their epidemiology, we have developed a tentative genotyping scheme, which was used to differentiate the viruses detected in a set of epidemiological studies. NLVs and SLVs were detected by generic RT-PCR in stool specimens from 5.1% and 2.4% of cases with acute gastroenteritis for which a general practitioner was consulted, and in 16.5% and 6.3% of community cases of gastroenteritis. In addition, NLVs were associated with more than 80% of reported outbreaks of gastroenteritis from 1994–1999. Typically, several genotypes of NLV co-circulate in the community. Occasionally, however, several consecutive outbreaks were caused by essentially the same virus, although an epidemiological link had not previously been noted. This was most pronounced in 1995/1996, when a Lordsdale-like variant was detected that subsequently was found worldwide. This epidemic spread suggests differences in virulence or mode of transmission. In addition, we found that related NLVs are highly prevalent in calves in The Netherlands, raising questions about their potential for zoonotic transmission.

2001 Gastroenteritis viruses. Wiley, Chichester (Novartis Foundation Symposium 238) p 197–218

Gastroenteritis due to viral infection of the intestinal tract is a common illness in humans, with a high morbidity reported worldwide. It is increasingly recognized that caliciviruses are a significant cause of this disease. The caliciviruses that infect humans are divided into two genera: the Norwalk-like viruses (NLVs), also known as small-round-structured viruses, and the Sapporo-like viruses (SLVs) or 'typical' caliciviruses (Kapikian & Chanock 1990). Both NLVs and SLVs cause acute self-limiting gastroenteritis with diarrhoea and vomiting. NLVs are readily transmitted via food, and are an important cause of outbreaks in institutions such as nursing homes (Green 1997).

Although caliciviruses cannot be grown in tissue culture, their entire genome has been sequenced directly from stool extracto (Jiang et al 1990, 1993, Lambden et al 1993, Dingle et al 1995, Liu et al 1995). This has led to the rapid development of diagnostic assays based on RNA amplification by reverse-transcriptase (RT)-PCR, enabling epidemiological studies at a larger scale (de Leon et al 1992, Jiang et al 1992, Green et al 1993). In our research, described in this paper, we are studying the importance of caliciviruses as a cause of illness in The Netherlands, in comparison with other enteric pathogens. We have developed methods for molecular typing of strains in order to study modes of transmission and to trace viruses through the population.

Detection of NLV and SLV by consensus RT-PCR

Several groups have developed RT-PCR-based detection methods following the cloning of prototype NLV strains. The first round RT-PCR assays, however, were suboptimal, as they had been optimized using one or a few prototype strains (Moe et al 1994). When it became clear that NLVs were highly variable (Lew et al 1994, Green et al 1993, Wang et al 1994, Ando et al 1994), we developed a single-round generic NLV-specific primer pair by empirically selecting primers targeting a highly conserved region of the genome, i.e. the viral RNA polymerase (POL). In our hands, the best results were obtained with an antisense primer close to the 5'-end of the coding region for the conserved YGDD motif (Vinjé & Koopmans 1996, Vinjé et al 1997). In its present format, the assay detects strains from at least 15 known genotypes with high specificity (100%). While the detection limit was found to be as low as 3–30 RNA-containing particles, it is likely to be different for viruses from different genetic clusters, given the high level of sequence heterogeneity even in this relatively conserved region of the viral genome. Although non-specific bands may occasionally be produced with RNA extracts from stool specimens due to the low stringency of the consensus PCR, specificity is determined by a high stringency probe hybridization assay using a mixture of probes. The assay is now used routinely in The Netherlands and some other European countries (Vinjé & Koopmans 1996, Vinjé et al 1997). Similar assays have been developed by other groups, and studies are underway to compare the diagnostic performance of these assays.

On the basis of the same principle, we have developed a generic or consensus RT-PCR assay for the SLVs within the family *Caliciviridae*. Again, primers are used which target the YGDD motif, with eightfold degeneracy and a low-stringency annealing step to allow for mismatches between the primer and its target sequence. So far, we were able to amplify RNA from 93% of a panel of 59 stool samples that had been collected over a 10-year period by electron microscopy (EM) evaluation of patients' stools in the UK and Sweden (Vinjé et al 2000a).

Genotyping as a tool for molecular epidemiological studies

In the absence of an *in vitro* culture system for these viruses, antigenic typing has been limited to studies with solid-phase immune EM (SPIEM), and — more recently — with recombinant capsid protein-based ELISA (Lewis et al 1995, Jiang et al 1996). Clearly, the human caliciviruses are antigenically quite variable, but little is known about the role of this variability in their epidemiology, e.g. are there differences in virulence or transmissibility, are certain variants associated with specific modes of transmission or geographic areas, and does infection with viruses belonging to one lineage induce cross-protection to viruses from other lineages? A complete study of these issues would require assays that allow us to discriminate strains on the basis of their antigenic properties, such as (a panel of) recombinant capsid-based antigenic typing ELISAs, or alternatives such as serotyping monoclonals, neither of which are available for NLV or SLV at present. Therefore, we have tried to develop an interim molecular typing scheme that correlates with antigenic typing in close collaboration with David Brown and Jon Green at Colindale. Regions across the genome of a broad range of antigenically and genetically distinct NLV strains have been sequenced, including the complete capsid gene. Our working criteria for defining genotypes are: (1) greater than 80% amino acid similarity when comparing complete capsid gene sequences; (2) at least 85% similarity based on the nucleotide sequence of the polymerase fragment for genogroup I (GGI), and 90% for GGII strains; (3) consistent clustering by phylogenetic analysis irrespective of which method is used for phylogeny reconstruction, with high bootstrap values for the lineages; and (4) one cluster being represented by at least two strains (Vinjé & Koopmans 2000, Vinjé et al 2000b, Green et al 2000).

From these studies, NLVs from the two genogroups have tentatively been grouped into 15 genotypes, and SLVs into four genotypes (Jiang et al 1997, Noel et al 1997b, Vinjé & Koopmans 2000, Vinjé et al 2000b, Koopmans et al 2000) (Table 1). Genotypes were named after the variants that had been reported first. Strains are quite distinct with homologies of the total capsid protein sequence between genogroups ranging from 37–44% for NLVs. Viruses from one genotype (Alphatron, Table 1) cluster almost equidistantly from GGI and GGII strains. They were grouped with GGII based on the conserved motifs at the start of the capsid gene, but might in fact belong to a third genogroup (Vinjé & Koopmans 2000). For SLV, maximum differences between capsid sequences reach up to 60% (between the London strain and other variants), suggesting that the SLV also can be divided into at least two genogroups (Jiang et al 1997). With few exceptions, clustering of strains was consistent, regardless which genomic region was used for the analysis (Vinjé et al 2000b, Green et al 2000). For strains belonging to 9 genotypes, SPIEM typing had also classified them as distinct, suggesting a

TABLE 1 Provisional classification scheme for genotyping of human caliciviruses, and examples of strains based on recent publications on strain diversity

Genus	GG	Genotype name[a]	CDC cluster[b]	Not assigned[c]	CPHL/RIVM cluster[d]	Other examples
NLV	I	Norwalk	1		Norwalk	KY/89/JPN
		Desert Shield	3		Desert Shield	Birmingham291
		Southampton	2		Southampton	White Rose, Crawley
		Queens Arms	4		Queens Arms	Valetta, Thistlehall
		Musgrove	5		*Musgrove*	Butlins
		Winchester		6	*Winchester*	LWymontley
		Sindlesham		7	*Sindlesham*	Mikkeli, Lord Harris
	II	Hawaii	1		Girlington	Wortley*
		Snow Mountain	2		Melksham	
		Mexico	3		Mexico	Toronto, Auckland, Rotterdam
		Lordsdale	4		Grimsby	Bristol, Camberwell, Pilgrim, SymGreen
		Hillingdon	5		*Hillingdon*	White river, Welterhof
			6			Seacroft/90/UK
		Leeds	7		*Leeds*	Gwynedd, Venlo, Creche
			8**			539
			9			378/Idaho Fall/96/US
			10**			Yat/94/UK
		Alphatron		11	*Alphatron*	
Tentative		Amsterdam		12		

Genus	GG	Genotype name	CDC cluster	CPR cluster[e]	RIVM cluster
SLV	III	Sapporo		Houston/86	Sapporo
		Houston	Parkville	Houston/90	Parkville
		Stockholm			*Stockholm*
	IV	London		London	London

Recently identified novel lineages are indicated in italics (based on Vinjé et al 2000a,b, Vinjé & Koopmans 2000, Green et al 2000).
*Wortley virus was classified as a distinct genotype by Green et al (2000), but with the more stringent criteria used by Vinjé et al (2000b) and Vinjé & Koopmans (2000) is clustered with Hawaii virus (83% amino acid similarity in the total capsid gene). ** = only based on partial capsid sequences (Ando et al 2000).
[a]Vinjé et al (2000b).
[b]Adapted to the classification scheme as proposed by the Centers for Disease Control and Prevention (CDC), Atlanta, GA, USA (Ando et al 2000).
[c]No corresponding genotype number proposed by Ando et al (2000).
[d]Central Public Health Laboratory (CPHL), London, UK and RIVM (Green et al 2000, Vinjé & Koopmans 2000, Vinjé et al 2000b).
[e]Center for Pediatric Research (CPR), Norfolk, VA, US (Jiang et al 1997).

TABLE 2   Diversity of GGI and GGII NLVs (A), and of SLVs (B) given as percentage nucleotide (*) or amino acid (**) diversity between strains belonging to the same (divergence within) or different genotypes (divergence between)

(A) NLVs

		ORF1	ORF2-N	ORF2-C	ORF2	ORF3
GGI	Size	140*	±278**	±130**	Complete**	97*
	Divergence within	87–100	87–100	30–100	80–100	89–100
	Divergence between	64–78	64–78		62–80	61–72
GGII	Size	202	±249	±130	Complete	138#/97
	Divergence within	91–100	81–100	26–100	80–100	89–100
	Divergence between	60–90	60–79		52–80	61–72

#138 in the Lordsdale cluster of viruses, 97 in the other clusters.

(B) SLVs

	ORF1	ORF2
Size	106**	complete**
Divergence within	Nk	80–100
Divergence between	68–80	62–80

'Size' indicates size of genome fragment on which analysis was based. ORF2-N = 5′end of capsid gene, ORF2-C = (hypervariable) central portion of capsid gene.

correlation between antigenic typing and our proposed genotyping scheme (Vinjé et al 2000b). Diversity is different for different genomic regions, with the central region of the capsid gene being hypervariable (Table 2). The conserved regions of the POL gene and the N-terminal region of the capsid gene are quite conserved, and can be used as target regions for genotyping studies (Table 2). The lower degree of sequence divergence in the polymerase gene, and the relative ease of combining diagnosis with molecular typing has led to the widespread use of POL-typing in molecular epidemiological studies (Vinjé & Koopmans 1996, Vinjé et al 1997, Ando et al 1995, Levett et al 1996, Fankhauser et al 1998, Maguire et al 1999, Schreier et al 2000).

At the time of the meeting, the CDC published a proposal for a numerical scheme of genotypes (Ando et al 2000). Comparative analysis was done between the capsid sequences generated by CDC, and representatives of the clusters described above (Table 1). From this comparison, the total number of currently recognized NLV genotypes appears to be as high as 19, although some CDC clusters were based on partial capsid sequences and therefore need to be confirmed. In the near future, a consensus should be reached on which scheme to use for genotyping.

Clearly, the cut-off points chosen for defining genotypes are arbitrary. For instance, Wortley virus and Venlo virus have been grouped with the Hawaii and Leeds genotype, respectively, by our criteria. They both are, however, quite distinct at 83.5 and 82% amino acid similarity with the reference strain for the genotype, based on the complete capsid sequence. Our classification may have to be revised with new insights obtained by antigenic typing, but until then may prove to be useful for comparison of data from different groups working on the molecular epidemiology of caliciviruses. To provide a standardized and easy-to-use genotyping method for diagnostic laboratories, we have developed a filter-based typing assay with specific probes for each of the currently known genotypes (reverse-line blot hybridization assay; RLB) (Vinjé & Koopmans 2000). The RLB method is easy to perform: it has a high throughput of strains, labelled membranes can be reused, new probes can be added, and standardization between laboratories is straightforward. Clearly, given the cut-off for genotype (at 10–15% nucleotide divergence) RLB can not be used to compare closely-related strains, for which nucleotide sequence analysis will remain the method of choice. However, the amount of sequencing can be reduced drastically by excluding dissimilar strains by use of RLB. At present, the use of the RLB in clinical virological laboratories is evaluated with special emphasis on detection limits for different genotypes and tolerance for mismatches within the probe region.

Do genotypes constitute serotypes?
Our attempts at tissue culture isolation of Norwalk-like caliciviruses

In order to compare the classification of strains into genotypes with a biologically relevant characteristic such as serotyping, it will be essential to grow caliciviruses *in vitro* or in an accessible animal model. So far, however, all attempts to do so have failed (Green 1997). Presumably, virus replication is dependent on factors present in the intestinal content and the origin and degree of differentiation of the intestinal (epithelial) cells. In the past year, we have tried to establish differentiated epithelial cell cultures. We cultured Detroit 562 cells as a model for pharynx epithelial cells, HuTu-80 for duodenal epithelial cells, Caco-2 cells for colonic cells with enterocytic features, and HCT-8 cells for colon epithelium. Prior to inoculation, the stool samples and/or cells were treated with artificially prepared intestinal contents containing α-amylase, pepsin, pancreatin, lipase, mucin and bile at physiological concentrations. So far, all inoculations were passaged at least five times without a cytopathogenic effect being observed in any of the samples, and viral RNA could not be detected in any of the culture conditions (Duizer et al 2000).

Genetic instability

At the first Calicivirus conference in Atlanta, USA, 1999, Dr Tamie Ando presented his analysis of currently used diagnostic RT-PCR primers and showed that the proportion of positives had gradually declined over the years, suggesting that the more recently detected caliciviruses were slightly different. In a similar analysis of our data, we have not observed such a decline, although the consensus sequence of Lordsdale-like strains found in 1999 differs by as much as 3% (nucleotides in polymerase gene fragment) from that of the 1996 strain. This drift suggests that indeed primers used in diagnostic RT-PCR assays will have to be re-evaluated critically at regular intervals.

For the majority of strains clustering is independent of the genomic region used for the clustering analysis, however, several exceptions were noted from our work (Rotterdam virus, Seacroft virus, Wortley virus, Vinjé et al 2000b, Vinjé & Koopmans 2000, Green et al 2000) as well as work by other groups (Snow Mountain Agent, Hardy et al 1997, possibly Goulburn valley virus, Seah et al 1999, Jiang et al 1999). The most likely explanation for these discrepancies is that strains have arisen by recombination. The above examples suggest that recombination may even be relatively common.

Epidemiological studies of infectious intestinal disease in The Netherlands

Physician-based study

The epidemiology of NLV infections in people who are sufficiently ill to visit their physician has been assessed in a physician-based case-control study that started in May of 1996, and ended May 1999 (de Wit et al 1997, 2001). Cases and controls were recruited through physicians that participate in the NIVEL network, covering approximately 1% of the population of The Netherlands. Detailed questionnaires were used to establish risk factors for acquisition of infection with a broad range of microorganisms (*Salmonella* spp., *Shigella* spp., *Campylobacter* spp., *Yersinia* spp., *E. coli* spp., *Giardia* spp., *Cryptosporidium* spp., *Dientamoeba*, *Entamoeba*, *Blastocystis*, *Cyclospora*, astrovirus, group A rotavirus, adenovirus types 40/41, and NLV) (de Wit et al 2001). In total, stools were tested for 857 cases and 574 controls. The overall incidence of gastroenteritis (corrected for non-response) was 79.7 per 10 000 person years. From May 1996 to May 1999,

NLVs were detected by a generic RT-PCR assay in stool specimens from 5.1% of cases with acute gastroenteritis for which a general practitioner was consulted, and in 1.1 % of otool specimens from control patients (de Wit et al 2001). The presence of SLV was assayed in the second half of the study (431 cases and 287 controls) and was found to be 2.4% in cases and 1.5% in controls. For comparison, rotavirus was found in 5.3% of cases and in 1.4% of controls. The incidence of NLV was significantly higher in young children, but remained at around 3–5% for all age groups, whereas SLV were found almost exclusively in children. The age distribution in children was different for different viruses: whereas NLV and rotavirus peaked in children < 1 year of age, followed by the 1–4 year olds, SLV and astrovirus were detected most commonly in 5–12 year old children, followed by 1–4 year olds (Table 3). An intriguing observation was that 20% of NLV positives were in people who had had symptoms for more than 2 weeks before consulting their physician. More than half of these had symptoms > 4 weeks, suggesting that prolonged shedding of NLV may occur.

Community study

In December 1998, we started a population-based cohort study with a nested case-control component (Abbink et al 1998). In this study, a randomized sample of people from the population area covered by physician practices was asked to enter the study cohort for a half year. All participants submitted questionnaires when they entered the cohort, and an additional questionnaire and stool specimens when having symptoms. At the onset of illness, two age- and sex-matched controls were recruited from the cohort. Comparative analysis of data from the physician-based study and this study will — among others — provide information on the severity of illness caused by specific microorganisms. Preliminary analysis of the data shows a very high incidence of NLV in people of all age groups (16.5% of cases, 113 positive out of 685 case episodes) (Koopmans et al 2000), with a slightly higher incidence in very young children (Table 4). Asymptomatic infections were also seen commonly, especially in the young children (overall 5% of controls, or 32 positives out of 641 control samples). Similarly, SLV were quite commonly found (6.3% of all cases, 1.6% of controls), with the highest incidence in youngest children (Table 4).

Outbreak investigations

In The Netherlands, outbreaks of gastroenteritis are reported to the municipal health services (MHS) or to food inspection services (FIS). Outbreaks are labelled NLV-associated if 50% or more stool specimens from patients are positive by RT-PCR, with a minimum number of five specimens analysed per

TABLE 3 Viruses in stool samples from cases and controls of different age groups in a physician-based study of gastroenteritis in The Netherlands from May 1996–May 1999

	Overall		<1 yr		1–4 yrs		5–14 yrs		15–29 yrs		30–59 yrs		60+ yrs	
	case	cont	case	cont	case	cont	case	cont	case	cont	case	cont	case	cont
N	857	574	32	17	136	69	96	58	170	72	313	244	102	102
Rotavirus	5.3[a]	1.4	21.2	0.0	15.2	4.4	1.0	0.0	4.1	1.4	1.9	1.6	2.9	0.0
Adenovirus	2.2	0.4	9.1	0.0	9.4	1.5	1.0	0.0	0.6	1.4	0.3	0.0	0.0	0.0
Astrovirus	1.5	0.4	0.0	0.0	1.5	0.0	4.2	0.0	0.6	0.0	0.6	0.0	3.9	2.0
NLV	5.1	1.1	15.2	0.0	8.7	1.5	3.1	1.7	5.9	1.4	3.9	0.8	1.0	1.0
SLV[b]	2.4	1.5	4.2	8.3	4.9	5.0	6.1	0.0	2.8	0.0	0.6	0.7	0.0	0.0
Total calicivirus	7.5	2.6	19.4	8.3	13.6	6.5	9.2	1.7	8.7	1.4	4.5	1.5	1.0	1.0

[a]Indicates percentage values.
[b]SLV: only tested in samples of 431 cases and 287 controls.
Adapted from de Wit et al (2001).

TABLE 4   Viruses in stool samples from cases and controls of different age groups in a community cohort study of gastroenteritis in The Netherlands from December 1990 – December 1999

	0–4 years		5–12 years		> 12 years	
	cases	controls	cases	controls	cases	controls
Rotavirus	9.8[a]	0.7	1.6	0.8	4.7	1.1
Adenovirus	5.0	0.5	1.6	0.0	0.0	2.2
Astrovirus	2.2	0.7	3.2	0.0	1.0	1.1
NLV	18.5	6.7	13.7	0.8	11.3	2.2
SLV	7.6	2.2	5.7	0.8	1.0	0.0
Total calicivirus	26.1	8.9	19.4	1.6	12.3	2.2

[a]Data indicate percentage values.
Adapted from de Wit et al (2001).

outbreak, and no other pathogen is present. Overall, NLV could be detected in more than 80% of all reported outbreaks of gastroenteritis from 1994–2000 (Vinjé et al 1997, Koopmans et al 2000). Since the outbreaks for which specimens are sent to RIVM are a biased selection, we have tried to get a more precise estimate of the proportion of NLV outbreaks by collecting samples from every outbreak of gastroenteritis reported to the MHS for the duration of 1 year in 1996. Again, the majority of these outbreaks (87%) were associated with NLV. Most outbreaks occurred in nursing homes (59%) and hospitals (25%), with high attack rates both in residents/patients (45%) and nursing staff (29%). The focus of investigation of outbreaks reported to the FIS is slightly different and microbiological assays are done on leftovers from implicated food items for microbiological tests. Since reliable tests for the detection of NLV in various food items are not yet available, the incidence of NLV in these outbreaks is not known. In addition, there is clearly underreporting for foodborne outbreaks of NLV. However, of the 26 foodborne outbreaks that have been investigated virologically by the RIVM since 1991, 77% (20) were caused by NLV.

Genetic diversity of strains recovered from humans

We have used the POL-based genotyping method since 1994 for typing of outbreak strains and since May 1996 for typing of strains from sporadic cases from the epidemiological studies. In these years we have observed that genogroup (GG) II strains by far outnumber the GGI strains, although the

TABLE 5 Distribution of GGI and GGII strains from 1996–1999 as detected in outbreaks or in population-based studies, and number of different genotypes detected per year for the different study populations

	Year	% GGI	Number of genotypes	% GGII	Number of genotypes
Outbreaks	1996	0	0	100	2
	1997	26	2 (1)	73	3
	1998	0	0	100	4 (1)
	1999	18	4 (1)	86*	6
Population	1996	22	2 (2)	77	3 (1)
	1997	7	1	94	5 (2)
	1998	13	2 (2)	87	4 (1)
	1999	22	3	80	6

*1 mixed outbreak. Numbers in brackets indicate number of genotypes uniquely detected in this population, e.g. for the 1997 outbreaks: 2 genotypes within GGI, 1 genotype found only in outbreaks.

percentages may vary from year-to-year (Table 5) (Vinjé & Koopmans 1996, Vinjé et al 1997). In most years, several lineages co-circulate in the community and cause outbreaks, with at least five genotypes circulating in the second half of 1996, 7 in 1997, 7 in 1998 and 9 in 1999 (Table 5; Figs 1, 2 and 3). However, in 1994, and especially in the 1995/1996 winter season a different pattern was observed, when sequential outbreaks were caused by strains that were indistinguishable based on the polymerase gene sequence. We observed a small 'epidemic' in 1994 caused by a Mexico-like virus (MxV), a large scale 'epidemic' from 1995– July 1996, when the same Lordsdale-like virus (LDV) with only few nucleotide changes was found in 53 consecutive outbreaks, and a third small 'epidemic' from September through December 1996 caused by a strain in the genotype Leeds (P1B cluster, Ando et al 1995). The last of these 'epidemic' strains (Venlo strain) was also found in the same period in sporadic cases from the physician-based study, although the variation of genotypes was greater in the stools from the NIVEL study (Table 6). In the years following these 'epidemics', the MxV and Venlo-like viruses have been detected occasionally. The LDV-like strain was found as the dominant variant in countries all over the world (Noel et al 1999), and is still commonly found though with a seemingly decreasing frequency (Fig. 4). In the past years, the majority of all outbreaks or cases were associated with strains from a limited number of genotypes. Overall genotype distributions were quite similar for outbreak data and for data from the population based studies, suggesting that outbreaks reflect most of the diversity seen in the endemic virus population. The discrepancies (e.g. as observed in 1996) are interesting, as they may indicate differences in mode of transmission or virulence characteristics. London strains were over-represented

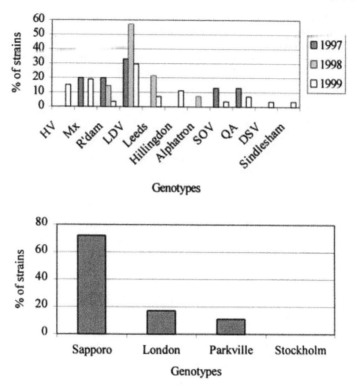

FIG. 1.   Distribution of genotypes of NLV (top) and SLV (bottom) in cases of gastroenteritis detected during a physician-based study in The Netherlands from 1996–1998. For genotype designations see Table 1.

in the community study, as was noted earlier from Sweden and the UK, suggesting that these strains are less virulent (Vinjé et al 2000a). In the near future we will analyse the epidemiological database in combination with genotyping information for such genotype-specific characteristics.

The sudden emergence and spread of a single strain raises important questions about the mode of transmission that allowed these events to occur, especially since no obvious epidemiological links were found between most outbreaks. Besides the possibility of large scale food- or waterborne transmission, the possible existence of an animal reservoir, or the existence of variants with altered tissue tropism (e.g. favoring spread by the respiratory route) are working hypotheses that need to be addressed in future studies. Recently, a European consortium with participants from nine countries has initiated a project aimed at developing standardized surveillance for enteric viruses in Europe, including a database that will be used as an early warning tool. Our goal is to thus provide a framework for studies addressing the above hypotheses.

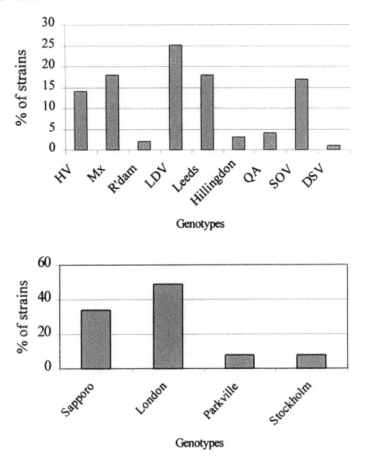

FIG. 2.   Distribution of genotypes of NLV (top) and SLV (bottom) in cases of gastroenteritis detected during a community cohort study in The Netherlands in 1999. For genotype designations see Table 1. Approximately two-thirds of the samples from the study have been analysed.

Investigation of animal caliciviruses
related to Norwalk-like caliciviruses

Until recently, the NLVs were considered to be pathogens with humans as the sole host. However, recent publications from Japan and the UK reported the presence of NLVs in some pigs and in some historic stool samples from calves (Sugieda et al 1998, Liu et al 1999, Dastjerdi et al 1999). The calf viruses, named Newbury agent and Jena virus, had been shown to be pathogenic for young calves under

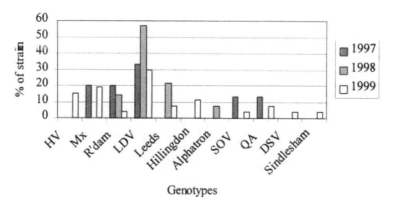

FIG. 3.   Distribution of genotypes of NLV in outbreaks of gastroenteritis reported to municipal health services in The Netherlands in 1997, 1998 and 1999 (until October).

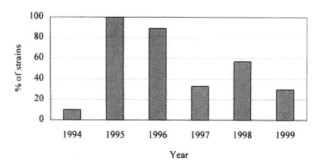

FIG. 4.   Proportion of outbreaks associated with the Lordsdale-like 'common' strain as percentage of all NLV outbreaks investigated in The Netherlands from 1994–1999.

experimental conditions and in field studies (Liu et al 1999, Dastjerdi et al 1999). The two bovine enteric caliciviruses were genetically distinct, but were most closely related with GGI NLVs, while the swine viruses were closely related with GGII NLVs. In a pilot study, we found that NLVs were widespread in cattle farms in The Netherlands, with 45% of the 74 calf herds testing positive for NLV by the generic RT-PCR designed for detection of NLV in humans. All Netherlands calf strains were tightly clustered and most closely related to the Newbury strains. The differences at the polymerase gene sequences, however, suggest that these viruses may be a distinct lineage of bovine NLV. This needs to be confirmed by capsid sequencing. All dairy herd samples were negative ($n=20$), and one pig herd out of 63 was found positive for a virus, which clustered with the published pig calicivirus sequences from Japan (van der Poel et al 2000). Preliminary data from

TABLE 6 Average proportion of the three most prevalent genotypes NLV in outbreaks (1997–1999), the NIVEL study (1996–1998), and the SENSOR study (1999) in The Netherlands

Study population	Genotypes	Average proportion (%)
Outbreaks 1997–1999	LDV	40
	LDV+Mx	53
	LDV+Mx + R'dam	66
NIVEL 1996–1998	LDV	32
	LDV+Mx	49
	LDV+Mx + Leeds	80
SENSOR 1999	LDV	25
	LDV+Mx	43
	LDV+Mx + Leeds	61

a three year surveillance of calf herds suggests that our initial observation reflects a common situation.

At this stage it is unclear if the animal NLVs form genetically distinct stable lineages, or are in fact part of a common pool of viruses circulating between animals and humans, although the finding of highly related strains in animals in different countries suggests the former. Studies are needed to solve this issue.

Conclusions

From the studies so far, caliciviruses are increasingly recognized as an important public health problem, with very high incidence rates in people of all age groups. By molecular epidemiological studies, we are now beginning to unravel the epidemiology of the different lineages of calicivirus. To advance our understanding of transmission routes and the mechanism behind the appearance of 'epidemic' strains a standardized international surveillance system is needed, which allows for rapid strain comparison from different sources in order to identify common strains early in the epidemic. Such an early warning system would allow the rapid recognition of supranational outbreaks, for which the sources then can be traced by a detailed outbreak investigation. Eventually, mapping these pathways will allow identification of risk factors (high-risk foods, processing methods, as well as high risk import/transport routes) which subsequently can be targeted by prevention programmes.

Acknowledgements

I would like to thank Dr Wim van der Poel, Reina van der Heide, Hanneke Deijl, Petra de Bree, the other members of the NIVEL team, the SENSOR team, the municipal infectious disease specialists (for their collections of outbreak specimens), and all the participating volunteers for their role in the work described here from our laboratories. I am grateful to Dr Tamie Ando for the comparative analysis of sequences from the RIVM/Colindale database with unpublished CDC sequences, the results of which have been used in Table 1. I would also like to acknowledge the stimulating discussions with our collaborators in Sweden (Dr Lennart Svensson, Dr K. O. Hedlund), UK (Dr David Brown, Dr Jon Green, Dr David Lewis), and our partners in the European consortium.

References

Abbink F, van Duynhoven YTHP, de Wit MAS, Koopmans MPG, van Leeuwen WJ, Kortbeek LM 1998 A population cohort study with a nested case-control study: a study design to estimate the incidence and aetiology of gastroenteritis in the Netherlands. 4th World Congress on Foodborne infections and intoxications, Berlin, June 1998, 171:P-A03

Ando T, Mulders MN, Lewis DC, Estes MK, Monroe SS, Glass RI 1994 Comparison of the polymerase region of small round structured virus strains previously classified in three antigenic types by solid-phase immune electron microscopy. Arch Virol 135:217–226

Ando T, Jin Q, Gentsch JR et al 1995 Epidemiologic applications of novel molecular methods to detect and differentiate small round structured viruses (Norwalk-like viruses). J Med Virol 47:145–152

Ando T, Noel JS, Fankhauser RL 2000 Genetic classification of NLVs. J Infect Dis 181:336–348

Dastjerdi AM, Green J, Gallimore CI, Brown DW, Bridger JC 1999 The bovine Newbury agent-2 is genetically more closely related to human SRSVs than to animal caliciviruses. Virology 254:1–5

de Leon R, Matsui SM, Baric RS et al 1992 Detection of Norwalk virus in stool specimens by reverse transcriptase-polymerase chain reaction and nonradioactive oligoprobes. J Clin Microbiol 30:3151–3157

de Wit MAS, de Kortbeek L, van Leeuwen N et al 1997 Interim report on a physician-based case-control study of acute gastro-enteritis in The Netherlands (NIVEL) 1996–1997. RIVM report 216852001 (in Dutch). RIVM, Bilthoven, The Netherlands

de Wit MAS, Koopmans M, Kortbeek LM, van Leeuwen W, Vinjé J, van Duynhoven Y 2001 Gastroenteritis in sentinel general practices in The Netherlands. Emerg Infect Dis 7:82–91

Dingle KE, Lambden PR, Caul EO, Clarke IN 1995 Human enteric Caliciviridae: the complete genome sequence and expression of virus-like particles from a genetic group II small round structured virus. J Gen Virol 76:2349–2355

Duizer E, Koopmans M 2000 Development of an *in vitro* method to culture human calicivirus. In: Cell biology of virus entry, replication and pathogenesis. Taos, New Mexico, February 29–March 5 (Keystone Symp) p 56

Fankhauser RL, Noel JS, Monroe SS, Ando T, Glass RI 1998 Molecular epidemiology of 'Norwalk-like viruses' in outbreaks of gastroenteritis in the United States. J Infect Dis 178:1571–1578

Green J, Norcott JP, Lewis D, Arnold C, Brown DWG 1993 Norwalk-like viruses: demonstration of genomic diversity by polymerase chain reaction. J Clin Microbiol 31:3007–3012

Green J, Vinjé J, Gallimore C, Koopmans M, Hale A, Brown D 2000 Capsid protein diversity among small round structured viruses. Virus Genes 20:227–236

Green KY 1997 The role of human caliciviruses in epidemic gastroenteritis. Arch Virol (suppl) 13:153–165

Hardy M, Kramer SF, Treanor JJ, Estes MK 1997 Human calicivirus genogroup II capsid diversity revealed by analysis of the prototype Snow Mountain Agent. Arch Virol 142:1469–1479

Jiang X, Graham DY, Wang KN, Estes MK 1990 Norwalk virus genome cloning and characterization. Science 250:1580–1583

Jiang X, Wang J, Graham DY, Estes MK 1992 Detection of Norwalk virus in stool by polymerase chain reaction. J Clin Microbiol 30:2529–2534

Jiang X, Wang M, Wang K, Estes MK 1993 Sequence and genomic organization of Norwalk virus. Virology 195:51–61

Jiang X, Matson DO, Cubitt WD, Estes MK 1996 Genetic and antigenic diversity of human caliciviruses (HuCVs) using RT-PCR and new EIAs. Arch Virol Suppl 12:251–262

Jiang X, Cubitt WD, Berke T et al 1997 Sapporo-like human caliciviruses are genetically and antigenically diverse. Arch Virol 142:1813–1827

Jiang X, Espul C, Zhong WM, Cuello H, Matson DO 1999 Characterization of a novel human calicivirus that may be a natural occurring recombinant. Arch Virol 144: 2377–2387

Kapikian AZ, Chanock RM 1990 Norwalk group of viruses. In: Fields BN, Knipe DM, Howley PM et al (eds) Fields' virology, 2nd edn. Raven Press, New York, p 671–693

Koopmans M, Vinjé J, de Wit M, van der Poel W, van Duynhoven Y 2000 Molecular epidemiology of caliciviruses in The Netherlands. J Infect Dis (suppl) 181:S262–S269

Lambden PR, Caul EO, Ashley CR, Clarke IN 1993 Sequence and genome organization of a human small round-structured (Norwalk-like) virus. Science 259:516–519

Levett PN, Gu M, Luan B et al 1996 Longitudinal study of molecular epidemiology of small round-structured viruses in a pediatric population. J Clin Microbiol 34:1497–1501

Lew JF, Kapikian AZ, Valdesuso J, Green KY 1994 Molecular characterization of Hawaii virus and other Norwalk-like viruses: evidence for genetic polymorphism among human caliciviruses. J Infect Dis 170:535–542

Lewis D, Ando T, Humphrey CD, Monroe SS, Glass RI 1995 Use of solid-phase immune electron microscopy for classification of Norwalk-like viruses into six antigenic groups from 10 outbreaks of gastroenteritis in the United States. J Clin Microbiol 33:501–504

Liu BL, Clarke IN, Caul EO, Lambden PR 1995 Human enteric caliciviruses have a unique genome structure and are distinct from the Norwalk-like viruses. Arch Virol 140: 1345–1356

Liu BL, Lambden PR, Gunther H, Otto P, Elschner M, Clarke IN 1999 Molecular characterization of a bovine enteric calicivirus: relationship to the Norwalk-like viruses. J Virol 73:819–825

Maguire AJ, Green J, Brown DW, Desselberger U, Gray JJ 1999 Molecular epidemiology of outbreaks of gastroenteritis associated with small round-structured viruses in East Anglia, United Kingdom, during the 1996–1997 season. J Clin Microbiol 37:81–89

Moe CL, Gentsch J, Ando T et al 1994 Application of PCR to detect Norwalk virus in fecal specimens from outbreaks of gastroenteritis. J Clin Microbiol 32:642–648

Noel JS, Ando T, Leite JP et al 1997a Correlation of patient immune responses with genetically characterized small round-structured viruses involved in outbreaks of nonbacterial acute gastroenteritis in the United States, 1990 to 1995. J Med Virol 53:372–383

Noel JS, Liu BL, Humphrey CD et al 1997b Parkville virus: a novel genetic variant of human calicivirus in the Sapporo virus clade, associated with an outbreak of gastroenteritis in adults. J Med Virol 52:173–178

Noel JS, Fankhauser RL, Ando T, Monroe SS, Glass RI 1999 Identification of a distinct common strain of 'Norwalk-like viruses' having a global distribution. J Infect Dis 179:1334–1344

Schreier E, Doring F, Kunkel U 2000 Molecular epidemiology of outbreaks of gastroenteritis associated with small round structured viruses in Germany in 1997/98. Arch Virol 145:443–453

Seah EL, Gunesekere IC, Marshall JA, Wright PJ 1999 Variation in ORF3 of genogroup 2 Norwalk-like viruses. Arch Virol 144:1007–1014

Sugieda M, Nagaoka H, Kakishima Y, Ohshita T, Nakamura S, Nakajima S 1998 Detection of Norwalk-like virus genes in the caecum contents of pigs. Arch Virol 143:1215–1221

van der Poel W, Vinjé J, van der Heide R, Herrera M, Vivo A, Koopmans M 2000 Norwalk-like calicivirus genes in faeces of farm animals. Emerg Infect Dis 6:36–41

Vinjé J, Koopmans M 1996 Molecular detection and epidemiology of small round structured viruses in outbreaks of gastroenteritis in The Netherlands. J Infect Dis 174:610–615

Vinjé J, Koopmans M 2000 Simultaneous detection and genotyping of Norwalk-like viruses by oligonucleotide array in a reverse-line blot hybridisation format. J Clin Microbiol 38:2595–2601

Vinjé J, Altena S, Koopmans M 1997 The incidence and genetic variability of small-round-structured viruses in outbreaks of gastroenteritis in The Netherlands. J Infect Dis 176:1374–1378

Vinjé J, Deijl H, van de Heide R et al 2000a Molecular detection and epidemiology of typical human caliciviruses. J Clin Microbiol 38:530–536

Vinjé J, Green J, Lewis D, Gallimore CI, Brown D, Koopmans M 2000b Genetic polymorphism across the three open reading frames of Norwalk-like caliciviruses. Arch Virol 145:223–241

Wang J, Jiang X, Madore HP et al 1994 Sequence diversity of small, round structured viruses in the Norwalk virus group. J Virol 68:5982–5990

DISCUSSION

Desselberger: You talked of genotypes, clades and lineages: could you clarify what you mean exactly by these terms?

Koopmans: For genotype, I like to use an arbitrary definition of genotype, which is 80% amino acid diversity of the complete capsid sequence. I don't use 'clades', but David Matson may be able to clarify the meaning of this term.

Matson: The issue is a bit complex. 'Clade' is a more generic term. A 'genotype' is a specific term that we sometimes use when we can't use 'serotype': it is a working handle until we can get a method for defining the serotype. 'Genotype' also is used when our primary focus is on the genome only.

Koopmans: In fact, the division between genogroups I and II is fading in our hands, in the sense that we have capsids that are almost equidistant between the two poles. We now have grouped these capsids with genogroup II strains on the basis of the presence of the conserved motifs that have been described. If you put them in phylogenetic trees they sit right in the middle, between genogroups I and II. They may actually constitute a new genogroup (Vinjé & Koopmans 2000).

Brown: We have been involved in some similar studies, although not of quite such a representative population. I would like your opinion on what this diversity means. We have looked at about 800 outbreaks over six years in a population of about 3 million in the north of the UK. We have found that the Lordsdale virus has caused about 60% of the outbreaks over that time. We found it at a similar rate in children. Given what we don't know about immunity, and given the sustained preponderance of one strain, I wonder what real questions we are asking by showing that there is lots of diversity.

Koopmans: The whole discussion with the Lordsdale-like variant has been concerned with whether this is a recent introduction or not. Why did this virus show up all over the world all of a sudden? Was it a variant that was normal to the population? So far I don't think anyone has conclusive answers, but I do think this parallel surveillance may give indications for this. It is intriguing that in 1997–1999, there was a similar representation of strains in the community versus strains in outbreaks, whereas in 1996 just one variant caused all outbreaks. To me, this suggests that there is something different about that virus. I don't know whether this is transmissibility related or due to a different mode of transmission, but this is the kind of information that we are getting.

Glass: You said that most of your outbreaks depended on person–person spread. In our hands, person–person is the diagnosis of exclusion except for a few unusual cases. Only 20% of your outbreaks are food-borne as opposed to over half in our studies. How certain are you that only 20% are food-borne, and could it be more?

Koopmans: I am not certain; it could be more. This is a passive outbreak surveillance with all the usual handicaps. Our health system has both municipal health services and food inspection services. They do not communicate much. The typical situation is that the municipal health services tend to look at people and collect samples, and this helps us make a diagnosis. The food inspection services are used to working with bacteria. They go in and are focused on hygienic inspection. They do not routinely take stool samples from people, which are the only samples from which we can make a diagnosis of NLV infection with certainty. We know that we therefore miss many of the food-borne outbreaks (Koopmans et al 2000).

Glass: When we were discussing rotavirus types earlier, the consensus was that tracing the unusual types can tell us a lot about epidemiology. In contrast, in the NLVs, where there is so much diversity, it is the identical types that are the most interesting, because they tell us about the common outbreaks that might be trans-European. You just mentioned the Lordsdale virus in the UK, but through this European collaboration have you found any identical strains that have spread right across Europe?

Koopmans: We have recently started looking for trans-European outbreaks. However, one of the first tasks is to standardize the assays: there are 11 groups each using their own favourite PCR assay and typing assay.

Glass: If you send everyone a common strain, such as the Lordsdale strain, would you get back data saying that it was an identical strain in an outbreak?

Koopmans: We hope this would be the case: we are trying to develop this. One of the other aspects of the study is that we will review what kind of surveillance data people have, and what the biases are. From this, we hope to develop a minimal surveillance system to obtain comparative estimates of the role of NLV infections across Europe. Retrospectively, we have seen some more examples of international outbreaks.

Estes: I think this is a great study. One of the nice aspects is that you have people looking for viruses in food as well as in clinical samples. As you are deciding what primers you are going to pick, everyone has their favourite, but it also makes a difference on what kind of sample you are analysing. Certainly, in the environmental samples the virus load is always much lower. Most people have not looked at the sensitivity of detection using a particular primer set. This will be an important issue: we may need different primers for different settings.

Clarke: In order to know when these strains such as the Lordsdale virus were emerging, you need to go back in time to see whether or not they were present. If they are not there, we need to ask where they are coming from. The obvious places are animal populations. Or are we just looking at a finite number of human strains? Have people ever found sequences that resemble animal NLV sequences in the human population?

Monroe: We have found no human strains with sequences that fall into the animal lineages.

Estes: Have we looked long and hard enough?

Brown: Our experience is the same. I don't know how long Lordsdale has been circulating in humans, but we can go back to 1990 and it has been the predominant strain since then.

Ramig: I was interested in the comment about the relationship between human and animal strains. Diagnostics have been available for a relatively short time. Those of us in the rotavirus field at a similar stage didn't see crossing of species barriers, but as we have gone more into underdeveloped areas, we have begun to see this. I wouldn't be surprised if you were to see this also.

Greenberg: Gastroenteritis takes its biggest toll on young children, and the second biggest toll is on the elderly. There is then a great middle ground for whom gastroenteritis is an inconvenience. Are people really focusing in on the elderly and especially the nosocomial infections of the elderly, which for me as a physician are frequently the most vexing? Are there data that I am not aware of that fit these viral causes into the elderly population?

Glass: We have an ongoing study on elderly patients, but it is very slow. Our recent funding has been tied to food-borne transmission, and we are fighting with the bacteriologists to get support for studies to look at food-borne outbreaks. We think that when these outbreaks are evaluated on an even level, the viruses will come out on top. Ultimately, the question will concern what we can do about them. If we can identify key foods or key practices that we can change, we can make an impact.

Greenberg: There have been several major epidemics in the elderly, in nursing homes. Do you have these data?

Glass: Not for the elderly as a group. We know that many of the outbreaks are in nursing homes.

Brown: In the UK we have a passive outbreak surveillance scheme, which is similar to that in The Netherlands. We recognize more than 400 outbreaks in the elderly involving more than 20 000 cases each year. This represents gross underascertainment and we don't have any precise data on sporadic cases. Of these reported outbreaks we may recognize perhaps 10 that are food linked.

Glass: Do you have hospitalization data?

Brown: Yes.

Ramig: One thing that has struck me listening to this discussion is a sense that people are beginning to think of this more in a population genetics sense. Ulrich Desselberger raised this idea earlier, and pointed out that rotavirus is really a quasi-species where on average every genome is going to differ from other genomes by a mutation. In this situation one then has to think, as one develops these phylogenetic trees, about building them from consensus sequences rather than individual clones that are sampled out of populations. The other thing we have to realize is that the consensus sequence in a quasi-species often will not reflect the phenotypes that are expressed by that quasi-species. There are things to be gained by looking at the problem as a population problem, but it is going to be complex in the short-term. Another question that comes up is that of the importance of reassortment in rotaviruses or recombination in NLVs. If you start looking at population genetics, genetic recombination or reassortment always increases the fitness of a virus population. We need to think along these lines. If a virus crosses into a heterologous species and recombines or reassorts with a virus that is homologous there, this virus is then going to be pitted in a fitness race against the other viruses in that quasi-species. With these acute viruses, in which replication takes place for a short time before the virus is transmitted, there may not be enough time for competition to allow these new recombinants or reassortants to dominate the population. This may be one of the reasons that we tend to see different strains persist.

Koopmans: It has taken a great amount of work to get to this point; however, I agree with you and I would like to go back to some of our human specimens and some of our animal specimens and look at the broadness of quasi-species and other such issues.

Monroe: We've looked at the diversity in the outbreaks that we analysed. In the USA we have a completely passive system that has much less comprehensive coverage than that of Marion Koopmans. Each quarter we see a different strain that is predominant except for the common strain in 1995/1996. We had a long-term absence of G1 strains to the point where the technician asked if she could stop doing the PCR for G1 strains because it was never positive; then of course the next three outbreaks were G1-type strains. Strains come and go. There is also the issue of stability. Now that we find G1 strains again, we find strains that are remarkably close to the 1968 Norwalk Ohio strain. There is tremendous diversity, but also stability. In any case where we have looked at person–person transmission, and the best we have gone is three cycles, the virus coming out of the last person is identical in the regions that we have sequenced to that of the first person. We don't see any evidence for short-term accumulation of changes. The diversity that we are seeing now is ancient: the viruses that we are seeing have been around for decades or millennia. They are reintroduced back into the population. In the little bit of serum work that we have done, looking at outbreak strains and comparing them, we have found much higher seroprevalance to the prototype Norwalk than to Toronto, suggesting that historically the former was more prevalent than the latter. We still see viruses that are remarkably close to Norwalk, so it is not like there is global immunity to that strain. It still shows up.

Holmes: I wanted to point out that the rotaviruses are predominantly enteric viruses in animals and people. The caliciviruses, in contrast, cause a wide variety of diseases in different species. Studying caliciviruses as if they only cause disease in humans and only cause enteric infection may be risky; we need to keep our minds open to the diversity of these caliciviruses.

Matson: I have some negative data. We looked at 100 tonsils with RT-PCR and a couple of primer pairs, and found no caliciviruses. Tonsils are usually taken from children of 10–12 years of age. We also looked at joint fluids from a few children with monoarticular arthritis and didn't find calicivirus. We looked in children with cancer who had aphthous ulcers and also had negative results.

References

Koopmans M, Vinjé J, de Wit M, van der Poel W, van Duynhoven Y 2000 Molecular epidemiology of caliciviruses in The Netherlands. J Infect Dis 181:S262–269

Vinjé J, Koopmans M 2000 Simultaneous detection and genotyping of Norwalk-like viruses by oligonucleotide array in a reverse-line blot hybridisation format. J Clin Microbiol 38: 2595–2601

Novartis 238: Gastroenteritis Viruses.
Copyright © 2001 John Wiley & Sons Ltd
Print ISBN 0-471-49663-4   eISBN 0-470-84653-4

Molecular biology of astroviruses: selected highlights

Suzanne M. Matsui, David Kiang, Nancy Ginzton, Teri Chew and
Ute Geigenmüller-Gnirke

Department of Medicine, Division of Gastroenterology, Stanford University School of Medicine, Stanford, CA 94305-5487, and Veterans Affairs Palo Alto Health Care System, 3801 Miranda Avenue, Palo Alto, CA 94304, USA

Abstract. Human astrovirus, the prototype of the *Astroviridae* family, is a non-enveloped positive-strand RNA virus with distinctive morphology. Initially named for a characteristic 5–6 point star evident on the surface of faecally shed viral particles by direct electron microscopy, a recent study using cryoelectron microscopy and image reconstruction indicates that viral particles consist of a smoothly rippled, solid capsid decorated with short spikes. Mechanisms underlying the assembly of these viral particles have not been fully elucidated. However, studies of two full-length cDNA clones of human astrovirus serotype 1 suggest that capsid residue Thr227 plays a critical role in the assembly of infectious viral progeny. The development of a full-length clone (pAVIC) from which infectious RNA can be transcribed has also facilitated studies of the viral 3C-like serine protease, encoded in ORF1a. These studies demonstrate that the full-length ORF1a product (101 kDa) is processed *in vitro* to an N-terminal 64 kDa fragment and a C-terminal 38 kDa fragment. Mutation of the predicted catalytic triad inhibits proteolysis. In other studies based on modifications of pAVIC, preliminary evidence supports the feasibility of developing a reporter cell line to facilitate astrovirus detection.

2001 Gastroenteritis viruses. Wiley, Chichester (Novartis Foundation Symposium 238) p 219–236

Human astrovirus is the prototype of the *Astroviridae*, a family of non-enveloped, positive-strand RNA viruses (reviewed in Matsui & Greenberg 2000). By direct electron microscopy, astroviruses recovered from stools display a distinctive surface star for which they were named. Since the star-like appearance is evident on approximately 10% of the viral particles of a given preparation, an experienced microscopist may be required to make a definitive identification on the basis of morphology alone. In addition, in a study of astroviruses propagated in cell culture, the surface star was not found, but could be induced by alkaline treatment (Risco et al 1995). In this study, electron micrographs of intact purified viral preparations (not alkaline-treated) showed particles that were round with spike-like protrusions from the surface and an external diameter of 41 nm.

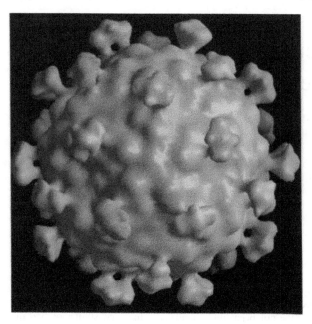

FIG. 1.   Human astrovirus serotype 1 map from negative stain (Yeager et al 2001). The result of image processing (Yeager et al 1990) of a negatively stained preparation of purified H-Ast1 virions is shown. Image processing requires digitization of micrographs, masking of individual particles, subtraction of background densities, and calculation of the Fourier transforms for each particle. Level of resolution is 24 Å. A particle, viewed along the fivefold axis of symmetry, is shown.

Recent structural analysis using cryoelectron microscopy shows some unique features of the astrovirus surface that cannot be appreciated in most routine images obtained by direct electron microscopy (Yeager et al 2001). Images of frozen-hydrated astrovirus particles, purified from a preparation of cell culture-adapted human astrovirus serotype 1 and stained with uranyl acetate, show spherical particles of uniform size with clearly visible surface spikes. 3D reconstruction from these cryoelectron microscopy images show a smoothly rippled, solid capsid shell with a diameter of 330 Å and 30 dimeric spikes, centred at the twofold axis of symmetry, that extend about 50 Å from the surface (Fig. 1). Inside the capsid, the genomic RNA appears to assume a partial icosahedral configuration.

Genome organization

The genome of astrovirus consists of plus-sense, single-stranded RNA, 6.8 kb in length, excluding the poly(A) tract at the 3′ end (Fig. 2). The messenger sense

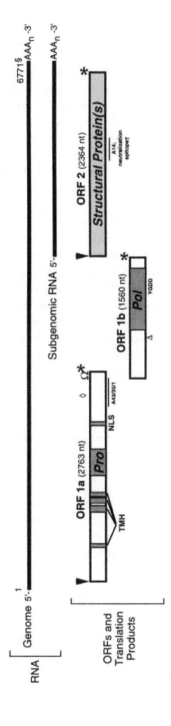

FIG. 2. Genome organization of human astrovirus serotype 1 (Oxford strain). Human astroviruses isolated directly in Caco-2 cells contain an additional 45 nt in ORF1a (Willcocks et al 1994b) at (Ω). Initiation and termination codons are indicated by black arrowheads and asterisks, respectively. The first potential initiation codon in ORF1b is shown by (Δ). The ribosomal frameshift signal located in the 70 nt overlap region between ORF1a and -1b is indicated by (◊). Motifs, including the protease (Pro), polymerase (Pol), transmembrane helices (TMH) and nuclear localization signal (NLS), are darkly shaded. Immunoreactive epitopes encoded in ORF1a and -2 are indicated by a thin bar. The A14 immunoreactive epitope (Matsui et al 1993) overlaps with the N-terminus of the VP26 (Sánchez-Fauquier et al 1994) neutralization domain (†). ORF2, lightly shaded, codes for the capsid precursor protein. Adapted from Matsui (1997), with permission.

genome consists of two modules in three open reading frames (ORFs). ORFs 1a and 1b at the 5' end encode motifs for non-structural proteins, including a viral protease and nuclear localization signal in ORF1a and an RNA-dependent RNA polymerase in ORF1b (Jiang et al 1993, Lewis et al 1994, Willcocks et al 1994a). ORF2, encompassing the 3' one-third of the genome, encodes an approximately 87 kDa structural protein that is the precursor of the capsid proteins of the mature virus (Monroe et al 1991, 1993, Lewis et al 1994, Bass & Qiu 2000).

Astroviruses display a number of notable features. First, the protease and polymerase are encoded in two separate reading frames, but are believed to be translated as a polyprotein. The first start codon (AUG) in ORF1b is found over 400 nucleotides (nts) into this reading frame, in a suboptimal context for initiation according to Kozak's rules (Kozak 1987). The 70 nt overlap region between ORF1a and -1b is highly conserved among human serotypes and suggests translation of ORF1b by the mechanism of ribosomal frame-shifting. This region contains a frame-shifting signal that consists of a shifty heptamer (AAAAAAC) and nearby downstream sequences capable of forming a stem–loop structure (Marczinke et al 1994, Lewis & Matsui 1995, 1996), both of which are features that are required for frame-shifting in retroviruses, to translate the protease and polymerase, and coronaviruses, to translate the protease (Jacks et al 1988, Brierley et al 1989). Unlike retroviruses and coronaviruses, human astrovirus does not appear to require more complex pseudoknot formation for this event to occur. Turkey astrovirus (Koci et al 2000) and avian nephritis virus (Imada et al 2000) also contain sequences that can be aligned with the shifty heptamer and stem–loop motifs of human astrovirus.

Second, during infection in cell culture, both full length (6.8 kb) genomic and ORF2-specific (2.4 kb) subgenomic RNAs are produced. Translation of the subgenomic RNA likely is used to produce large amounts of structural proteins to assemble progeny viruses efficiently, a strategy that is well characterized for alphaviruses (Schlesinger & Schlesinger 1996).

Third, astroviruses lack an identifiable RNA helicase domain. According to Kadaré & Haenni (1997), it is highly unusual for positive-strand RNA viruses, with genomes greater than 5.8 kb, to not encode such a domain. It is not known how astroviruses compensate for this apparent deficiency.

Characterizing the virally encoded 3C-like serine protease motif

Currently available astrovirus protease motif sequences (Jiang et al 1993, Lewis et al 1994, Willcocks et al 1994a, GenBank accession AF141381 and Protein accessions AAF18462 and BAA92848) can be aligned with the motifs defined for other viruses (Fig. 3). Prominent features include a putative catalytic triad of His461, Asp489 and Ser551 (numbering according to serotype 1, Oxford strain)

```
HAST1   447 GTGFFSG.ND IV..TAAHVV ..GNNTFVNV CY..EGLMYE AK.....V.R YM........ P...E.KDI. 495
HAST2   447 GTGFFSG.ND IV..TAAHVV ..GNNTFVNV CY..EGLMYE AK.....V.R YM........ P...E.KDI. 495
HAST3   447 GTGFFSG.ND IV..TAAHVV ..GNNTFVNV CY..EGLMYE AK.....V.R YM........ P...E.KDI. 495
ANV     510 GVGFRLG.NY IY..TAGHVV ..GRAKIAKI TW..KGLTSQ AK.....VLG HI........ ELPLF.TDTL 559
TAST    586 GVGFRFM.NY IL..TAEHVV ..QGSDIATL KN..GSVSVK SK.....VIK TI........ PIFES.VDNV 635
EAV    1089 ..VWTRN.NE VVVLTASHVV GRANMATLKI .....G...D AMLTLTFK.K .......... .....NGDF. 1136
HCV    1075 .....NG... .VCWTVYH.. GAGTRTIASP ....KGPVIQ .......... .M........ Y...TNVD.. 1110


TEV    2071 GIGF..G.PF II..TNKHLF RRNNGTLLVQ SL..HG.VFK VKNTTTLQ.Q HL........ I...DGRDM. 2123
MHV      31 .......WLD DKVYCPRHVI CSSAD..... .......... ........M.T DPDYPNLLCR V...TSSDF. 70
HAV    1551 ......GVKD DWLLVPSHAY KFEKDYEMME FYFNRGGTYY SISAGNV... ..VIQSLDVG .....FQDV. 1609
HRV14  1564 ....GLGIHD RVCVIPTHAQ PGD.DVLVNG QKIRVKDKYK LVDPENIN.L ELTVLTLDRN E...KFRDI. 1627
                       *                                                           *


HAST1   496 A.FVTCPGDL HP.TARLKLS KNP...DYS. CVTVMAYVN. .EDL...... VVS....... TAAAMVHGNT 546
HAST2   496 A.FITCPGDL HP.TARLKLS KNP...DYS. CVTVMAYVN. .EDL...... VVS....... TAAAMVHGNT 546
HAST3   496 A.FITCPGDL HP.TARLKLS KNP...DYS. CVTVMAYVN. .EDL...... VVS....... TAAAMVHGNT 546
ANV     560 A.RLEIPKPF QQ.LPVFRLA KSS...END. YVQMVCFDNQ LQNV...... VTF....... SGWANIDGDY 616
TAST    636 A.VLKLPPEL NS.VKPIKLA KKV...QSD. YLTLTAYDPN FQHA...... ATF....... TGWCIIDGNW 692
EAV    1137 AEAVTTQSEL PGNWPQLHFA Q.PTTGPAS. WCTATG.... .DEE....G LLS......G EVC....... 1188
HCV    1111 QDLVGWPA.. .PQGSR...S LTPCT..... CGSSDLYLV. .TRHA....D VIP......V RRRGDSRG.S 1158


TEV    2114 I.IIRMPKDF PPFPQKLKF. REPQREERI. CLVTTNFQT. .KSMS....S MVS......D TSCTFPSSDG 2180
MHV      61 CVM....... ...SGRMSLT VMSYQMQGCQ LVLTVTLQN. .PNTPKYSFG VVKPGE.TFT VLAAYNGRPQ 124
HAV    1600 VLMKVPTIPK FRDITEHFIK KGDVPRALNR LATLVTTVN. .G.TP....M LISEGPLKME EKATYVHKKN 1666
HRV14  1618 .......... .....RGFIS E.DL.EGVD. .ATLVVHSN. .NFTN.....T ILEVGPVTM. ..AGLINLSS 1668


             ▼▼▼   ●                        ▼ ▼▼
HAST1   547 ......L..S YAV....RTQ DGMSGAP..V CDK...YGRV LAVHQTN 569
HAST2   547 ......L..S YAV....RTQ DGMSGAP..V CDK...YGRV LAVHQTN 569
HAST3   547 ......L..S YAV....RTQ DGMSGAP..V CDK...YGRV LAVHQTN 569
ANV     617 ......L..N APF....ETY AGTSGSP..I INR...DGRM LGVHFGS 639
TAST    693 ......L..N NSF....DTK FGNSGAP..Y CDH...DGRL VGIHLGT 715
EAV    1189 ......LA.. .......WTT SGDSGSA.VV ..Q...GDAV VGVHTGS 1201
HCV    1159 ......LLSP RPI....SYL KGSSGGP.LL CPA....GHA VGIFRAA 1183
                                    *
TEV    2181 ......IFWK HWI....QTK DGQCGSP.LV STR...DGFI VGIHSAS 2207
MHV     125 GAFHVTLRSS H..TIKGSFL CGSCGSVGYV LTGDSV..RF VYMHQLE 166
HAV    1667 DGTTVDLTVD QAWRGKGEGL PGMCGGA.LV SSNQSIQNAI LGIHVAG 1712
HRV14  1669 TPTNRMIRYD Y......ATK TGQCGGV.LC ATGK.....I FGIHVGG 1700
                             *  **
```

FIG. 3.   Alignment of the astrovirus 3C-like serine protease motif with those of other viruses. The predicted 3C-like serine protease motif of human astrovirus serotypes 1–3 ([HAST1, 2 and 3], GenBank accession numbers L23513, Z25771; L13745; and AR141381) were aligned with the 3C-like protease motifs of avian astroviruses (turkey astrovirus [TAST], AF206663; avian nephritis virus [ANV], protein accession number BAA92848), hepatitis C virus (HCV, P26664), tobacco etch virus (TEV Nia, P04517), murine hepatitis virus (MHV, 453423), hepatitis A virus (HAV, p26580), and human rhinovirus type 14 (HRV14, P03303) using the Pileup program. Motifs with Ser in the catalytic triad are shown in the upper panel and those with Cys (instead of Ser) are shown in the lower panel. Asterisks indicate residues that are conserved in all motifs compared. A filled circle indicates the amino acids (also shown in bold) predicted to form the catalytic triad, an inverted triangle represents predicted substrate binding amino acids (also underlined) and periods denote gaps. The single letter amino acid code is used.

and substrate binding residues (Fig. 3). Given that this alignment strongly suggests that a protease is encoded within ORF1a, our studies sought to prove the functional significance of the protease motif. ORF1a constructs (Fig. 4A) were expressed in an *in vitro*, cell-free, transcription-translation system (Kiang & Matsui 2001). Derived products were immunoprecipitated with antibodies specific for various epitopes encoded by ORF1a (Fig. 4A), separated by SDS-PAGE, and visualized by autoradiography.

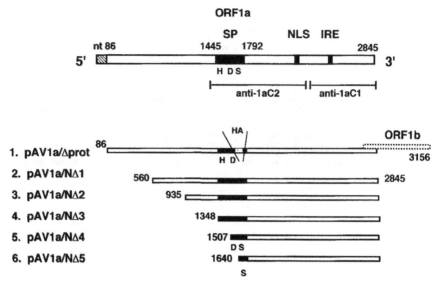

FIG. 4. (A) ORF1a-specific antibodies and constructs. The upper panel shows a schematic representation of ORF1a of human astrovirus serotype 1, with epitopes for the 3C-like serine protease (SP), nuclear localization signal (NLS) and immunoreactive epitope (IRE) indicated. The predicted catalytic triad residues His461, Asp489 and Ser551 are shown as HDS. The regions to which antibodies anti-1aC2 and anti-1aC1 are directed are shown below the top bar. In the lower panel, the construct 1 (pAV1a/Δprot) product contains a nine amino acid substitution by an unrelated nonapeptide (HA) in the region around the predicted catalytic serine. Constructs 2–6 encode progressively larger N-terminal deletions. The distance (in nucleotide length) from the 5' end at which each of these constructs begins is indicated to the left of the respective bar.

The full-length ORF1a construct, designated pAV1a, was mutated in several ways (Fig. 4A). In pAV1a/Δprot, the region encoding amino acids (aa) 546–554 that contained Ser551 of the predicted catalytic triad and two probable substrate-binding residues (Thr546 and Gln547) was substituted by a cassette encoding an unrelated nonapeptide. Three additional constructs were made in which each residue of the catalytic triad was mutated individually by site-directed mutagenesis (His461Leu, Asp489Val and Ser551Ala).

Immunoprecipitation of the pAV1a product by C-terminal antibodies (anti-1aC1 and anti-1aC2) yielded two major products, p101 (a 101 kDa full-length product) and p38 (a 38 kDa fragment) (data not shown). Products of 48 and 41 kDa (p48 and p41, respectively) were also immunoprecipitated. Similar evaluation of the pAV1a/Δprot product yielded the p101 product primarily and only a faint band at 38 kDa, suggesting that mutation of at least one residue of the catalytic triad and nearby substrate binding residues interferes with the

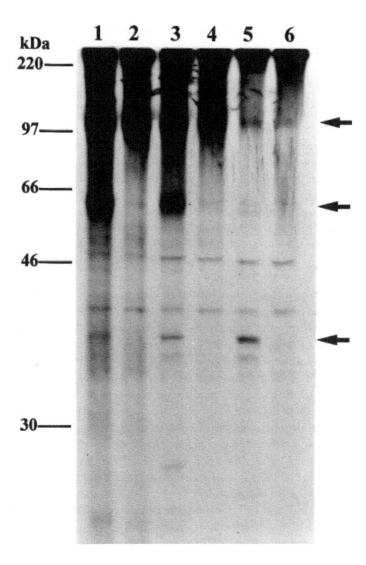

FIG. 4. (B) Proteolytic processing of the ORF1a product. ORF1a constructs pAV1a (wild-type) and pAV1a/Δprot (with mutated protease motif) were modified to include an eight amino acid FLAG epitope at the N-terminus (pAV1aFLG and pAV1aFLG/Δprot, respectively). Products from pAV1aFLG lysates (lanes 1, 3 and 5) and pAV1aFLG/Δprot (lanes 2, 4 and 6) were immunoprecipitated with anti-FLAG antibody (lanes 1 and 2), anti-1aC2 (lanes 3 and 4) and anti-1aC1 (lanes 5 and 6). Upper arrow points to the full-length ORF1a product (p101), middle arrow to N-terminal cleavage fragment p64 and lower arrow to C-terminal cleavage fragment p38. Molecular size markers in kDa are indicated on the left.

processing of p101. The intensities of p48 and p41 did not change, suggesting that these products were not derived by 3C-like protease-dependent processing of p101. Altering individual residues of the catalytic triad gave similar results, suggesting the importance of each of the residues in proteolytic processing of p101.

The marked hydrophobicity of the N-terminus of the ORF1a product made it difficult to synthesize adequate quantities of substrates for antibody production. To circumvent this problem, a cassette encoding an 8 aa FLAG epitope (Sigma) was inserted at the 5′ end of ORF1a and ORF1a/Δprot (pFLGAV1a and pFLGAV1a/Δprot, respectively). Anti-FLAG monoclonal antibody (Sigma) was used to detect N-terminal cleavage products of p101 catalysis. Immuno-precipitation of pFLGAV1a with anti-FLAG antibody and anti-1aC2 yielded two major products, p101 and a 64 kDa protein (p64) (Fig. 4B). Substantial reduction in the intensity of p64 was observed when pFLGAV1a/Δprot was expressed and immunoprecipitated with anti-FLAG antibody. The intensity of both p64 and p38 was significantly reduced when the pFLGAV1a/Δprot product was immuno-precipitated with anti-1aC2 antibody.

Five N-terminal deletion constructs were designed to estimate the N-terminal boundary required to preserve proteolytic activity, as indicated by wild-type levels of p38. N-terminal truncations that did not impinge on the predicted protease motif (deletions of up to 420 N-terminal residues) yielded p38 levels comparable to wild-type (data not shown). However, p38 could no longer be detected with further truncations of 474 and 518 N-terminal residues, suggesting that an intact catalytic triad is required for processing to occur.

In summary, these data suggest that the full length ORF-1a product, p101, is processed *in vitro* to two fragments: p64 at the N-terminus that includes the protease motif and p38 at the C-terminus that includes the nuclear localization signal (NLS) (Jiang et al 1993, Willcocks et al 1999) and an immunoreactive epitope (Matsui et al 1993). The precise cleavage site has not been determined, but is predicted to be between aa 550 and 600. The predicted catalytic triad appears to be an essential component of the protease motif and plays a role in the processing of p101. Baseline levels of processing are maintained with constructs containing N-terminal deletions of up to 420 aa that do not impinge on the predicted protease motif. However, processing is significantly diminished when constructs with larger N-terminal deletions or site-specific mutation of His461, Asp489 or Ser551 were studied.

Astrovirus infectious RNA and a determinant of infectivity

We have demonstrated that RNA extracted from virions is infectious (Geigenmüller et al 1997a). That is, when purified viral RNA is introduced into

BHK cells by transfection, progeny virus particles are produced and can be used to infect Caco-2 cells, in the presence of trypsin, to levels comparable to wild-type. This two-step, two-cell-line procedure is necessary since BHK cells are easily transfectable and will support astrovirus infection once RNA is introduced into the cells, while Caco-2 cells are readily infectable, but not easily transfectable.

Infectious RNA can also be transcribed from a full-length cDNA clone of human astrovirus serotype 1 (pAVIC; Geigenmüller et al 1997a). Two silent point mutations in the 3′ end of ORF1a were introduced into pAVIC to distinguish progeny of this clone from wild-type. In BHK cells transfected with RNA transcribed from pAVIC, replication, production of subgenomic RNA, translation of structural proteins and typical viral aggregates were demonstrated. The lysate of these cells could be used to infect Caco-2 cells and viral progeny bearing the signature silent mutations of pAVIC were isolated. Prior to construction of pAVIC, an initial full-length astrovirus cDNA clone had been obtained (Geigenmüller et al 1997b). When RNA transcribed from the initial clone was transfected into BHK cells, replication could be demonstrated, subgenomic RNA was produced and structural proteins were detectable by *in situ* immunostaining. However, when these cells were examined by electron microscopy, no clear, well-ordered aggregates of viral particles, a hallmark of astrovirus-infected cells, could be visualized; occasional amorphous clusters of possible virus-like particles were observed instead. In addition, lysates of the transfected cells could not infect Caco-2 cells. These findings suggested that the lack of infectivity of the 'viral progeny' was due to aberrant capsid assembly.

To identify the sequence(s) responsible for the phenotypic difference between the viral progeny derived from the initial full-length clone (non-infectious) and pAVIC (infectious), sequences were compared. Four point mutations were found in ORF2: one mutation was silent, while the other three (nt 5006, 5586 and 5745) resulted in amino acid changes. By systematically introducing single nucleotide changes at the latter sites on either the non-infectious clone background, or infectious clone (pAVIC) background, the critical nucleotide was shown to reside at position 5006 (Table 1). This was the only site at which a specific mutation could change the phenotype of the progeny viruses from noninfectious to infectious and vice versa. In addition, if nt 5006 was mutated to T in pAVIC, resulting in a conservative amino acid change from Thr to Ser at aa 227, the phenotype of the progeny virus was no longer infectious. Thus, it appears that this site is highly sensitive to amino acid substitutions. The important role of Thr227 in proper virion assembly through effects on capsid protein processing or capsid-capsid interactions remains to be elucidated. For the picornavirus coxsackie B4, Thr129 of the capsid protein VP1 has been identified as the determinant of the virulent phenotype in an animal model (Caggana et al 1993). Using the three-dimensional structure of poliovirus type 1 (Hogle et al 1985) and

TABLE 1   Identification of a determinant of H-Ast-1 infectivity by mutational analysis

	Nucleotide (nt) and amino acid (aa) position						
	nt	aa	nt	aa	nt	aa	
Clone	5006	227	5586	420	5745	473	Phenotype[a]
AVIC	A	Thr	C	Ala	A	Asp	Infectious
Mutant TAA	A	Thr	C	Ala	G	Gly	Infectious
Mutant AV	A	Thr	T	Val	A	Asp	Infectious
Mutant TA[b]	G	Ala	C	Ala	A	Asp	Not infectious
Mutant TS[b]	T	Ser	C	Ala	A	Asp	Not infectious
Noninfectious	G	Ala	T	Val	G	Gly	Not infectious
Mutant Asp	G	Ala	T	Val	A	Asp	Not infectious
Mutant VA	G	Ala	C	Ala	G	Gly	Not infectious
Mutant AT[b]	A	Thr	T	Val	G	Gly	Infectious

[a]Phenotype of viral progeny: infectious, lysate of transfected BHK cells infects Caco-2 cells; not infectious, lysate of transfected BHK cells cannot infect Caco-2 cells.
[b]Mutation that results in phenotype change compared to background clone.

sequence alignments, Thr129 mapped to the large loop that connects beta strands D and E of VP1, adjacent to Ile143 of poliovirus which is a determinant of attenuation (Ren et al 1991).

Development of a reporter cell line for astrovirus detection

The CDC has identified as a priority the need for 'simple detection methods that are more sensitive and more specific than the current EIA' (Glass et al 1996). Such methods would permit larger scale epidemiological studies and improve understanding of astrovirus infection and immunity. To enhance detection of astrovirus, we propose development of a reporter cell line. Such cell lines have been described for several other viruses (Rocancourt et al 1990, Kimpton & Emerman 1992, Stabell & Olivo 1992, Olivo et al 1994), and their design depends on the replication strategy of the virus to be detected.

The replication and transcription scheme postulated for astrovirus is inferred from the well characterized life cycle of alphaviruses such as Sindbis virus. Astroviruses have a similar genome organization (5'-non-structural–structural-3') and structural protein translation strategy (subgenomic RNA) to alphaviruses (Schlesinger & Schlesinger 1996). Upon infection, the non-structural proteins are translated from the input positive strand viral genome. The non-structural proteins then participate in transcribing a full-length negative strand RNA which subsequently serves as the template for the transcription of new genomic and subgenomic RNAs. The capsid precursor protein is finally produced by translation of the subgenomic RNA. Detection of newly synthesized capsid protein indicates viral replication has occurred.

On the basis of this strategy, development of a reporter cell line for astrovirus requires, first, assembly of a reporter construct, a cDNA copy of a defective astroviral genome that is deficient in some transreplication function (Fig. 5). The construct carries the reporter gene for green fluorescent protein (GFP) inserted in-frame into ORF2. Subsequently, the construct is stably inserted into the genome of Caco-2 cells, under the control of a Rous sarcoma virus promoter which should give rise to constitutive expression of a replication- and transcription-deficient astroviral reporter construct in the uninfected cell. In this state, no subgenomic RNA is expected to be transcribed due to the defect in a critical non-structural protein. In addition, it is unlikely that any GFP reporter protein will be translated directly from the defective genomic RNA since that would require internal ribosomal initiation. When the reporter cells are infected with a wild-type astrovirus, functional non-structural proteins translated from the infecting virus should complement in *trans* the defective replication and transcription of the reporter construct, leading to transcription of a subgenomic RNA and, ultimately, expression of GFP. The infected reporter cells should be detectable by their green fluorescence when observed with an optical fluorescence microscope.

This assay has several potential applications, including the determination of whether a clinical or field sample contains infectious astrovirus. In the laboratory, this assay could be used in place of the plaque assay to quantify the infectious titre of a viral sample, purify astrovirus or isolate neutralization escape mutants.

Our preliminary reporter construct is based on the ability to complement ORF1b function (U. Geigenmüller & S. M. Matsui, unpublished data). The construct, pΔT3329-10GFP (shown in Fig. 5), displays two important features. First, the deletion of a single nucleotide at position 3329 introduces a premature stop codon in the ORF1b product that results in production of a non-functional RNA-dependent RNA polymerase and impairment of RNA transcription. This defect can be complemented in *trans* by intact ORF1b product supplied by wild-type astrovirus. Second, ORF2 is modified to encode a capsid–GFP fusion protein in which the first 10 N-terminal amino acids of the astrovirus capsid are preserved and fused in-frame with GFP. This capsid–GFP fusion construct (10GFP) was selected among several others which were designed with longer stretches of retained astrovirus capsid sequence, because of the consistently strong green fluorescence demonstrated by this construct. Transcription of the subgenomic RNA, and hence expression of the capsid–GFP fusion protein, is dependent on the provision of functional ORF1b product by wild-type virus.

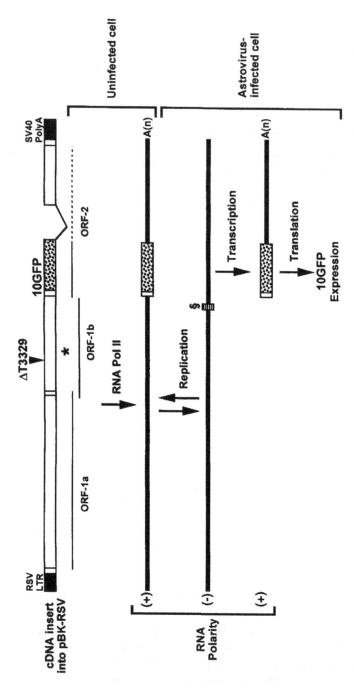

FIG. 5.   Defective human astrovirus serotype 1 cDNA (pΔT3329) with GFP reporter gene insert, and replication of its transcribed RNA. Black boxes at both ends indicate important plasmid features that surround the defective H-Ast1/reporter gene construct. Astrovirus sequence is shown in white, with the defect in ORF1b indicated by the black arrowhead and the premature stop codon it introduces indicated by (*). The GFP reporter gene is indicated by the box with the speckled pattern. The astrovirus subgenomic promoter, which is functional only in the negative strand and preserved in this construct, is denoted under the symbol (§).

A line of Caco-2 cells that has been stably transformed with pΔT3329-10GFP has been developed. No expression of GFP was detectable in these cells when uninfected. This cell line was then incubated with a cell culture-adapted strain of human astrovirus serotype 1, and successfully infected cells were detected with astrovirus group-specific monoclonal antibody 8E7 (Herrmann et al 1988) and Texas red. Initial examination by confocal microscopy revealed only a few cells with green fluorescence. By adjusting the brightness over these cells to a higher level, GFP expression was observed in every infected cell. Green fluorescence colocalized in the cytoplasm with expressed astrovirus capsid antigen (red). Green signal was also detected in the nucleus and nucleoli of infected cells since the 28.2 kDa capsid–GFP fusion protein is sufficiently small to diffuse freely between the nuclear and cytoplasmic compartments.

The most significant findings of our reporter cell line study were that GFP is expressed in every infected cell, lending support to the principle of complementation in *trans* upon which this assay is based, and that expression of GFP from the reporter construct is strictly dependent on *trans*-complementation. This pilot study is encouraging for the development of a simple, rapid and accurate detection assay for astrovirus infection, although many aspects of this system require further optimization. Of utmost importance is the need to improve sensitivity, if this test is to have practical applications for clinical and epidemiological studies.

In conclusion, the development of the astrovirus genomic clone pAVIC has enabled systematic exploration of many aspects of the molecular biology of astrovirus, by allowing the targeted introduction of mutations into the viral genome. At the level of the non-structural astroviral proteins, we have been able to show that the protease, encoded by ORF1a, is involved in the processing of the ORF1a translation product itself. We have also demonstrated that the function of the RNA-dependent RNA polymerase, encoded by ORF1b, can be complemented in *trans*. With regard to the structural viral proteins, we found that most of ORF2 can be replaced by a foreign gene, such as the GFP reporter gene, and display efficient expression of GFP in transfected cells. These findings suggest the use of astrovirus as a human expression vector and demonstrate the feasibility of establishing a reporter cell line for astrovirus. Finally, by introducing mutations into ORF2, we are studying requirements for viral assembly and formation of infectious viral particles.

Acknowledgements

This work was supported by a Department of Veterans Affairs Merit Review grant and National Institutes of Health grant R21 AI43513 (to S.M.M.). The Molecular and Cellular Biology Core Facilities of the Stanford Digestive Disease Center (National Institutes of Health grant DK 38707) were used. D.K. is supported by National Institutes of Health grant 1F32 DK09829.

References

Bass DM, Qiu S 2000 Proteolytic processing of the astrovirus capsid. J Virol 74:1810–1814

Brierley I, Digard P, Inglis SC 1989 Characterization of an efficient coronavirus ribosomal frameshifting signal: requirement for an RNA pseudoknot. Cell 57:537–547

Caggana M, Chan P, Ramsingh A 1993 Identification of a single amino acid residue in the capsid protein VP1 of coxsackievirus B4 that determines the virulent phenotype. J Virol 67: 4797–4803

Geigenmüller U, Ginzton NH, Matsui SM 1997a Construction of a genome-length cDNA clone for human astrovirus serotype 1 and synthesis of infectious RNA transcripts. J Virol 71: 1713–1717

Geigenmüller U, Ginzton NH, Oshiro LS, Matsui SM 1997b Identification and characterization of a non-infectious mutant of human astrovirus serotype 1. Scientific Program and Abstracts of the American Society for Virology. 16th Annual Meeting, Bozeman, MT, p 98

Glass RI, Noel J, Mitchell D et al 1996 The changing epidemiology of astrovirus-associated gastroenteritis: a review. Arch Virol (Suppl)12:287–300

Herrmann JE, Hudson RW, Perron-Henry DM, Kurtz JB, Blacklow NR 1988 Antigenic characterization of cell-cultivated astrovirus serotypes and development of astrovirus-specific monoclonal antibodies. J Infect Dis 158:182–185

Hogle JM, Chow M, Filman DJ 1985 Three-dimensional structure of poliovirus at 2.9 Å resolution. Science 229:1358–1365

Imada T, Yamaguchi S, Mase S, Tsukamoto K, Kubo M, Morooka A 2000 Avian nephritis virus (ANV) as a new member of the family *Astroviridae* and construction of infectious ANV cDNA. J Virol 74:8487–8493

Jacks T, Power MD, Masiarz FR, Luciw PA, Barr PJ, Varmus HE 1988 Characterization of ribosomal frameshifting in HIV-1 gag-pol expression. Nature 331:280–283

Jiang B, Monroe SS, Koonin EV, Stine SE, Glass RI 1993 RNA sequence of astrovirus: distinctive genomic organization and a putative retrovirus-like ribosomal frameshifting signal that directs the viral replicase synthesis. Proc Natl Acad Sci USA 90:10539–10543

Kadaré G, Haenni A-L 1997 Virus-encoded RNA helicases. J Virol 71:2583–2590

Kiang D, Matsui SM 2001 Proteolytic processing of a human astrovirus nonstructural protein. submitted

Kimpton J, Emerman J 1992 Detection of replication-competent and pseudotyped human immunodeficiency virus with a sensitive cell line on the basis of activation of an integrated β-galactosidase gene. J Virol 66:2232–2239

Koci MD, Seal BS, Schultz-Cherry S 2000 Molecular characterization of an avian astrovirus. J Virol 74:6173–6177

Kozak M 1987 An analysis of 5'-noncoding sequences from 699 vertebrate messenger RNAs. Nucleic Acids Res 15:8125–8148

Lewis TL, Matsui SM 1995 An astrovirus frameshift signal induces ribosomal frameshifting *in vitro*. Arch Virol 140:1127–1135

Lewis TL, Matsui SM 1996 Astrovirus ribosomal frameshifting in an infection-transfection transient expression system. J Virol 70:2869–2875

Lewis TL, Greenberg HB, Herrmann JE, Smith LS, Matsui SM 1994 Analysis of astrovirus serotype 1 RNA, identification of the viral RNA-dependent RNA polymerase motif, and expression of a viral structural protein. J Virol 68:77–83

Marczinke B, Bloys AJ, Brown TDK, Willcocks MM, Carter MJ, Brierley I 1994 The human astrovirus RNA-dependent RNA polymerase coding region is expressed by ribosomal frameshifting. J Virol 68:5588–5595

Matsui SM 1997 Astrovirus. In: Richman DD, Whitley RJ, Hayden FG (eds) Clinical virology. Churchill Livingstone, New York, p 1111–1121

Matsui SM, Greenberg HB 2000 Astroviruses. In: Knipe DM, Howley PM, Griffin D et al (eds) Fields' Virology, 4th edition. Lippincott Williams & Wilkins, Philadelphia, PA, in press

Matsui SM, Kim JP, Greenberg HB et al 1993 Cloning and characterization of human astrovirus immunoreactive epitopes. J Virol 67:1712–1715

Monroe SS, Stine SE, Gorelkin L, Herrmann JE, Blacklow NR, Glass RI 1991 Temporal synthesis of proteins and RNAs during human astrovirus infection of cultured cells. J Virol 65:641–648

Monroe SS, Jiang B, Stine SE, Koopmans M, Glass RI 1993 Subgenomic RNA sequence of human astrovirus supports classification of *Astroviridae* as a new family of RNA viruses. J Virol 67:3611–3614

Olivo PD, Frolov I, Schlesinger S 1994 A cell line that expresses a reporter gene in response to infection by Sindbis virus: a prototype for detection of positive strand RNA viruses. Virology 198:381–384

Ren R, Moss EG, Racaniello VR 1991 Identification of two determinants that attenuate vaccine-related type 2 poliovirus. J Virol 65:1377–1382

Risco C, Carrascosa JL, Pedregosa AM, Humphrey CD, Sánchez-Fauquier A 1995 Ultrastructure of human astrovirus serotype 2. J Gen Virol 76:2075–2080

Rocancourt D, Bonnerot C, Jouin H, Emerman M, Nicolas JF 1990 Activation of a β-galactosidase recombinant provirus: application to titration of human immunodeficiency virus (HIV) and HIV-infected cells. J Virol 64:2660–2668

Sánchez-Fauquier A, Carrascosa AL, Carrascosa JL et al 1994 Characterization of a human astrovirus serotype 2 structural protein (VP26) that contains an epitope involved in virus neutralization. Virology 201:312–320

Schlesinger S, Schlesinger MJ 1996 Togaviridae: the viruses and their replication. In: Fields BN, Knipe DM, Howley PM et al (eds) Fields' virology. Lippincott-Raven, Philadelphia, PA, p 825–841

Stabell EC, Olivo PD 1992 Isolation of a cell line for rapid and sensitive histochemical assay for the detection of herpes simplex virus. J Virol Meth 38:195–204

Willcocks MM, Brown TDK, Madeley CR, Carter MJ 1994a The complete sequence of a human astrovirus. J Gen Virol 75:1785–1788

Willcocks MM, Ashton N, Kurtz JB, Cubitt WD, Carter MJ 1994b Cell culture adaptation of astrovirus involves a deletion. J Virol 68:6057–6058

Willcocks MM, Boxall AS, Carter MJ 1999 Processing and intracellular location of human astrovirus non-structural proteins. J Gen Virol 80:2607–2611

Yeager M, Dryden KA, Olson NH, Greenberg HB, Baker TS 1990 Three-dimensional structure of rhesus rotavirus by cryoelectron microscopy and image reconstruction. J Cell Biol 110:2133–2144

Yeager M, Tihova M, Nowotny N, Matsui S 2001 Icosahedral design of human astrovirus. Submitted

DISCUSSION

Arias: Is the 3C-like protease encoded by ORF1 also responsible for processing the ORF2 polyprotein?

Matsui: We haven't really looked at that, although we plan to. We also want to look at whether this protease is responsible for processing the polyprotein S1 derived from the ORF1a/1b fusion. This may be more likely than processing of the capsid.

Carter: We have coexpressed the protease and capsid protein in baculovirus-infected insect cells. We don't get cleavage of the capsid protein ORF.

Suzanne, have you looked at the synthesis of ORF1a in cells? When we have done this we have never seen the 68 kDa protein that you referred to. We have always seen smaller proteins, and we suspect the N-terminus is chopped earlier, presumably by a cellular enzyme.

Matsui: We have some evidence from the vaccinia virus system and it appears that there is an ORF1a protease-independent process that cleaves off 18–19 kDa of protein. There may be a few more cleavages, but these need to be verified.

Green: Might there be a VPg protein in astroviruses, or a methyl transferase region?

Matsui: Steve Monroe and his collegues at CDC described a possible VPg protein, based on sequence analysis (Jiang et al 1993).

Monroe: The VPg motif was identified by Eugene Koonin when we were first looking at ORF1a sequences (Jiang et al 1993). I don't think there is any experimental evidence that there is a VPg in astrovirus.

Green: In your transfection studies, was that RNA from virus or from infected cells? Did you try protease K treatment, like in the classical calicivirus studies?

Matsui: Both purified viral RNA and RNA from infected cells were tested. We don't have data on the effect of protease K treatment on RNA infectivity since this intervention had an adverse effect on the cells.

Clarke: When you transfected the cells, did you just use naked RNA without modifying it?

Matsui: The transcribed RNA was capped.

Monroe: You showed in your diagram the production of the subgenomic RNA and the minus-strand intermediate. Years ago we did blotting and I was convinced that there was a minus-strand equivalent of the subgenomic, which would denote a mechanism different from that of the alphaviruses. We have never really followed up on this.

Estes: But your reporter cell line theoretically wouldn't work.

Monroe: It could work. You have to make the minus-strand somehow, either from the full-length plus strand or from something else. But it would suggest that you could put a minus strand in as your reporter, and that this would be replicated.

Desselberger: Do you have any idea whether this vital amino acid 227 in the capsid protein determines the ability of the virus to interact with the receptor?

Matsui: Amino acid 227 is in the part of the ORF2 product that is quite highly conserved among the different serotypes. The first 400 or so amino acids are highly conserved between serotypes. The threonine 227 residue also is conserved among other serotypes. We don't know for sure, but is likely that the spikes are encoded in a more variable part of ORF2, beyond amino acid 415 or so.

Carter: Some time ago John Herrmann produced a monoclonal antibody that reacted broadly with all the astroviruses (Herrmann et al 1988). We have recently been mapping the site of where this antibody binds. We find that it is a bipartite site: it binds to two areas separated by about 150 nucleotides. Both are needed to get good antibody binding. Amino acid 227 is just at the start of the second site. This suggests that 227 is part of the conserved region of the genome because of this pan-reactivity, but it must also be located towards the surface of the capsid.

Greenberg: Have you tried to make an infectious clone incorporating your GFP construct?

Matsui: We have not. Incorporating GFP in the capsid sequence, for example, may adversely distort the conformation of the capsid proteins.

Green: How well does trypsin prime infectivity?

Matsui: Trypsin is required for the astrovirus to infect susceptible cells, such as Caco-2. We therefore routinely add trypsin to the BHK lysates when we test for infectivity in Caco-2 cells. The system of BHK cells transfected with infectious RNA may be a good way to look at intracellular viral maturation, because it doesn't require trypsin.

Green: What do you think the nuclear localization signal is doing?

Matsui: We have not studied this, but Mike Carter and Margaret Willcocks have.

Carter: We always assumed that it was there to do something, so we did some two-hybrid work and pulled out a load of clones with which it seemed to react. Some were quite suggestive, but we weren't able to confirm that any were real.

Green: Have you tried mutagenizing that region in the infectious clone?

Matsui: No.

Carter: The capsid is found in the nucleus as well.

Matsui: There is capsid antigen transiently in the nucleus during viral infection.

Carter: You said your cryoelectron microscopy was done with cell culture-grown virus. Alicia Sanchez believes that the spiky form can be converted to the more condensed smooth form. Have you ever tried that?

Matsui: We haven't tried that. What she reported in 1995 was that serotype 2 human astrovirus grown in cell culture exhibited surface spikes and that these spiked particles were infectious (Risco et al 1995). Treatment with high pH buffers (about pH 10 for 10 mins) yielded particles with a star-like morphology. If she exposed them to pH 10.5 there was a rapid disassembly of the viral particles. The 'star-like' morphology found in a fraction of astroviruses shed in faeces may reflect the effect of the faecal milieu on viral particle morphology.

Estes: How do you intend to use your reporter cell system for diagnostics or field studies?

Matsui: Hopefully, we could take field samples, put a drop on the reporter cells, and determine whether they contain infectious astrovirus by looking for cells that fluoresce green. In addition, since we have difficulty plaquing astrovirus, we thought that this might be a way to identify 'plaques' of astrovirus.

Greenberg: How many molecules of polymerase will you need to get a green colour?

Matsui: We haven't titred this out.

References

Herrmann JE, Hudson RW, Perron-Henry DM, Kurtz JB, Blacklow N 1988 Antigenic characterisation of cell cultivated astrovirus serotypes and development of astrovirus-specific monoclonal antibodies. J Infect Dis 158:182–185

Jiang B, Monroe SS, Koonin EV, Stine SE, Glass RI 1993 RNA sequence of astrovirus: distinctive genomic organization and a putative retrovirus-like ribosomal frameshifting that directs the viral replicase synthesis. Proc Natl Acad Sci USA 90:10539–10543

Risco C, Carrascosa JL, Pedregosa AM, Humphrey CD, Sánchez-Fauquier A 1995 Ultra-structure of human astrovirus serotype 2. J Gen Virol 76:2075–2080

Novartis 238: Gastroenteritis Viruses.
Copyright © 2001 John Wiley & Sons Ltd
Print ISBN 0-471-49663-4   eISBN 0-470-84653-4

Molecular epidemiology of human astroviruses

Stephan S. Monroe*, Jennifer L. Holmes*† and Gaël M. Belliot*‡

Viral Gastroenteritis Section, Division of Viral and Rickettsial Diseases, National Center for Infectious Diseases, Centers for Disease Control and Prevention, Atlanta, GA 30333, USA, †Oak Ridge Institute for Science and Education, Oak Ridge, TN, USA, and ‡Atlanta Research and Education Foundation, Atlanta, GA 30033, USA

Abstract. Human astroviruses (HAstVs) are associated with 5–9 percent of cases of gastroenteritis in young children. Seven serotypes (HAstV-1 to -7), which correlate with genotypes, have been defined by using immune typing methods. We have used partial nucleotide sequence information from the capsid protein gene for molecular typing of 29 unique human astrovirus strains obtained from prospective studies of children with gastroenteritis in Egypt and Malawi. HAstV-1 was the most commonly detected strain, consistent with previous studies, but a surprising variety of strains were identified in both collections. An eighth astrovirus type, HAstV-8, has been defined on the basis of the complete capsid protein gene sequence and was detected in both collections analysed in this study. Although HAstV-8 and HAstV-4 strains segregate into well resolved clades by analysis of sequences from the region encoding protein P2 (VP32), the pair-wise distances between these types are less than those between strains of the other serotypes. In contrast, analysis of sequences from the region encoding protein P3 unambiguously resolve HAstV-4 and HAstV-8 strains, consistent with their classification as distinct serotypes. Overall, strains representing six of the eight serotypes were detected in two collections of samples from prospective studies of gastroenteritis in young children indicating that multiple astrovirus types are frequently co-circulating within communities.

2001 Gastroenteritis viruses. Wiley, Chichester (Novartis Foundation Symposium 238) p 237–249

Astroviruses were first detected in 1975 during examination of the faeces of infants with diarrhoea by using electron microscopy (Madeley & Cosgrove 1975, Appleton et al 1977). The viruses were described as 28–30 nm particles with a smooth outer edge and a surface star appearance and were given the name astrovirus. Particles with similar structural features were subsequently detected in the faeces of a variety of animal species (reviewed in Matsui & Greenberg 1996). Cultivation of human astroviruses was originally achieved in primary human embryonic kidney cells, with a stringent requirement for trypsin in the growth medium (Lee & Kurtz 1981). Direct isolation of human astroviruses from clinical specimens was later reported using a continuous human colon carcinoma cell line, Caco-2 (Willcocks et al 1990), allowing for routine isolation of strains from well characterized collections.

Our awareness of the importance of astroviruses as a cause of infantile diarrhoea has changed as more sensitive detection methods have been developed in recent years. The concentration of astrovirus shed during infection is lower than that observed for many other enteric viruses (e.g. rotavirus and adenovirus) and initial studies, which relied on detection by relatively insensitive electron microscopy, reported astrovirus in less than 3% of cases of childhood diarrhoea (Lew et al 1990, Monroe et al 1991, reviewed in Glass et al 1996). The generation of a group-reactive monoclonal antibody (Herrmann et al 1988) allowed for the development of more sensitive enzyme immunoassays (EIAs) for detection of astrovirus in clinical specimens (Herrmann et al 1990). Using these more sensitive methods, astrovirus was found to be associated with 3–9% of cases in several prospective studies of childhood diarrhoea (Herrmann et al 1991, Kotloff et al 1992, reviewed in Glass et al 1996). The determination of the complete nucleotide sequence of two human astrovirus isolates (Jiang et al 1993, Willcocks et al 1994) allowed for the development of highly sensitive reverse transcriptase (RT)-PCR detection assays (Major et al 1992, Jonassen et al 1993, 1995, Mitchell et al 1995). A direct comparison of the detection efficiency of EIA and RT-PCR using samples from an outbreak in a day care setting demonstrated the increased sensitivity of RT-PCR and documented asymptomatic shedding of astrovirus in older children (Mitchell et al 1995).

Serotypes of human astrovirus have historically been defined on the basis of immunoelectron microscopy, immunofluorescence, neutralization assays and type-specific EIA (Lee & Kurtz 1994, Noel et al 1995, Koopmans et al 1998). Type-specific rabbit antisera, generated by Dr John Kurtz and Terry Lee at the Public Health Laboratory in Oxford, UK, have been used as the reference reagents for most of the assay formats (Kurtz & Lee 1984). Seven serotypes of human astrovirus (HAstV1–7) have been fully characterized (Lee & Kurtz 1994), with an eighth serotype suggested on the basis of nucleotide sequence information available in GenBank (Z66541). The independence of HAstV-8 as a distinct serotype was questioned, however, by the observation of partial one-way reactivity with HAstV-4 by using standard immunoelectron microscopy assays (J. Kurtz, personal communication). Studies on the relative prevalence of astrovirus serotypes in various populations have demonstrated that HAstV-1 is the type most commonly detected, while HAstV types 6 and 7 are rarely detected (Lee & Kurtz 1994, Noel & Cubitt 1994, Noel et al 1995).

The astrovirus genome consists of a single-stranded RNA of positive polarity encoding three open reading frames (ORFs) (Jiang et al 1993, Willcocks et al 1994, Matsui & Greenberg 1996, Matsui et al 2001, this volume). ORFs 1a and 1b encode proteins involved in virus replication and their expression involves generation of an ORF1a–1b fusion protein via a ribosomal frameshift (Marczinke et al 1994, Lewis & Matsui 1996). ORF2 encodes the capsid protein precursor (Monroe et al 1993) which is processed to the mature capsid proteins by a pathway that remains to be rigorously established (Sánchez-Fauquier et al 1994, Bass & Qui 2000). All serotypes contain at least three capsid proteins, P1, P2 and P3, with the P2 protein encoding group-reactive epitopes, and the P3 protein encoding serotype-specific epitopes (Belliot et al 1997a).

With the development of RT-PCR assays for detecting astroviruses came the potential for typing strains by comparison of nucleotide sequence information. The usefulness of this approach was demonstrated when genetic types inferred by phylogenetic analysis of sequences from a region within ORF2 were shown to correlate precisely with antigenic types determined by type-specific EIA (Noel et al 1995). Surprisingly, a similar analysis of sequences from within ORF1a resulted in a different grouping of strains (Belliot et al 1997b). Strains from types 1–5 clustered in one distinct group, termed genogroup A, while those from types 6 and 7 clustered in genogroup B. While it was possible to clearly separate strains into these two well resolved genogroups by using either analysis of nucleotide sequence information or the results of probe hybridization experiments, it was not possible to separate strains within a genogroup into individual serotypes by using these techniques (Belliot et al 1997b).

We have recently participated in characterizing astrovirus strains from two studies of gastroenteritis in young children, one in Egypt (Naficy et al 1999) and another in Malawi (Cunliffe et al 1998). The details of the study designs and the methods for astrovirus detection and characterization will be presented elsewhere (Holmes et al 2001). In brief, astrovirus positive samples identified by group-reactive EIA were genetically typed by analysis of RT-PCR products generated from the P2 region of ORF2 (Noel et al 1995). On the basis of unique sequences of the amplification products, 17 distinct astrovirus strains were identified in the samples from Egypt and 12 in the samples from Malawi (Fig. 1). Interestingly, each collection contained samples clustering with six of the eight serotypes, including the recently described HAstV-8. These results confirm our previous work, and that of more recent studies, which indicated that multiple astrovirus serotypes co-circulate in communities within a few years (Noel et al 1995, Mustafa et al 2000).

We next examined the clustering of strains based upon analysis of sequences of RT-PCR products generated from ORF1a (Belliot et al 1997b). As previously reported, the strains segregated into two well resolved genogroups, A and B (Fig. 2). Consistent with the higher overall similarity in this region of the genome compared to ORF2, several of the strains that were distinguishable on the basis of sequences in ORF2 contained identical sequences in the region of ORF1a analysed. As noted previously, it was not possible to unambiguously

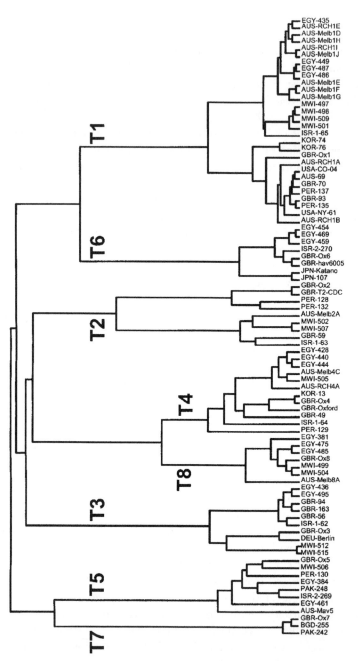

FIG. 1. Relationship of astrovirus strains based upon partial sequences from ORF2. Distances were calculated based on the 348 nucleotide amplification products from ORF2 by using the distances program of the GCG package. The country of origin of each strain is indicated by three letter ISO3166 code. All strains of an individual serotype fall within a single lineage, indicated T1–T8.

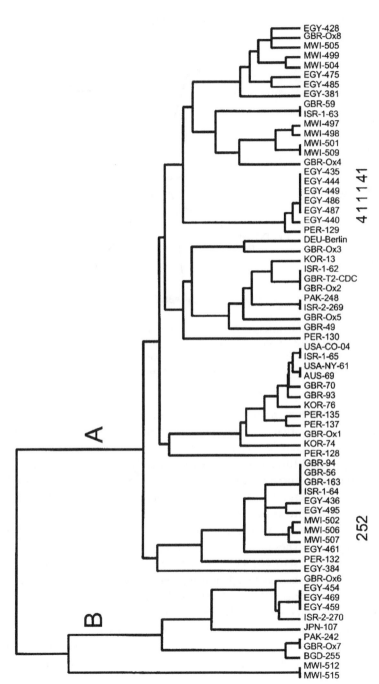

FIG. 2. Relationship of astrovirus strains based upon partial sequences from ORF1a. Distances were calculated based on the 214 nucleotide amplification products from ORF1a by using the distances program of the GCG package. The country of origin of each strain is indicated by a three letter ISO3166 code. All strains of serotypes 1–5 and 8 are clustered in genogroup A, while those of serotypes 6 and 7 are clustered in genogroup B. Within genogroup A, strains belonging to different serotypes (indicated by numbers) may have very similar, or identical, ORF1a sequences.

P2 (324 aa)   P3 (273 aa)

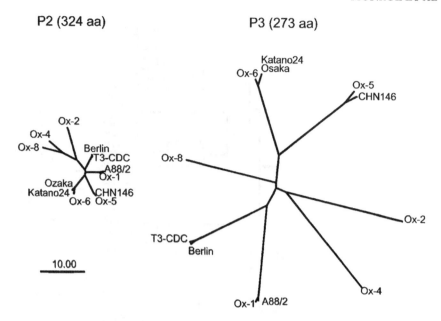

FIG. 3. Relationship of astrovirus strains based upon complete amino acid sequences. Distances were calculated based on predicted amino acid sequences for the P2 and P3 proteins from twelve strains for which complete ORF2 sequences were available in GenBank. The dendrograms are plotted to the same scale with the bar representing 10 amino acid changes.

assign strains to individual serotypes on the basis of sequences in ORF1a. Furthermore, it appeared that sequences in this region of ORF1a were more likely to cluster by geographic location than by serotype. For example, four samples from Egypt and three from Malawi had nearly identical sequences in their ORF1a amplicons, despite clustering as different serotypes in ORF2 (Fig. 2). These results suggest that although conserved regions of ORF1a are useful targets for RT-PCR assays designed to efficiently detect all astrovirus types, one cannot use analysis of sequence information from this region of the genome to assign genetic types that correlate with antigenic types.

The finding of multiple serotype 8 strains in these two collections prompted us to re-examine the issue of the genetic relationship between HAstV serotypes 4 and 8. Analysis of partial sequences from ORF2 indicates that strains from these serotypes fall into distinct clusters, but the pair-wise distances between the serotypes are less than some of the distances between strains within other serotypes (e.g. HAstV2, Fig. 1). To examine this relationship in more detail, we compared predicted amino acid sequences for 12 astrovirus strains for which complete ORF2 sequences were available. The close genetic relationship between serotypes 4 and 8 was observed when we compared predicted amino acid sequences for the P2 proteins (Fig. 3). In contrast, when we compared predicted amino acid sequences for the P3 proteins from the same 12 strains, the absolute distances between serotypes were greater, and those between serotypes 4 and 8 were comparable to those between the other serotypes (Fig. 3). These findings are consistent with a model wherein the relatively conserved P2 proteins of serotypes 4 and 8 contain shared epitopes, which were detected in the immunoelectron microscopy assay, while the divergent P3 proteins contain serotype-specific epitopes distinguishable on the basis of predicted amino acid sequences.

The recent application of molecular diagnostics has firmly established that astroviruses are a common cause of acute gastroenteritis in young children. Genetic analysis of amplification products can be a useful technique for determining astrovirus strain types and this approach has revealed a surprising diversity of strains co-circulating within relatively isolated populations. Additional studies are needed to assess the severity of astrovirus infections as the basis for a careful cost–benefit analysis of a potential vaccination program. Additionally, the role of astroviruses as a cause of outbreaks of gastroenteritis, both in children and adults, needs to be more fully investigated as the basis for formulating recommendations for public health interventions to interrupt transmission.

Acknowledgements

We would like to thank our collaborators Abdollah Naficy, Stephen Savarino, and John Clemens from the Pediatric Infectious Diseases and Vaccines Section, NIH, and their co-workers at NAMRU-2, and C. Anthony Hart and Nigel Cunliffe from the Department of Medical Microbiology, University of Liverpool.

References

Appleton H, Buckley M, Thom BT, Cotton JL, Henderson S 1977 Virus-like particles in winter vomiting disease. Lancet i:409–411
Bass DM, Qui S 2000 Proteolytic processing of the astrovirus capsid. J Virol 74:1810–1814
Belliot G, Laveran H, Monroe SS 1997a Capsid protein composition of reference strains and wild isolates of human astroviruses. Virus Res 49:49–57
Belliot G, Laveran H, Monroe SS 1997b Detection and genetic differentiation of human astroviruses: phylogenetic grouping varies by coding region. Arch Virol 142:1323–1334
Cunliffe NA, Bresee JS, Gondwe J, Hart CA 1998 The epidemiology of diarrhoeal disease in children at Queen Elizabeth Central Hospital, Blantyre, Malawi, 1994–1997. Malawi Med J 11:21–25
Glass RI, Noel J, Mitchell D et al 1996 The changing epidemiology of astrovirus-associated gastroenteritis: a review. Arch Virol Suppl 12:287–300
Herrmann JE, Hudson RW, Perron-Henry DM, Kurtz JB, Blacklow NR 1988 Antigenic characterization of cell-cultivated astrovirus serotypes and development of astrovirus-specific monoclonal antibodies. J Infect Dis 158:182–185

Herrmann JE, Nowak NA, Perron-Henry DM, Hudson RW, Cubitt WD, Blacklow NR 1990 Diagnosis of astrovirus gastroenteritis by antigen detection with monoclonal antibodies. J Infect Dis 161:226–229

Herrmann JE, Taylor DN, Echeverria P, Blacklow NR 1991 Astroviruses as a cause of gastroenteritis in children. N Engl J Med 324:1757–1760

Holmes JL, Belliot G, Cunliffe NA et al 2001 Genetic diversity of human astroviruses from Egyptian and Malawian children. Submitted

Jiang B, Monroe SS, Koonin EV, Stine SE, Glass RI 1993 RNA sequence of astrovirus: distinctive genomic organization and a putative retrovirus-like ribosomal frameshifting signal that directs the viral replicase synthesis. Proc Natl Acad Sci USA 90:10539–10543

Jonassen TO, Kjeldsberg E, Grinde B 1993 Detection of human astrovirus serotype 1 by the polymerase chain reaction. J Virol Methods 44:83–88

Jonassen TO, Monceyron C, Lee TW, Kurtz JB, Grinde B 1995 Detection of all serotypes of human astrovirus by the polymerase chain reaction. J Virol Methods 52:327–334

Koopmans MP, Bijen MH, Monroe SS, Vinjé J 1998 Age stratified seroprevalence of neutralizing antibodies to astrovirus types 1 to 7 in humans in The Netherlands. Clin Diagn Lab Immunol 5:33–37

Kotloff KL, Herrmann JE, Blacklow NR et al 1992 The frequency of astrovirus as a cause of diarrhea in Baltimore children. Pediatr Infect Dis J 11:587–589

Kurtz JB, Lee TW 1984 Human astrovirus serotypes. Lancet ii:1405

Lee TW, Kurtz JB 1981 Serial propagation of astrovirus in tissue culture with the aid of trypsin. J Gen Virol 57:421–424

Lee TW, Kurtz JB 1994 Prevalence of human astrovirus serotypes in the Oxford region 1976–1992, with evidence for two new serotypes. Epidemiol Infect 112:187–193

Lew JF, Glass RI, Petric M et al 1990 Six-year retrospective surveillance of gastroenteritis viruses identified at ten electron microscopy centers in the United States and Canada. Pediatr Infect Dis J 9:709–714

Lewis TL, Matsui SM 1996 Astrovirus ribosomal frameshifting in an infection-transfection transient expression system. J Virol 70:2869–2875

Madeley CR, Cosgrove BP 1975 Viruses in infantile gastroenteritis. Lancet ii:124

Major ME, Eglin RP, Easton A J 1992 3' terminal nucleotide sequence of human astrovirus type 1 and routine detection of astrovirus nucleic acid and antigens. J Virol Methods 39:217–225

Marczinke B, Bloys A J, Brown TD, Willcocks MM, Carter M J, Brierley I 1994 The human astrovirus RNA-dependent RNA polymerase coding region is expressed by ribosomal frameshifting. J Virol 68:5588–5595

Matsui SM, Greenberg HB 1996 Astroviruses. In: Fields BN, Knipe DM, Howley PM et al (eds) Fields Virology. 3rd edn, vol 1. Lippincott-Raven, Philadelphia, PA, p 811–824

Matsui SM, Kiang D, Ginzton N, Chew T, Geigenmüller-Gnirke U 2001 Molecular biology of astroviruses: selected highlights. In: Gastroenteritis viruses, Wiley, Chichester (Novartis Found Symp 238) p 219–236

Mitchell DK, Monroe SS, Jiang X, Matson DO, Glass RI, Pickering LK 1995 Virologic features of an astrovirus diarrhea outbreak in a day care center revealed by reverse transcription-polymerase chain reaction. J Infect Dis 172:1437–1444

Monroe SS, Glass RI, Noah N et al 1991 Electron microscopic reporting of gastrointestinal viruses in the United Kingdom, 1985–87. J Med Virol 33:193–198

Monroe SS, Jiang B, Stine SE, Koopmans M, Glass RI 1993 Subgenomic RNA sequence of human astrovirus supports classification of *Astroviridae* as a new family of RNA viruses. J Virol 67:3611–3614

Mustafa H, Palombo EA, Bishop RF 2000 Epidemiology of astrovirus infection in young children hospitalized with acute gastroenteritis in Melbourne, Australia, over a period of four consecutive years, 1995–1998. J Clin Microbiol 38:1058–1062

Naficy AB, Abu-Elyazeed R, Holmes JL et al 1999 Epidemiology of rotavirus diarrhea in Egyptian children and implications for disease control. Am J Epidemiol 150:770–777

Noel J, Cubitt D 1994 Identification of astrovirus serotypes from children treated at the Hospitals for Sick Children, London 1981 to 1993. Epidemiol Infect 113:153–159

Noel JS, Lee TW, Kurtz JB, Glass RI, Monroe SS 1995 Typing of human astroviruses from clinical isolates by enzyme immunoassay and nucleotide sequencing. J Clin Microbiol 33:797–801

Sánchez-Fauquier A, Carrascosa AL, Carrascosa JL et al 1994 Characterization of a human astrovirus serotype 2 structural protein (VP26) that contains an epitope involved in virus neutralization. Virology 201:312–320

Willcocks MM, Carter MJ, Laidler FR, Madeley CR 1990 Growth and characterisation of human faecal astrovirus in a continuous cell line. Arch Virol 113:73–81

Willcocks MM, Brown TDK, Madeley CR, Carter MJ 1994 The complete sequence of a human astrovirus. J Gen Virol 75:1785–1788

DISCUSSION

Arias: We recently adapted a type 8 human astrovirus strain to grow in tissue culture, and sequenced its genome. Comparison of the ORF2 amino acid sequence of this virus with the corresponding sequences from other astrovirus serotypes showed that the N-terminal half of the protein is very conserved among the various serotypes, while the C-terminal half is much more variable. The phylogenetic trees that can be constructed from these two regions are not superimposable. Do you have an idea of why this could be? Could it be the result of genetic recombination or maybe the consequence of different selection pressures along the protein?

Monroe: I'm not sure I can directly address this. We do see different tree morphology depending on which parts of the virus we are looking at. In working with these viruses and the caliciviruses, one thing that is strikingly different to me is that the ORF1 sequences in astroviruses, including ORF1a and ORF1b, are amazingly conserved between serotypes. There is a difference in the order of 12% maximum. In contrast, in ORF2 they are very different, particularly at the C-terminus. In the caliciviruses the polymerase is more conserved than the capsid protein, but the relative difference is not nearly so great. As for the fundamental question of whether there are different rates of evolution in ORF1 versus ORF2, something is definitely different there. I don't know how this relates to the biology of the virus.

Koopmans: I can picture different pressures and different rates of evolution across a single genome. There is a diversity of capsid types and serotypes with one genotype. How does the second genogroup come into play?

Monroe: I can understand that the enzymes might be more conserved, but even if there was extreme pressure to conserve the polymerase amino acid sequence, I would expect to see more variation in the nucleotide sequence. This appears to be a bit out of whack to me. We speculate that the two different genogroups could have arisen by recombination. In fact, the differences between strains in genogroup A or B are very small indeed. It doesn't seem possible that this is a linear evolution from one to the other. This raises the whole issue of recombination: only when we get more sequences from animal astroviruses will we be able to see whether our genogroups A and B are both human types, or whether there is an animal type in here.

Matson: I think we have a recombinant astrovirus that is between types 5 and 7. The recombination junction is between the non-structural proteins and the capsid. We found it in Mexico and Houston.

Desselberger: Could you bring us up to date with serotype 8? When I talked to John Kurtz recently he said he only had a single isolate.

Monroe: As Roger Glass mentioned, when we get involved in many of these collections, it is the unusual ones we tend to focus on. It was striking that we found serotype 8 in both of these collections. The fundamental question is whether this strain arose just recently, and if so, could this be why we are detecting it. I don't think so. I didn't show the overall numbers, but in all the studies that have looked at serotypes the predominant theme is that serotype 1 is 40–50% of the strains; the other strains end up being about 10% each, equally distributed. In the trees, all the serotypes are equally divergent from each other. From just a pure evolutionary sense this would mean that they have all been around for the same period. I don't know why serotype 8 hasn't been seen before. Perhaps it has a different clinical presentation.

Arias: A comment about the frequency of type 8 astroviruses. We recently characterized 25 astrovirus strains by sequence from six different cities in Mexico. We found that three of those strains were type 8. Interestingly, all three type 8 viruses came from the city of Mérida, Yucatán, where they represented 40% of the isolates. Thus they don't seem to be rare in this region.

Matson: We also found type 8 in South Africa.

Koopmans: We have done a seroprevalence study looking at age-related acquisition of antibodies to the different serotypes. We found striking differences for types 1–4, seen mainly in young children, whereas type 5 is not seen until adulthood. This suggests that either their epidemiology is different, or they are picked up when people start travelling (Koopmans et al 1998). Do you have any indication of regional differences?

Monroe: No. In these collections the only type that didn't show up was type 7. In the earlier collections that Jackie Noel looked at, this is also the case.

Desselberger: Dr Koopmans, didn't your data also show that there were subsequent infections with different astrovirus types? You said there were sera containing antibodies against different astrovirus types.

Koopmans: Yes, there are neutralizing antibodies to multiple serotypes. We are not sure that these antibodies that are induced are completely monoreactive. The serotyping of the viruses, as we have done it, has been done with rabbit reference sera and using a 20-fold difference as an indicator for serotype specificity. By this approach, we concluded that the astrovirus types are indeed true serotypes. But this does not mean that there is no cross-reactive antibody following infection in humans. We addressed this issue by looking for correlations between antibody levels in individual sera. We found no cross-reactivity (Koopmans et al 1998).

Monroe: We use the same rabbit sera as a group-reactive sera at low dilution in ELISA, and as a type-specific sera at high dilution in the same ELISA. Clearly they are cross-reactive.

Desselberger: Dr Koopmans, your percentage values didn't give the titre distribution.

Koopmans: We have also looked at that. The titres are highest in the youngest children, but there is also a distinct peak in the 25–35 year olds.

Carter: You didn't put any animal strains on your phylogenetic trees. Presumably this is because there aren't many sequences available. If you look just at the variable region in ORF2, then several sequences are available, including strains from pig, lamb and turkey. If you do the tree this way, you find that all the human viruses cluster together with the exception of type 4, and all the animal viruses are down the other end with type 4 on the fringe. I know this is suggestive and controversial, but what about zoonotic infections in astroviruses?

Monroe: I think it is the same for any of these viruses, particularly when you are talking about young kids crawling around in the dirt and having pets or husbandry animals nearby, where the chance for co-infection is great. As Timo Vesikari has shown, there is a lot of co-infection with other human viruses. Type 4 is a little bit weird, and it wouldn't surprise me if it didn't quite come along with the others.

Carter: It may have come out of animals some time ago. Certainly, we got quite interested in this and started looking for evidence of infection in humans by the feline astrovirus. We think we have some evidence of seroconversion that appears to be specific to the feline astrovirus. Interestingly, the feline virus will actually replicate in Caco-2 cells, churning out loads of particles all of which are non-infectious. There is antigen production, but not actually growth of infectious virus as such in Caco-2 cells. I did wonder whether it might be possible to get at least abortive replication from some animals.

Estes: Ruth Bishop told us earlier that genetic lineages have respectability, but I'm still unclear as to the difference between genotype, lineage, cluster and clade. We have heard that clades are a more specific definition. I find reading the literature confusing.

Matson: A clade is simply a branch. A sequence that differs by only one amino acid doesn't tell you whether you are in a serotype or a genus or a family.

Estes: So is this a useful term?

Matson: It is when you are not sure what you are talking about! We have brought into the literature terms like genotype, for which there is really not any consensus as to what it is, at least within the caliciviruses. Whether the clades that are called genotypes have any biological significance is uncertain. They may have epidemiological significance because one can track a particular strain through an outbreak.

Estes: I think I understand what a genotype is; the question is what is the difference between a genotype and a lineage, or are they just two words for the same thing?

Patton: The definition of a clade seems quite artificial. Two persons looking at the same phylogenetic tree can differ in their interpretation of branch points and numbers of clades. From reviewing the literature, it is not clear that investigators working with different groups of viruses would agree on the definition of a clade.

Matson: A clade is applicable to the analysis that is being performed for that consensus sequence. Within that analysis, we say there are this number of clades. If you do another region of the genome, the clades will be different. It is dependent upon the analysis. It is clear from the capsid regions of the *Astroviridae* that different tree patterns are produced from sequences of different regions. Clade is a generic term for a branch; clusters are clades that seem to group together in a particular way. Genotype is an attempt to say serotype when serotype would not be accepted, or may be used when genomic regions are compared. The danger is using genotype to imply serotype when the biological meaning of genotype is unknown.

Greenberg: I disagree. There used to be a definition of serotype, which was a 20-fold difference between homotypic and heterotypic reaction. As you are all aware in the rotavirus field, when things did not work properly, we changed the definition. As long as a serotype definition is applied consistently, it is a fair thing to do. But for VP4, various people have used various definitions, from 20-fold to eightfold to fourfold. It seems to be similar for genotype: how much diversity are we going to classify as distinct? I don't think anyone in this room thinks that genotype is a substitute for serotype. It sometimes cosegregates with serotype, and sometimes doesn't: it is a different tool. In the HIV field, clades is used as an interchangeable term for genotype, I think.

Monroe: The point is that there is no scale. If you took all retroviruses or lentiviruses, all HIV would be one clade: this is a different scale. If you take all caliciviruses, all the NLVs are one clade.

Greenberg: What about all *Reoviridae*?

Monroe: The same thing applies. There is no scale implied in the word clade. In order for us to be able to communicate between laboratories about NLVs, we need to decide what the definitions are for genotype, and then apply those rules. We almost need to do the same as researchers in fields like hepatitis A have done, where, for instance, they say that a genotype is more than 12% using these nucleotides analysed by this method.

Reference

Koopmans M, Bijen M, Monroe SS, Vinjé J 1998 Age-stratified seroprevalence of neutralizing antibodies to astrovirus types 1–7 in The Netherlands. Clin Diagn Lab Immunol 5: 33–37

General discussion II

Matson: I have a comment about heterotypic protection to rotavirus. We did a study in daycare centres where kids were monitored for two rotavirus seasons, with at least one weekly stool specimen (O'Ryan et al 1994). We only detected G1 and G3 viruses. Then we looked at the antibody levels using an epitope-specific antibody assay for G1–G4, and the monoclonals we used were neutralizing monoclonals used for typing. We found that as the children had an increasing number of infections, children exposed to types 1 and 3 also had increasing levels of type-specific antibody for types 2 and 4. These levels would be considered to be protective. The simple conclusion is that two non-type G2/G4 infections are sufficient to induce protective levels of type 2 and 4 antibody.

Greenberg: We have just seen structures of astroviruses that look different to the structures that I am used to looking at for other viruses. Dr Prasad, you are the walking encyclopaedia of structures; is there some weird plant virus for instance that looks like this?

Prasad: No. It looks like it is 180 molecules of something. One common feature that I see between caliciviruses and astroviruses is a smooth shell. Then the protrusions are more elaborate in the case of caliciviruses and Norwalk-like viruses (NLVs), whereas here the protrusions are tiny. Although the length seems to be 50 Å, similar to that in caliciviruses, the dimensions seem to be small. If you take the shell, this would account for only about 35 kDa, so there must be a lot more protein that is either cleaved, or inside.

Matsui: It is probably cleaved, because it was grown in trypsin.

Prasad: What is the molecular weight of the structural protein? Was there one structural protein making up the capsid?

Matsui: Astroviruses are believed to have at least two structural (capsid) proteins that are derived from the capsid precursor protein (ORF2 product): ∼ 35 kDa and ∼ 29–35 kDa, depending on serotype. We have done some volume calculations based on these values.

Prasad: Volume calculations would work only if you knew what the molecular weight was. You would know the volume from the 3D reconstructions. You could use the density, and calculate the molecular weight. Unless you know the molecular weight of the protein that makes up the capsid, it will be difficult to interpret in terms of where the RNA is.

Glass: One issue that Stephan Monroe addressed concerning serotype diversity is that in developing countries, the diversity of viruses is much greater and mixed infections are more common. He looked at a small collection of astrovirus strains from Malawi and Egypt and found six of the eight predominant serotypes. Similarly, in Lucknow, India, we found seven different strains among only 25 specimens of rotavirus examined. A further issue is the case fatality rate. One of the issues with astrovirus is where do we go with it? Is there enough astrovirus to consider it to be a public health threat? There are some data, such as the early study by John Herrmann in Thailand, where 8% of the children hospitalized in Bangkok had astroviruses (Herrmann et al 1991). We have an interesting rate of hopitalization, but what we don't know is whether this 8% of hospitalizations for severe disease translates to 8% of deaths. 8% of diarrhoeal deaths equals 200 000 deaths per year, and this would be a reasonable target for interventions. However, if we were to find the more severe the disease, the less frequently it is caused by astroviruses, we could put this aside completely. I am still uncomfortable with the study of Cruz et al (1992) in Guatemala and the studies in Thailand, which suggest that astrovirus is present at a significant level in hospitalized patients. We need more data.

Kapikian: As you know, a question I have asked for years concerns the importance of astrovirus as an aetiological agent for diarrhoea severe enough to require admission to hospital. I recall in 1995 at the viral gastroenteritis meeting in Japan, you (Roger Glass) laid down a challenge to me after my presentation in which I had noted a very small percentage of severe cases due to astroviruses, saying that with the new tools for detection available, astroviruses would be detected more frequently than I had shown. The studies from Guatemala and Thailand you mentioned certainly were of great interest. However, the answer to my question appears to be elusive. I think it is important with the new techniques that the relative importance of astroviruses in the aetiology of severe diarrhoea be ascertained and its role thus be established.

Glass: One of the directions in all these studies, whether it is with caliciviruses, astroviruses or group C rotaviruses, is to firmly establish the disease burden. For each of these we have the same problem of adequacy of diagnostics that can be easily applied. We have an ELISA for astroviruses, which is good but not great. When you look at the Doug Mitchell studies, you get quite a different picture of the epidemiology when you use a more sensitive assay (RT-PCR) (Mitchell et al 1995) than if you just use the ELISA (Mitchell et al 1993). Anything done with ELISA will give an underestimate of the true disease incidence. We need to automate the PCR in some way so it is more user-friendly for field studies on the significance of astrovirus, calicivirus and group C rotavirus infections. We have been interested in the group C rotaviruses for a long time. We know that they exist in the US, but we don't have an ELISA that can be easily applied for routine surveillance, nor do we have shedding at the same level of rotavirus. One of the real challenges of this field is to have more sensitive diagnostics applied. For calculations of rotavirus disease burden we have always extrapolated from hospitalized patients with severe disease to deaths. Whether this is a proper extrapolation or not, or whether malnutrition, tuberculosis and other diseases are co-factors in those deaths, is unknown. When we make the extrapolation with rotavirus that there are 600 000 deaths, there are no autopsy studies that allow us to be sure. This is another priority.

Kapikian: We don't know the exact number, but we do know that consistently rotaviruses are the single most important aetiological agents of severe diarrhoea in infants and young children, both in developed and developing countries.

Green: There are people who say that half of the diarrhoeal deaths are due to malnutrition.

Kapikian: For severe diarrhoea illnesses in children, consistently about 35–50% are associated with rotavirus infection anywhere in the world. The role of astroviruses has been examined by various groups more recently, and their role as an aetiological agent of severe diarrhoea appears to be low. All I'm saying is that I think that the time has come with the wonderful techniques that we have available to try to answer a few of these questions. Otherwise we will be going around in circles for the next 10 years without achieving a firm conclusion.

Clarke: There is a study in the UK looking at community acquired infections where astroviruses, group A and C rotaviruses and caliciviruses are being surveyed. David Brown may be able to comment on the prevalence of astrovirus infection in the community in the UK.

Brown: The IID study was a large study that used electron microscopy (EM) for all viral diagnosis, so it suffered from underdiagnosis due to the low sensitivity of EM. Astroviruses were found at a lower prevalence than rotaviruses and NLVs in a similar way to that Timo Vesikari described earlier. The severity of illness in different virus infections is an important question. The rotavirus vaccine studies are the ideal place to examine the severity of infection using that material. The problem with UK hospitalization data, and we have seen some quite high incidences of astrovirus infection, is that admission criteria vary depending on the community served. So although hospitalization is a broad proxy for severity, it is not always as precise as we would like.

Estes: Why is there not a good diagnostic test for group C rotavirus? The antigen that Jean Cohen has expressed in baculovirus cross-reacts with human group C rotavirus. There is no reason why within a 2 month period you couldn't make good antibodies.

Clarke: We produced one (James et al 1998), and the human group C ELISA exists and works well.

Greenberg: Is group C rotavirus shed in amounts that would make it reliably detectable by ELISA?

Clarke: Yes. We have sometimes detected group C antigen in samples where there are no obvious virions.

Saif: At least in animals, especially when we have found group C rotavirus in adult cattle we have missed it consistently by EM, antigen methods and PAGE, but we have detected it consistently by RT-PCR (Chang et al 1999). Screening just using ELISA or PAGE could be missing quite a few.

Holmes: What is the significance in different parts of the world of dual infection with different kinds of diarrhoea viruses?

Koopmans: From our studies we have found mixed infections in 2–3% of cases, but this is usually a combination of a virus and a bacterium or parasite. The combinations are not consistent. This is just with the routine diagnostics (de Wit et al 2000).

Desselberger: From the data I surveyed in my paper the general impression is that there are more dual infections in collections from developing countries than in developed countries. The patient group in which there are dual or even multiple infections are immunocompromised children.

Saif: If we are talking about future directions, it seems that there are several important areas here. We might want to target rotavirus vaccines to 6 week old infants. What seems to be missing is more studies in neonates, including studies in neonatal animal models. It is recognized in the literature that the neonatal immune response differs from the adult immune response in terms of being lower in magnitude and in some cases hyporesponsive. If we are going to vaccinate six week old infants, in developing countries are maternal antibodies going to play a bigger role when oral live vaccines are used? Studies in pigs given maternal antibodies to human rotavirus suggest that these antibodies could pose a problem for the efficacy of live oral vaccines in infants (Hodgins et al 1999, Parreno et al 1999). A third issue is that of innate immune responses to rotavirus. These responses are interconnected with the acquired response. Perhaps this explains some of the responses we get with the infectious agent versus trying to use inactivated virus.

Vesikari: The only good study in neonates is one we did in 1984–87 (Ruuska et al 1990). We gave a single dose of bovine rotavirus vaccine to neonates. To cut a long story short, it effectively cut off the severe rotavirus disease in much the same way as was found in Ruth Bishop's study of natural neonatal rotavirus infection (Bishop et al 1983). If the goal of rotavirus vaccination is limited to the elimination of severe rotavirus disease, this can be reached with a single dose of rotavirus vaccine, and I would say probably with any rotavirus vaccine. It does not reduce the incidence of symptomatic rotavirus illness, but it eliminates the really severe cases. Probably because the neonates don't have a lot of lymphoid tissue or germinal centres in the gut, my guess is that there might not be any intussusception in this age group. The strongest argument against neonatal immunization is that this doesn't fit the US immunization schedule, which is a sacred cow: no pharmaceutical company would consider developing a rotavirus vaccine that could not be given according to the current US immunization schedule.

Greenberg: I think Linda Saif was correct: as we look for rotavirus vaccine, something that we don't know about is the ontogeny of the immune response in the newborn. I have made a living with animal models, but I think that in this area, above all others, that the human will be the most likely place to get meaningful data. The ontogeny of the immune response varies from species to species.

Patton: The live attenuated vaccines under development for respiratory syncytial virus and the parainfluenza viruses are proposed to be administered to neonates. If these vaccines are to be effectively used, then the US immunization schedule will have to be modified. And if this is accomplished, it would seem possible that the schedule might also be altered to allow a rotavirus vaccine to be given earlier than 6 months.

Green: Mary Estes, would you update us on the NLV virus-like particle (VLP) vaccine candidate?

Estes: The article on Norwalk virus vaccines will be out in another week (Estes et al 2000). There is controversy about whether there is a need for a calicivirus vaccine. As the epidemiology has changed there has been increasing interest in having a calicivirus vaccine. The group that at the moment is the most interested in a vaccine is the military, because it is clear that as the Navy deploys people on aircraft carriers, which are in effect big floating cities, and they have a significant amount of diarrhoeal disease. There have been enteritis problems in areas such as Kuwait which they thought were bacterial, but when they looked there was more calicivirus disease than had been anticipated. We have given two doses of our VLPs in a phase I trial to adult volunteers, 250 μg per dose given orally in water. All the volunteers had an immune response and there were no side-effects. No one has been challenged yet to look at efficacy.

Offit: What were you measuring?

Estes: Boosts of serum IgG. We have recently made a new challenge pool of Norwalk virus. We are doing the paperwork to try to file an IND to get approval to test this. Assuming that this goes through, sometime in the next year we will be testing this and will then be able to test efficacy. We have done one other study in which we expressed the NLV capsid protein in potatoes in collaboration with Charlie Arntzen, to see whether an edible vaccine might work. Potato was used as a model; not because we think this is what we would use in the future. The potatoes were fed to volunteers and antibody responses were monitored as well as circulating antibody-secreting cells at the University of Maryland under Carol Tacket's direction (Tacket et al 2000). One of the problems with the edible vaccines is that we don't always know exactly what the dose was, but the majority of the volunteers had both antibody secreting cells or an antibody response of one isotype or another.

Offit: What are the data, if any, that natural infection with NLV confers subsequent protection to reexposure?

Estes: These are from the early volunteer studies where volunteers were given one dose of NLV and then at different times after were rechallenged (Parrino et al 1977). It was clear from those studies that there can be short term immunity of up to six weeks. It was less clear whether there was long-term immunity, although a few individuals showed this. Two doses were never given followed by challenge in the long-term situation. The sort of timing and testing that would be used for an optimal vaccine was never done.

Greenberg: This was following natural infection. One natural rotavirus infection gives protection equal to three vaccinations from the data in Mexican children published by Dr Matson and colleagues (Velázquez et al 1996).

Estes: But one natural infection with rotavirus doesn't give long-term immunity.

Matson: There is transient faecal IgA and the titre achieved in the convalescent period never falls to the preinfection level. But it does fall.

Estes: There is certainly evidence for short-term immunity; whether there will be long term immunity is not certain.

Saif: Following up on the Norwalk virus volunteer studies that were done some time ago at NIH, has anything been done subsequently on the observation that high antibody titres were more like a risk factor for disease, or is this not true? Where are we with this?

Estes: In the studies that we did, people with higher preexisting antibody titres to NLV had a greater chance of getting clinical disease after infection, but we don't know what those antibodies were directed to (Gray et al 1994). I would argue that they are not neutralizing antibodies.

Matson: They were both serum and faecal.

Greenberg: They were both mucosal and serum, and published in a non-peer reviewed publication, *Perspectives in Virology* (Greenberg et al 1981). This was the only place my data ever appeared. There is also an article by Suzanne Matsui and myself in the *Journal of Infectious Diseases* that summarizes all this old literature (Matsui & Greenberg 2000). At least for me, the best interpretation is that the higher the antibody level in an adult patient, the more likely that this person had been infected previously. Rather than antibody causing illness, the antibody is an indicator of susceptibility. No one has a good handle on why some adults appear to be more susceptible to infection and illness than others. There is something in the equation above and beyond immunity that varies between adults as far as susceptibility to infection is concerned.

Kapikian: The paradoxical effect of antibody in protection against Norwalk virus was highlighted for me in an immunoelectron microscopy (IEM) experiment in which I carried out, on selected sera under code, the serological portion of a study by Neil Blacklow and colleagues in which 12 volunteers were challenged with the Norwalk virus twice, 27–47 months apart. Six of the volunteers developed illness after the first challenge and again became ill after the second challenge, 27–42 months later. However, the other six volunteers did not become ill following the initial challenge and after challenge 31–34 months later. When I tested the selected sera by IEM for antibody to Norwalk virus, I found that the volunteers who did not become ill had little, if any antibody to Norwalk virus in prechallenge serum and also failed to develop a serological response. Volunteers who became ill after each challenge developed a serological response after each challenge. I thought that there was a mix up of the coding of the specimens and asked Neil to provide another aliquot of the volunteers' sera. The results of the selected sera to be sent were confirmed once again (Parrino et al 1977). Later on, the IEM studies were essentially confirmed by Harry Greenberg using the RIA-BL assay (Greenberg et al 1981).

Koopmans: There is also a study by Christine Moe, who showed that in volunteers with NLV as the challenge, depending on whether or not they had preexisting NLV-specific antibodies, the people who did have them had a much steeper dose–response curve. This is with type specific, up-to-date assays (Moe et al 1998, 1999).

References

Bishop RF, Barnes GB, Cipriani E, Lund JS 1983 Clinical immunity after neonatal rotavirus infection: a prospective longitudinal study in young children. N Engl J Med 309:72–76

Cruz JRA, Bartlett AV, Herrmann JE, Caceres P, Blacklow NR, Cano F 1992 Astrovirus-associated diarrhea among Guatemalan ambulatory rural children. J Clin Microbiol 30:1140–1144

Chang KO, Nielsen PR, Ward LA, Saif LJ 1999 Dual infection of gnotobiotic calves with bovine strains of group A and porcine-like group C rotaviruses influences the pathogenesis of a group C rotavirus. J Virol 73:9284–9293

de Wit MAS, Koopmans MPG, Kortbeek TM, van Leeuwen NJ, Vinjé J, van Duynhoven YTHP 2001 Gastroenteritis in sentinel general practices in the Netherlands. Emerg Infect Dis 7:82–91

Estes MK, Ball JM, Guerrero RA et al 2000 Norwalk virus vaccines: challenges and progress. J Infect Dis 181:S367–S373

Gray JJ, Cunliffe C, Ball J, Graham DY, Desselberger U, Estes MK 1994 Serological responses in adult volunteers challenged with Norwalk virus: detection of IgM, IgA and IgG Norwalk virus-specific antibodies by indirect ELISA with baculovirus-expressed Norwalk virus capsid antigen. J Clin Microbiol 32:3059–3063

Greenberg HB, Wyatt RG, Kalica AR et al 1981 New insights into viral gastroenteritis. Perspect Virol 11:163–187

Herrmann JE, Taylor DN, Echeverria P, Blacklow NR 1991 Astroviruses as a cause of gastroenteritis in children. N Engl J Med 324:1757–1760

Hodgins DC, Kang S-Y, deArriba L et al 1999 Effects of maternal antibodies on protection and the development of antibody responses to human rotavirus in gnotobiotic pigs. J Virol 73:186–197

James V, Lambden PR, Caul EO, Clarke IN 1998 Enzyme-linked immunosorbent assay based on recombinant human group C rotavirus inner capsid protein (VP6) to detect human group C rotaviruses in faecal specimens. J Clin Microbiol 36:3178–3181

Matsui SM, Greenberg HB 2000 Immunity to calicivirus infection. J Infect Dis 181(Suppl 2):S331–S335

Mitchell DK, Van R, Morrow AL et al 1993 Outbreaks of astrovirus gastroenteritis in day care centers. J Pediatr 123:725–732

Mitchell DK, Monroe SS, Jiang X et al 1995 Virologic features of an astrovirus diarrhea outbreak in a day care center revealed by reverse transcriptase polymerase chain reaction. J Infect Dis 172:1431–1444

Moe C, Rhodes D, Pusek S et al 1998 Determination of Norwalk virus dose–response in human volunteers. Poster #C-384. Abstracts of the 98th Annual Meeting of the American Society for Microbiology, May 1998, Atlanta, GA

Moe CL, Sobsey MD, Stewart PW, Crawford-Brown D 1999 Estimating the risk of human calicivirus infection from drinking water. Poster P4-6, First International Calicivirus Workshop, March 1999, Atlanta, GA

O'Ryan ML, Matson DO, Estes MK, Pickering L 1994 Acquisition of serum isotype-specific and G type-specific antirotavirus antibodies among children in day care centers. Pediatr Infect Dis J 13:890–895

Parreno V, de Arriba L, Kang S et al 1999 Serum and intestinal isotype antibody responses to Wa human rotavirus in gnotobiotic pigs are modulated by maternal antibodies. J Gen Virol 80:1417–1428

Parrino TA, Schreiber DS, Trier JS, Kapikian AZ, Blacklow NR 1977 Clinical immunity in acute gastroenteritis caused by the Norwalk agent. N Engl J Med 297:86–89

Ruuska T, Vesikari T, Delem A, André FE, Beards GM, Flewett TH 1990 Evaluation of RIT 4237 bovine rotavirus vaccine in newborn infants: correlation of vaccine efficacy to season of birth in relation to rotavirus epidemic period. Scand J Infect Dis 22:269–278

Tacket CO, Mason HS, Losonsky G, Estes MK, Levine MM, Arntzen CJ 2000 Human immune responses to a novel Norwalk virus vaccine delivered in transgenic potatoes. J Infect Dis 182:302–305

Velázquez FR, Matson DO, Calva JJ et al 1996 Rotavirus infection in infants as protection against subsequent infections. N Engl J Med 335:1022–1028

Novartis 238: Gastroenteritis Viruses.
Copyright © 2001 John Wiley & Sons Ltd
Print ISBN 0-471-49663-4 eISBN 0-470-84653-4

Enteric infections with coronaviruses and toroviruses

Kathryn V. Holmes

Department of Microbiology, B-175, University of Colorado Health Sciences Center, 4200 East 9th Avenue, Denver, CO 20862, USA

Abstract. Many enteric viruses are difficult or impossible to propagate in tissue culture. Coronaviruses and toroviruses are large, enveloped, plus-strand RNA viruses in the order Nidovirales that cause enteric disease in young pigs, cows, dogs, mice, cats and horses. Two different serogroups of mammalian coronaviruses cause frequent respiratory infections in humans, and coronaviruses and toroviruses have been implicated in human diarrhoeal disease by immunoelectron microscopy. However, there is as yet no consensus about the importance of these enveloped viruses in human diarrhoea, and little is known about their genetic variability. The large spike (S) glycoprotein is an important determinant of species specificity, tissue tropism and virulence of coronavirus infection. To infect enterocytes, both S glycoproteins and the viral envelope must resist degradation by proteases, low and high pH, and bile salts. One specific site on the S glycoprotein of bovine coronavirus must be cleaved by an intracellular protease or trypsin to activate viral infectivity and cell fusion. S glycoprotein binds to specific receptors on the apical membranes of enterocytes, and can undergo a temperature-dependent, receptor-mediated conformational change that leads to fusion of the viral envelope with host membranes to initiate infection. Analysing spike–receptor interactions may lead to new ways to propagate these enteric viruses as well as new strategies for development of novel antiviral drugs.

2001 Gastroenteritis viruses. Wiley, Chichester (Novartis Foundation Symposium 238) p 258–275

Viruses that cause gastroenteritis must be resistant to inactivation in the hostile environment of the enteric tract where they are exposed to proteolytic enzymes, bile salts, mucus, bacterial products and extremes of pH. Each type of gastroenteritis virus is optimized for replication in one or more types of specialized cells in the enteric tract. The virus must be able to bind to specific receptors on the membranes of the target cell, and the viral genome must encode an apparatus that allows the virion or its nucleocapsid to penetrate through the plasma membrane or endosomal membranes to initiate infection. The virus must be optimized for efficient replication in the specialized cells of the gastroenteric tract. In the infected cells, sufficient progeny virus must be made to infect other cells or be shed from the infected animal before the infected cell is killed either by virus infection or immune responses, or by apoptosis due to differentiation of the enterocytes. Many enteric viruses must survive in the external environment in water or soil long enough to initiate infection by the faecal–oral route. Some viruses that cause enteric diseases are transmitted by the respiratory route, and the enteric tract is infected subsequent to virus replication in the respiratory tract.

Most viruses that infect the enteric tract are non-enveloped viruses with naked nucleocapsids designed to withstand the hostile environment in the enteric tract. In the *Coronaviridae* family of the order Nidovirales (Cavanagh et al 1993, Cavanagh 1997, Siddell & Snijder 1998), members of the coronavirus and torovirus genera cause enteric diseases of many species of domestic animals and possibly of humans. These are plus-strand RNA viruses that have envelopes as an essential component of the virions. The viral envelopes consist of lipoprotein bilayers and several virus-encoded envelope proteins or glycoproteins (Duckmanton et al 1998, Lai & Cavanagh 1997, Lai & Holmes 2000). In coronaviruses, the virion glycoprotein, S, which is found in the large trimeric spikes on the envelope is specialized for binding to specific receptors on enteric epithelial cells and for inducing receptor-mediated fusion of the viral envelope with host cell membranes that introduces the viral nucleocapsid into the cytoplasm of the target cell (Lai & Holmes 2000). The mechanisms by which these enveloped viruses survive in the enteric tract and bind to and enter their target cells are being explored.

Results and Discussion

Enteric diseases

Coronaviruses and toroviruses that cause enteric diseases and their natural host species are listed in Table 1 (Cavanagh et al 1993, Koopmans & Horzinek 1994). In general, most of these viruses cause disease only in one host species, and disease is more severe in infant animals than in adults. Inapparent infection is common in adults. Shedding of virus in the faeces may persist for weeks after inoculation. Animals can be infected by oral inoculation. Several of these viruses can replicate in the epithelial cells of the respiratory tract as well as the enteric tract, and they can be transmitted by the respiratory route.

Virion structure and assembly

Coronaviruses have a helical nucleocapsid that consists of a 27–32 kb plus-strand RNA genome encapsidated by the nucleocapsid phosphoprotein N. The structure of torovirus nucleocapsids is unique. Thin sections of torovirus virions show that the electron-dense nucleocapsid is shaped like a doughnut or torus. No RNA-dependent RNA polymerase protein is found in virions of coronaviruses or

TABLE 1   Coronaviruses and toroviruses that cause enteric disease

Coronaviridae genera	Host species
Coronavirus	
Bovine coronavirus (BCoV)	Cattle
Mouse hepatitis virus (MHV)	Mice
Haemagglutinating encephalomyelitis virus (HEV)	Swine
Transmissible gastroenteritis virus (TGEV)	Swine
Feline enteric coronavirus (FCoV)	Cats
Canine coronavirus (CCoV)	Dogs
Human enteric coronavirus (HECoV)	Humans (?)
Torovirus	
Berne virus (ETV)	Horses
Breda virus (BoTV)	Cattle
Porcine torovirus (PoTV)	Swine
Human torovirus (HTV)	Humans

toroviruses because immediately after uncoating in the infected cell, the plus-strand RNA genomes are translated to make the viral polymerase polyprotein.

Coronaviruses do not bud from the plasma membrane. Instead, coronavirus envelopes are acquired by budding of the nucleocapsid at membranes of a pre-Golgi complex called the budding compartment where viral glycoproteins S, M, E and, in some coronaviruses, HE, are incorporated into the viral envelope (Bos et al 1997). The intracellular localization of the viral membrane glycoprotein, M, appears to play a key role in determining the site of coronavirus budding. The small envelope glycoprotein, E, is required for virus budding (Bos et al 1996). The lipid composition of the coronavirus envelope reflects that of the membranes of the budding compartment, which is different from the lipid composition of the plasma membrane of the same cells (van Genderen et al 1995). The unusual lipid composition of coronavirus envelopes may play a role in making these viral envelopes more resistant to degradation by bile salts than envelopes of unrelated viruses that bud from the plasma membrane.

TGEV virions treated with non-ionic detergent release a spherical core that contains the viral nucleocapsid and M protein, but lacks the viral spike glycoprotein, S. Although virions of coronaviruses appear spherical while budding and soon afterwards, they mature and change to a flattened disk shape after being released into the lumen of the intracytoplasmic vesicles (Salanueva et al 1999, Holmes et al 1984). The vesicles filled with virions apparently fuse

TABLE 2   Coronavirus receptors

Virus	Receptor
MHV	Murine CEACAM1a and related murine glycoproteins
BCoV	9-O-acetylated sialic acid moieties
HCoV-OC43	9-O-acetylated sialic acid moieties
TGEV	Porcine aminopeptidase N (pAPN)
FCoV	Feline aminopeptidase N (fAPN)
HCoV-229E	Human aminopeptidase N (hAPN)
CCoV	Canine APN (cAPN) (?)

with the plasma membrane to release virions by an exocytosis-like process. In polarized epithelial cell lines grown on filters, coronaviruses can be released either at apical or basolateral membranes, or both, depending on the virus and the cell line (Rossen et al 1997).

Spike glycoprotein interactions with virus receptors

The spike (S) glycoproteins of coronaviruses bind to specific cell membrane glycoproteins that serve as virus receptors and induce fusion of the viral envelope with host cell membranes. At least three types of membrane molecules are used as receptors for various coronaviruses as shown in Table 2. The S glycoproteins of MHV strains utilize as receptors murine glycoproteins in the carcinoembryonic antigen (CEA) family of glycoproteins in the immunoglobulin superfamily (Holmes & Dveksler 1994). The prototype receptor CEACAM1a (formerly called MHVR or Bgp1a) is expressed on apical membranes of endothelial cells and many epithelial cells including respiratory, enteric, and thymic epithelial cells, and on hepatocytes, macrophages, B cells and activated T lymphocytes (Godfraind et al 1995). Transfection of non-murine cells with cDNA encoding murine CEACAM1a renders the cells susceptible to MHV infection (Dveksler et al 1991).

Carbohydrate moieties, principally 9-O-acetylneuraminic acid, are recognized by both the haemagglutinin-esterase glycoprotein (HE) expressed on the envelopes of some coronaviruses including BCoV, HEV, some strains of MHV and toroviruses, and by the S glycoproteins of some coronaviruses (Schultze & Herrler 1993, Duckmanton et al 1999). Removal of the carbohydrate moiety from susceptible cells by treatment with neuraminidase or esterase markedly reduces the infectivity of the virions, but does not eliminate infection altogether (Vlasak et al 1988). It is not yet certain whether the binding of HE or S glycoprotein to 9-O-acetylneuraminic acid can directly mediate membrane fusion, or whether an unidentified co-receptor may be required for virus entry.

The third type of receptor used by coronaviruses is aminopeptidase N (APN), a large Class II membrane metallo-glycoprotein expressed on the apical membranes of respiratory and enteric epithelial cells, macrophages, and at synaptic junctions (Yeager et al 1992, Delmas et al 1992, Wessels et al 1990). The coronaviruses in antigenic group I, including TGEV, HCoV-229E, FCoV and probably CCoV, apparently all utilize APN proteins as receptors (Tresnan et al 1996, Benbacer et al 1997). TGEV uses pAPN, but not hAPN, and HCoV-229E uses hAPN, but not pAPN as a receptor. Thus the specificity of receptor interactions can determine the species specificity of coronavirus infection. All four viruses in serogroup 1 can utilize feline APN as a receptor in cell culture, suggesting that this may have been the original receptor for group I coronaviruses (Tresnan et al 1996). It is likely that conserved elements of the S glycoproteins of these viruses bind to conserved elements of APN. Mapping of the sites on APN that determine the species specificity of virus receptor activity was done using chimeric porcine and human APN glycoproteins (Benbacer et al 1997). Substitution of an eight amino acid region near the N-terminus of hAPN for the corresponding region of the pAPN glycoprotein conferred susceptibility to HCoV-229E. In contrast, a region in the C-terminal domain determines receptor activity for porcine, feline and canine coronaviruses (Hegyi & Kolb 1998). Possibly these two regions are adjacent in the as yet unknown three-dimensional structure of APN. Site directed mutagenesis that introduced a single N-linked glycosylation site at amino acid 291 of human APN, similar to that found in the corresponding region of porcine APN, was sufficient to block infection by HCoV-229E (D. Wentworth & K. Holmes, unpublished results). Thus, genetic drift among APN glycoproteins of different species that serve as coronavirus receptors can affect host susceptibility to coronavirus infection.

The S glycoproteins of coronaviruses and toroviruses are highly glycosylated. A coiled-coil in the stem of the spike glycoprotein mediates the formation of trimers of S on the viral envelope. For some coronaviruses, including MHV and BCoV, the coiled-coil domain of S is required for membrane fusing activity, as shown for fusion glycoproteins of unrelated enveloped viruses (Hernandez et al 1996, Baker et al 1999). In MHV and BCoV virions, near the middle of each molecule of S protein in the spikes, a single trypsin cleavage site is exposed. Cleavage at this site by trypsin extracellularly or by a furin-like protease inside the Golgi yields the S1 and S2 glycoproteins (Lai & Holmes 2000, Lai & Cavanagh 1997). The N-terminal domain of S1 is required for receptor binding (Suzuki & Taguchi 1996), and the S2 domain is required for membrane fusion. This cleavage event activates coronavirus-induced membrane fusion and viral infectivity for some cell lines (Storz et al 1981), but is not essential for viral infectivity since mutants of these viruses and different coronaviruses that lack the protease cleavage site are infectious (Bos et al 1997, Hingley et al 1998). In the small intestine, trypsin is available to cleave the viral S glycoprotein if the cleavage site is available. By analogy with other viral fusion glycoproteins such as HA of influenza, HN of Sendai virus, and gp120/41 of HIV1, it is likely that the cleavage event that forms S1 and S2, also induces a conformational change of the coronavirus spike glycoprotein that poises it to undergo further conformational changes leading to membrane fusion in response to alkaline pH or receptor binding.

Fusion glycoproteins of HIV, Ebola virus and influenza A undergo programmed conformational changes in response to receptor binding or low pH like that found in endosomes (Weissenhorn et al 1999). The receptor-binding domain swings aside, uncovering a hydrophobic fusion peptide at the new N-terminus of the coiled-coil domain that was generated by protease cleavage. The coiled-coil domain extends and the fusion peptide inserts into the cell membrane. A second conformational change follows which brings the transmembrane anchor in the viral envelope into close proximity to the fusion peptide anchored in the cell membrane, and then fusion of the lipid bilayers occurs leading to virus infection. Our laboratory showed that for the enterotropic murine coronavirus MHV, binding to purified soluble CEACAM1a receptor glycoprotein at 37 °C neutralized viral infectivity (Zelus et al 1998). Neutralization by soluble receptor was accompanied by an increase in hydrophobicity of virions shown by strong association with liposomes in sucrose density gradients (B. D. Zelus & K. Holmes, unpublished results). This did not occur when virions and soluble receptor were incubated at 4 °C. The temperature-dependent, receptor-dependent change in viral hydrophobicity was associated with a conformational change in the S2 protein that made it susceptible to cleavage by trypsin at 4 °C. Virions incubated with or without soluble receptor at 37 °C were then incubated with trypsin at 4 °C and the protease-resistant S peptides were detected by immunoblotting with monoclonal antibodies to S1 or S2. We found that incubation of virions with soluble receptor at 37 °C, but not at 4 °C, caused a conformational change in the S2 glycoproteins that made them susceptible to degradation to protease at 4 °C, while the S1 proteins were not digested by trypsin. Conformational change in the MHV S2 glycoprotein was also observed in virions treated at pH 8.0 and 37 °C in the absence of soluble receptor. This alkaline pH-dependent, temperature-dependent conformational change in the coronavirus spike protein may be facilitated by the high pH in the small intestine. MHV infection of mouse intestine results in formation of multinucleate giant cells on the tips of villi. Thus, the murine coronavirus S glycoprotein is ideally designed to be activated by proteases and/or the mildly alkaline pH in the small intestine to induce membrane fusion leading to virus entry and cell-to-cell spread of virus infection by cell fusion. MHV strains differ significantly in the amino acid sequences of the S glycoprotein, in epitopes expressed on S1 and S2, in susceptibility to protease cleavage at the S1/S2 boundary, in the stability of the interactions between S1 and S2, in the ability of S2 to induce cell fusion, and in the stability of viral infectivity under different host conditions. These variations in S are important determinants of the tissue tropism and virulence of the MHV strains in mice (Phillips et al 1999).

Role of coronaviruses and toroviruses in human enteric disease

Coronaviruses of many animal species have been shown to cause diarrhoea in their natural hosts following oral inoculation. Many, but not all, of these animal coronaviruses can be isolated from faeces of infected animals using cell lines from the natural host species or HRT18 cells, a human rectal tumour cell line. Presumably these cells must express the appropriate receptor for the virus. Addition of trypsin to the culture medium sometimes facilitates virus isolation and cytopathic effects of some primary coronavirus isolates such as BCoV (Storz et al 1981). The enzyme probably potentiates the temperature-dependent, receptor-induced or alkaline pH-induced conformational changes in the S protein that lead to membrane fusion and virus entry. Enteric infection is confirmed by isolation of the infectious virus from faeces, detection in faeces of viral RNA by RT-PCR, virus-encoded proteins by immunolabelling, or virions by immunoelectron microscopy using antibodies directed against viral envelope glycoproteins, or convalescent sera from patients or animals (Tsunemitsu et al 1999).

Human coronaviruses have been implicated in the aetiology of viral diarrhoea by several lines of evidence. Coronavirus-like particles were observed by immunoelectronmicroscopy in the faeces of humans, particularly infants, with diarrhoea. However, in negatively stained preparations, the pleiomorphic coronaviruses with their large petal-shaped spikes strongly resemble other enveloped viruses such as toroviruses, and also fragments of intestinal brush border membranes studded with cellular glycoproteins that are released into the intestinal lumen. Coronavirus antigens in human diarrhoeal stools in sporadic small outbreaks of enteric disease have most often been associated with HCoV-OC43 (Battaglia et al 1987). However, viral antigens can also be detected in some healthy contacts of infected individuals, making it difficult to unequivocally implicate the virus in the aetiology of the enteric disease. Isolation of human enteric coronaviruses has been more difficult than isolation of many animal coronaviruses. Some isolates could only be propagated for one round of replication, suggesting that some essential elements of the cell culture were not appropriate for serial propagation of the virus (Clarke et al 1979). A report of isolation from an infant with necrotizing enterocolitis of a human enterotropic coronavirus in primary organ cultures of human fetal intestine has not yet been confirmed in other labs (Resta et al 1985). Several isolates of putative human enteric coronaviruses in cell cultures were subsequently found to be very similar to BCoV, suggesting that either the patient had acquired a bovine virus infection, the samples were contaminated with bovine virus, or a BCoV-like virus circulates in the human population (Zhang et al 1994). Serological studies have not unequivocally proven the existence of a human enterotropic coronavirus. Because people are repeatedly infected with respiratory coronaviruses, adults usually have antibody to coronaviruses related to HCoV-229E and HCoV-OC43. To prove that a viral isolate is the aetiological agent of the enteric disease from which the virus inoculum was obtained, it is necessary to demonstrate a rise in titre of specific anti-viral antibody. Quantitative data are required for a reliable clinical assay. Based on enteric coronavirus infections of other species, infants are the likeliest population to show serious coronavirus-induced enteric disease. However, the immune response to coronaviruses in infants is not robust, so it is often difficult to use serology to prove coronavirus infection in infants. RT-PCR has been used to detect coronavirus RNA in faecal samples of infected animals, and such assays are also likely to be useful for the study of human enterotropic coronaviruses, particularly since the nucleotide sequences of human coronaviruses have been determined. New and sensitive assays to detect HCoV infection will soon be available to aid in studies on the incidence, epidemiology and pathogenesis of enterotropic HCoV infection in infants.

Toroviruses were first discovered in rectal swabs of a horse, yielding the prototype Berne strain which can be propagated in cell culture (Weiss et al 1983). Subsequently, similar viruses or virus-like particles have been observed in bovine, porcine and human diarrhoeal stools by electron microscopy although these viruses cannot be grown in cell culture (Duckmanton et al 1997, Jamieson et al 1998). Torovirus virions or VLPs aggregated by convalescent antibody or antibodies directed against glycoproteins encoded by S or HE open reading frames on the viral genome can be detected by immunoelectron microscopy (Jamieson et al 1998, Krishnan & Naik 1997). Nucleotide sequences of genes of several toroviruses have been determined, virus-encoded proteins have been expressed and used to raise antibodies, and these are now being used to develop sensitive diagnostic tests for torovirus infection in the enteric tract (Koopmans et al 1993, Duckmanton et al 1998, 1999). Bovine and porcine torovirus antigens and RNAs have been detected in diarrhoeal stools, and at much lower frequency in control stools, by immunoblotting and RT-PCR (Koopmans et al 1993). Antibodies directed against bovine torovirus cross-react with antigens in virions of human toroviruses (Koopmans et al 1997, Duckmanton et al 1998). In a case-control study, toroviruses were identified in 35% of paediatric gastroenteritis cases

TABLE 3 Possible mechanisms for survival of enveloped coronaviruses and toroviruses in the intestinal lumen

Resistance to	Possible mechanism
Bile salts	Lipid bilayer of viral envelope is derived from intracellular membranes
Proteases	Extensive glycosylation blocks numerous potential protease sites. This protects spikes from degradation, but allows one specific protease site to be cleaved, activating membrane fusion for some viruses
pH changes	Programmed pH-dependent conformational changes in structure and function of S glycoprotein is associated with membrane fusion
Mucus	Haemagglutinin-esterase activity of HE glycoprotein removes potential receptor moieties from glycoproteins in mucus and aids virus elution

and 14.5% of controls. Patients shedding torovirus in their stools were more frequently imunocompromised than patients shedding astroviruses or rotaviruses (Jamieson et al 1998). These data suggest that toroviruses may be an important cause of diarrhoea in children, particularly in immunocompromised patients.

While it is clear that enveloped coronaviruses and toroviruses commonly cause enteric infection in a variety of species, the molecular mechanisms that allow these enveloped viruses to survive and replicate in the enteric system have not yet been elucidated. Several possible specializations of the coronavirus and torovirus envelopes and S and HE envelope glycoproteins that may play key roles in survival of virions in the intestine are suggested in Table 3. When reverse genetics systems become available for coronaviruses and toroviruses, these hypotheses can be directly tested by mutational studies on the viral envelope glycoproteins.

Summary

New techniques for isolation in cell cultures of human enterotropic coronaviruses and toroviruses from diarrhoeal stools will elucidate the importance of these agents in human enteric diseases. Sensitive and specific diagnostic tests are becoming available to analyse the roles of these two types of viruses in human enteric diseases and to compare the viruses associated with different outbreaks of disease. Experiments that focus on the interactions between viral envelope glycoproteins and their cellular receptors are likely to elucidate the molecular mechanisms by which these enveloped viruses can cause enteric diseases.

Acknowledgements

The author is grateful for discussions with Bruce Zelus, David Wentworth, Dianna Blau, Jeanne Schickli, Aurelio Bonavia, Larissa Thackray and Brian Turner. This work was supported by NIH grant #AI 25231.

References

Baker KA, Dutch RE, Lamb RA, Jardetzky TS 1999 Structural basis for paramyxovirus-mediated membrane fusion. Mol Cell 3:309–319

Battaglia M, Passarani N, Di Matteo A, Gerna G 1987 Human enteric coronaviruses: further characterization and immunoblotting of viral proteins. J Infect Dis 155:140–143

Benbacer L, Kut E, Besnardeau L, Laude H, Delmas B 1997 Interspecies aminopeptidase-N chimeras reveal species-specific receptor recognition by canine coronavirus, feline infectious peritonitis virus, and transmissible gastroenteritis virus. J Virol 71:734–737

Bos EC, Luytjes W, van der Meulen HV, Koerten HK, Spaan WJ 1996 The production of recombinant infectious DI-particles of a murine coronavirus in the absence of helper virus. Virology 218:52–60

Bos EC, Luytjes W, Spaan WJ 1997 The function of the spike protein of mouse hepatitis virus strain A59 can be studied on virus-like particles: cleavage is not required for infectivity. J Virol 71:9427–9433

Cavanagh D 1997 Nidovirales: an new order comprising *Coronaviridae* and *Arteriviridae*. Arch Virol 142:629–633

Cavanagh D, Brian DA, Brinton MA et al 1993 The *Coronaviridae* now comprises two genera, coronavirus and torovirus: report of the *Coronaviridae* Study Group. Adv Exp Med Biol 342:255–257

Clarke SK, Caul EO, Egglestone SI 1979 The human enteric coronaviruses. Postgrad Med J 55:135–142

Delmas B, Gelfi J, L'Haridon R et al 1992 Aminopeptidase N is a major receptor for the entero-pathogenic coronavirus TGEV. Nature 357:417–420

Duckmanton LM, Luan B, Devenish J, Tellier R, Petric M 1997 Characterization of torovirus from human fecal specimens. Virology 239:158–168

Duckmanton LM, Tellier R, Liu P, Petric M 1998 Bovine torovirus: sequencing of the structural genes and expression of the nucleocapsid protein of Breda virus. Virus Res 58:83–96

Duckmanton LM, Tellier R, Richardson C, Petric M 1999 The novel hemagglutinin-esterase genes of human torovirus and Breda virus. Virus Res 64:137–149

Dveksler GS, Pensiero MN, Cardellichio CB et al 1991 Cloning of the mouse hepatitis virus (MHV) receptor: expression in human and hamster cell lines confers susceptibility to MHV. J Virol 65:6881–6891

Godfraind C, Langreth SG, Cardellichio CB et al 1995 Tissue and cellular distribution of an adhesion molecule in the carcinoembryonic antigen family that serves as a receptor for mouse hepatitis virus. Lab Invest 73:615–627

Hegyi A, Kolb AF 1998 Characterization of determinants involved in the feline infectious peritonitis virus receptor function of feline aminopeptidase N. J Gen Virol 79:1387–1391

Hernandez LD, Hoffman LR, Wolfsberg TG, White JM 1996 Virus–cell and cell–cell fusion. Annu Rev Cell Dev Biol 12:627–661

Hingley ST, Leparc-Goffart I, Weiss SR 1998 The spike protein of murine coronavirus mouse hepatitis virus strain A59 is not cleaved in primary glial cells and primary hepatocytes. J Virol 72:1606–1609

Holmes KV, Dveksler GS 1994 Specificity of coronavirus-receptor interactions. In: Wimmer E (ed) Cellular receptors for animal viruses. Cold Spring Harbor Press, Cold Spring Harbor, NY, p 403–443

Holmes KV, Frana MF, Robbins SG, Sturman LS 1984 Coronavirus maturation. Adv Exp Med Biol 173:37–52

Jamieson FB, Wang EE, Bain C, Good J, Duckmanton L, Petric M 1998 Human torovirus: a new nosocomial gastrointestinal pathogen. J Infect Dis 178:1263–1269

Koopmans M, Horzinek MC 1994 Toroviruses of animals and humans: a review. Adv Virus Res 43:233–273

Koopmans M, Petric M, Glass RI, Monroe SS 1993 Enzyme-linked immunosorbent assay reactivity of torovirus-like particles in fecal specimens from humans with diarrhea. J Clin Microbiol 31:2738–2744

Koopmans MP, Goosen ES, Lima AA et al 1997 Association of torovirus with acute and persistent diarrhea in children. Pediatr Infect Dis J 16:504–507

Krishnan T, Naik TN 1997 Electronmicroscopic evidence of torovirus like particles in children with diarrhoea. Indian J Med Res 105:108–110

Lai MMC, Cavanagh D 1997 The molecular biology of coronaviruses. Adv Virus Res 48:1–100

Lai MMC, Holmes KV 2000 Coronaviridae and their replication. In: Knipe DM, Howley PM, Griffin D et al (eds) Fields' virology, 4th edition. Lippincott-Raven, New York, in press

Phillips JJ, Chua MM, Lavi E, Weiss SR 1999 Pathogenesis of chimeric MHV4/MHV-A59 recombinant viruses: the murine coronavirus spike protein is a major determinant of neurovirulence. J Virol 73:7752–7760

Resta S, Luby JP, Rosenfeld CR, Siegel JD 1985 Isolation and propagation of a human enteric coronavirus. Science 229:978–981

Rossen JW, Strous GJ, Horzinek MC, Rottier PJ 1997 Mouse hepatitis virus strain A59 is released from opposite sides of different epithelial cell types. J Gen Virol 78:61–69

Salanueva IJ, Carrascosa JL, Risco C 1999 Structural maturation of the transmissible gastroenteritis coronavirus. J Virol 73:7952–7964

Schultze B, Herrler G 1993 Recognition of N-acetyl-9-O-acetylneuraminic acid by bovine coronavirus and hemagglutinating encephalomyelitis virus. Adv Exp Med Biol 342:299–304

Siddell SG, Snijder EJ 1998 Coronaviruses, toroviruses and arteriviruses. In: Mahy BWJ, Collier L (eds) Topley and Wilson's microbiology and microbial infections. Edward Arnold, London, p 463–484

Storz J, Rott R, Kaluza G 1981 Enhancement of plaque formation and cell fusion of an enteropathogenic coronavirus by trypsin treatment. Infect Immun 31:1214–1222

Suzuki H, Taguchi F 1996 Analysis of the receptor-binding site of murine coronavirus spike protein. J Virol 70:2632–2636

Tresnan DB, Levis R, Holmes KV 1996 Feline aminopeptidase N serves as a receptor for feline, canine, porcine, and human coronaviruses in serogroup I. J Virol 70:8669–8674

Tsunemitsu H, Smith DR, Saif LJ 1999 Experimental inoculation of adult dairy cows with bovine coronavirus and detection of coronavirus in feces by RT-PCR. Arch Virol 144:167–175

van Genderen IL, Godeke GJ, Rottier PJ, van Meer G 1995 The phospholipid composition of enveloped viruses depends on the intracellular membrane through which they bud. Biochem Soc Trans 23:523–526

Vlasak R, Luytjes W, Leider J, Spaan W, Palese P 1988 The E3 protein of bovine coronavirus is a receptor-destroying enzyme with acetylesterase activity. J Virol 62:4686–4690

Weiss M, Steck F, Horzinek MC 1983 Purification and partial characterization of a new enveloped RNA virus (Berne virus). J Gen Virol 64:1849–1858

Weissenhorn W, Dessen A, Calder LJ, Harrison SC, Skehel JJ, Wiley DC 1999 Structural basis for membrane fusion by enveloped viruses. Mol Membr Biol 16:3–9

Wessels HP, Hansen GH, Fuhrer C et al 1990 Aminopeptidase N is directly sorted to the apical domain in MDCK cells. J Cell Biol 111:2923–2930

Yeager CL, Ashmun RA, Williams RK et al 1992 Human aminopeptidase N is a receptor for human coronavirus 229E. Nature 357:420–422

Zelus BD, Wessner DR, Williams RK et al 1998 Purified, soluble recombinant mouse hepatitis virus receptor, Bgp1(b), and Bgp2 murine coronavirus receptors differ in mouse hepatitis virus binding and neutralizing activities. J Virol 72:7237–7244

Zhang XM, Herbst W, Kousoulas KG, Storz J 1994 Biological and genetic characterization of a hemagglutinating coronavirus isolated from a diarrhoeic child. J Med Virol 44:152–161

DISCUSSION

Greenberg: Is the mechanism of diarrhoea in animals with coronavirus presumed to be lysis of cells and loss of absorptive epithelium? Is there any other putative mechanism for diarrhoea for the coronaviruses?

Holmes: Not yet. We actually stumbled on the receptor story while we were looking for a viral enterotoxin years ago. What you mention is the generally accepted model for viral diarrhoea, but I don't think we know all there is to know about the pathophysiology of viral diarrhoea.

Greenberg: Coronaviruses have a genome that could easily encode a toxin.

Koopmans: The difference is, though, that in infected animals you readily find antigen in many epithelial cells.

Greenberg: Rotavirus is found in epithelial cells in large amounts.

Saif: TGEV is found throughout the entire small intestine, and it wipes out the entire intestinal epithelium (Saif & Wesley 1999).

Farthing: About 15–16 years ago, Professor Mathan in Vellore identified coronaviruses in the faeces of patients with tropical sprue. However, when he looked at control patients without diarrhoea, he found the same prevalence of coronaviruses. I guess from your talk that you are cautious about saying whether this is a pathogen in humans or not. It clearly is a pathogen in animals: there is tremendous homology between these viruses, particularly between pig and human intestine. They are virtually identical. Can you speculate on why there are these clear differences?

Holmes: I'm glad that you asked that question. There is no question that the human coronaviruses HCoV-229E and HCoV-OC43 cause respiratory infections. They cause up to 30% of colds in people. The question is whether they can also cause enteric infection. The porcine coronavirus, TGEV, is a very efficient cause of diarrhoea, particularly in young animals. A naturally occurring variant of TGEV, called PRCoV, has deletions of more than 200 amino acids in the receptor binding domain of the viral spike glycoprotein (Ballasteros et al 1995). PRCoV causes only respiratory infection. It may serve as a natural vaccine to protect animals from fatal enteric infection. HCoV-229E, the human coronavirus that we are working with, is one of only a handful of human coronavirus strains that are available for study. The sequence of the S gene of HCoV-229E resembles this porcine respiratory coronavirus. Possibly the region of S that is present in TGEV but is absent in PRCoV may have something to do with a difference in the stability of these viruses in the enteric tract. The feline coronavirus doesn't have that deletion in S, and grows very nicely in the cat enteric tract.

Saif: There is more to this story. PRCoV is largely avirulent, and TGEV is highly virulent (Saif & Wesley 1999). There are two major mutations: one is in the region you showed in the spike, which seems to relate to tissue tropism, but there is also a change in mRNA 3. Since Dr Luis Enjuanes of Spain has an infectious clone for TGEV we can now clearly address these two scenarios with the coronaviruses. One is the tissue tropism and the other is the virulence. I think these studies will be extremely interesting in the future. I was wondering, Kay, whether you could comment on the mechanism of persistence of these coronaviruses?

Holmes: Persistence of mouse hepatitis virus (MHV), particularly the enterotropic strains, usually occurs in mice that are immunosuppressed, such as nude mice or infants (Compton et al 1993). The viruses that are isolated from mice or murine cells with persistent MHV infection have mutations in the gene that encodes the spike glycoprotein (S) such that the cleavage between S1 and S2 is much less likely to occur, and therefore the virus particles are more stable. I think that a combination of viral factors and host factors are required for coronavirus persistence.

Bishop: What was the source of your human coronavirus?

Holmes: It is a human respiratory coronavirus. There have been a few reports of human enteric coronaviruses being propagated in cell culture, but several of them have turned out to be very closely related to or identical to bovine coronavirus strains (Moscovici et al 1980, Zhang et al 1994).

Kapikian: I remember at the meeting here on novel diarrhoea viruses in 1986 (Ciba Foundation 1987), there was great excitement because Dr Sylvia Resta and Dr James Luby had described the growth and passage of a human coronavirus from stools of infants with necrotizing enterocolitis in human intestinal culture. The agent was serially passaged and further characterized (Resta et al 1985). We were unable to obtain this virus. I believe that you are the only person I know who received the virus from Dr Luby's group. What has happened to this virus?

Holmes: We were never able to grow that virus in any cell line. Dr Resta had grown it in human fetal intestinal organ cultures. We tried to adapt it to many different cell lines without success. We could not show the cross-reactivity of the amount of material that we got with HCoV-OC43, HCoV-229E or animal coronaviruses. Dr Luby has recently made the putative human enterotropic coronavirus available to people through the ATCC (Luby et al 1999). Perhaps unfortunately, this was done after adapting this virus to a mouse macrophage cell line and a mosquito cell line. I have not studied that variant strain yet. It will be important to obtain nucleotide sequence information from this isolate.

Kapikian: Coronaviruses and their association with human gastroenteritis have been a very difficult area of research. In 1982, a report from France described the detection by electron microscopy (EM) of coronavirus in stools of newborns with necrotizing enterocolitis (Chany et al 1982). As noted in the proceedings of the Novel diarrhoea viruses symposium (Ciba Foundation 1987), it was later thought that this virus was a bovine coronavirus. I am not aware that a human coronavirus has been associated conclusively with enteric disease.

Holmes: Dr Storz's lab recently isolated a virus from a child with diarrhoea in Louisiana (Zhang et al 1994). This also looks like a bovine coronavirus. It may be that some of these coronaviruses from animals can cause disease in human contacts, but there appears to be no serial transmission of these viruses in humans.

Saif: There is a report from France in which the fifth cell culture passage (in HRT-18 cells) of coronavirus-like particles from a child with necrotizing enterocolitis caused diarrhoea in a calf, typical of a bovine coronavirus infection (Patel et al 1982). Coronavirus was re-isolated from the faeces and coronavirus-positive immunofluorescence was observed in the colon and rectum, suggesting that either the human enteric coronavirus infects cattle or that it was a bovine coronavirus strain that infected the child. In addition, there is a report of a lab worker infected with bovine coronavirus who developed diarrhoea and shed coronavirus particles in faeces (Storz & Rott 1981). In some recent work I have done with Mo Saif, we gave his student a well characterized DB2 strain of bovine coronavirus that we had isolated, passaged in gnotobiotic calves and adapted to cell culture. His student put this virulent calf-passaged bovine coronavirus into some turkey poults and baby chickens, and it caused diarrhoea in the turkeys but not the chicks (Ismail et al 2000).

There may be a less restrictive host specificity for bovine coronaviruses that means they can sometimes infect other hosts, including humans and turkeys. Perhaps this relates to their possession of a haemagglutinin with a high sequence homology to the haemagglutinin of influenza C viruses, which is also present on the human respiratory coronavirus, OC43 (Parker et al 1989, Zhang et al 1992).

Holmes: There is a coronavirus of elk that is very much like bovine coronavirus (BCoV; Daginakatte et al 1999). Perhaps they share pastures. The BCoV is one of the coronaviruses that binds to the 9-O-acetylated sialic acid. Perhaps this common receptor moiety gives the virus a broader host range.

Saif: We isolated coronaviruses antigenically indistinguishable from bovine coronaviruses from the faeces of wild ruminants with a dysentery-like diarrhoea syndrome (Tsunemitsu & Saif 1995). These species included white-tailed deer, sambar deer and a waterbuck. Mule and white-tailed deer also had antibodies to bovine coronavirus. The coronavirus isolates infected and caused diarrhoea in inoculated calves suggesting that wild ruminants harbour coronaviruses antigenically similar to bovine strains and transmissible to cattle.

Glass: We have seen lots of examples of rotaviruses and caliciviruses transmitted between animals and humans. Do any group of animal handlers such as veterinarians have antibodies against coronavirus that might suggest exposure? I ask this because in 1991, we had an EM conference in Atlanta. Al Kapikian was there with Owen Caul and Laura Aurelian who each saw coronaviruses frequently. We said that we wouldn't call something seen by EM a coronavirus ever again unless we had an independent confirmatory assay such as the ELISA that Marion Koopmans has worked on. This was nine years ago, and we still don't have consistent, confirmed cases that we are certain about. At some point we either need the confirmatory assays or we have to say we don't think that there are enteric coronaviruses in humans. Antibodies in veterinarians or livestock handlers would take us a step further.

Saif: I'm not sure that anyone has ever looked at that.

Holmes: Wallace Rowe found antibodies in humans to MHV, a murine coronavirus (Hartley et al 1964), which were probably antibodies to the antigenically related human coronavirus HCoV-OC43.

Saif: There is the problem of cross-reactivity in both groups. There is the HCoV-OC43 human coronavirus that cross-reacts with bovine coronavirus and there is the HCoV-229E human coronavirus that cross-reacts with the porcine TGEV coronavirus.

Holmes: As people are beginning to sequence more and more coronavirus genomes, they have found naturally occurring recombinants between canine and feline coronaviruses, where there is a cross-over in the spike protein that allows a dog virus to adapt to cats. I think that jumping species is something that we should be concerned about with coronaviruses. There are five animal species in which fatal neonatal diarrhoea can be caused by coronaviruses. Some of these Elvis-like sightings of coronavirus have been seen in human infant diarrhoeal samples. It is possible that they could jump, but it is unlikely.

Koopmans: Martin Petric has gathered data about human toroviruses. He has obtained sequences from some of the torovirus-like particles, and finds almost identical sequences in some regions to the equine toroviruses. The problem with these data is that they are not reproducible in other labs. He speculates about zoonotic transmission (Jamieson et al 1998, Duckmanton et al 1997).

Holmes: He is looking by immunoelectron microscopy at fecal specimens of children with diarrhoea that are hospitalized. He finds torovirus-like particles in 20–30%. The RT-PCR and sequencing of other regions of the viral genome may tell the tale.

Koopmans: I have spent some time at CDC trying to figure out what was going on with fringed particles in stools (Koopmans et al 1993). We did a blinded study where Martin collected stool samples containing viruses that he felt resembled toroviruses on the basis of the pictures that we have been sending him. We ran gradients in parallel with the animal torovirus, and tested those gradient fractions by ELISA using hyperimmune sera from cattle. From this it was clear that there is something in human faecal samples that in gradients, co-migrates with the animal toroviruses and is immunoreactive with the animal sera. We also found them in association with clinical symptoms in a study in Brazil (Koopmans et al 1997). This is as far as those studies got. We have also tried to amplify some of the genomes from this work. This never worked, but Martin has described that from similar particles they have genomic information (Duckmanton et al 1997). The difficulty is that a lot of the fringed particles were not confirmed as something that looks like a torovirus. I think that some of the fringed particles are viral but a lot of them aren't.

Holmes: We were interested in looking by EM at the interaction of beautiful coronaviruses, which have characteristic large, petal-shaped spikes, with brush border membrane vesicles that we have isolated from mouse small intestine. We first examined virus preparation and the membrane vesicles separately. We were surprised that we couldn't tell the coronaviruses and membrane vesicles apart because the brush border membranes have some large oligomeic protein complexes, such as amino peptidase N, that stick out from the membrane and look just like viral spikes.

Koopmans: I have looked at many toroviruses by EM but still wouldn't dare to diagnose them by this technique.

Glass: David Brown, do you still have the EM surveillance in the UK that would allow you to identify sightings?

Brown: We have a network of EMs, and two to three times a year someone sends in a micrograph showing fringed particles that could be coronavirus or torovirus. I had the good fortune to spend a year working with Professor V. I. Mathan in Vellore. It gets very hot in Vellore, and I found that I did develop an enthusiasm for EM because it was the only room in the hospital that had air conditioning. I spent a long time trying to characterize these particles. I think that these fringed particles were mostly bits of brush border and cell membrane. We do see them, but I have not seen convincing evidence that these are human torovirus or coronavirus. There is no serological evidence of infection in humans, either with the toroviruses or with the bovine coronavirus.

Holmes: Martin Petric has serological evidence from immunoelectron microscopy.

Brown: Immune EM on fringed particles is a difficult technique to interpret, because the particles do tend to stick together in any case. Perhaps Al Kapikian would be able to comment on this. When I was working with Tom Flewett in Birmingham, we did try to do immune EM on fringed particles, and I wouldn't advocate it as a way to spend your life.

Kapikian: You are right that they can spontaneously aggregate. However, we did detect a putative new human respiratory coronavirus using immune EM (Kapikian et al 1973). We were able to show that the particles characteristically aggregated following incubation with a convalescent serum. EM studies with fringed particles have been particularly difficult and require careful evaluation. I commend Martin Petric in his studies with the toroviruses. He has been extremely cautious, meticulous and careful in his studies with these fringed viruses. I was at a meeting in Montreal and he presented his data cautiously with so many caveats that the chairperson said, 'You have wonderful data, why all these concerns?' Martin replied, 'You don't know my colleagues in the gastroenteritis field!'

Saif: We routinely use immune EM to discriminate in bovine faecal specimens between Breda virus (a torovirus) and coronavirus. This is the only way we can do it, because of their morphogenetic similarity but antigenic distinctiveness.

Farthing: Were all your receptor studies done with intestinal epithelium?

Holmes: Those that I showed were done with cloned soluble receptor proteins purified from cultured cells. The anchored proteins are expressed on the apical brush border membranes of the epithelium.

Farthing: Is there a receptor on the bronchial epithelium?

Holmes: Yes, the same receptor glycoprotein is on apical membranes of respiratory epithelium.

Estes: I was interested in your concept that these viruses may be resistant to bile salts because of the intracellular membranes that they have picked up. Is there any evidence that these are associated with lipid rafts? Are they resistant to cold Triton X100?

Holmes: No, they are not resistant to Triton X100 as the virus envelope can be solubilized by it. Enteric coronaviruses are apparently resistant to bile salts, which would be found in the intestine. The pH 8 in the small intestine may help to activate the spike proteins of these viruses for entry into epithelial cells.

References

Ballasteros ML, Sanchez CM, Martin-Caballero J, Enjuanes L 1995 Molecular basis of tropism in the PRU46 cluster of transmissible gastroenteritis coronaviruses. Adv Exp Med Biol 380:557–562

Ciba Foundation 1987 Novel diarrhoea viruses. Wiley, Chichester (Ciba Found Symp 128)

Chany C, Moscovici O, Lebon P, Rousset S 1982 Association of coronavirus infection with neonatal necrotizing enterocolitis. Pediatrics 69:209–214

Compton SR, Barthold SW, Smith AL 1993 The cellular and molecular pathogenesis of coronaviruses. Lab Anim Sci 43:15–28 (erratum: 1993 Lab Anim Sci 43:203)

Daginakatte GC, Chard-Bergstrom C, Andrews GA, Kapil S 1999 Production, charecterization, and uses of monoclonal antibodies against recombinant nucleoprotein of elk coronavirus. Clin Diagn Lab Immunol 6:341–344

Duckmanton L, Luan B, Devenish J, Tellier R, Petric M 1997 Characterization of torovirus from human fecal specimens. Virology 239:158–168

Hartley JW, Rowe WP, Bloom HH, Turner HC 1964 Antibodies to mouse hepatitis viruses in human sera. Proc Soc Exp Biol Med 115:414–418

Ismail MM, Cho KO, Ward LA, Saif LJ, Saif YM 2000 Experimental bovine coronavirus infection of turkey poults and young chickens. Avian Dis, submitted

Jamieson FB, Wang EE, Bain C, Good J, Duckmanton L, Petric M 1998 Human torovirus: a new nosocomial gastrointestinal pathogen. J Infect Dis 178:1263–1269

Kapikian AZ, James HD, Kelly SJ, Vaughn AL 1973 Detection of coronaviruses by immune electron microscopy. Infect Immun 7:111–116

Koopmans M, Petric M, Glass RI, Monroe SS 1993 ELISA reactivity of torovirus-like particles in fecal specimens from humans with diarrhea. J Clin Microbiol 31:2738–2744

Koopmans MPG, Goosen ESM, Lima AAM et al 1997 Association of torovirus with acute and persistent diarrhea in children. Ped Inf Dis 16:504–507

Luby JP, Clinton R, Kurtz S 1999 Adaptation of human enteric coronavirus to growth in cell lines. J Clin Virol 12:43–51

Moscovici O, Chany C, Lebon P, Rousset S, Laporte J 1980 Association of coronavirus infection with hemorrhagic enterocolitis in newborn infants. CR Séances Acad Sci D 290:869–872

Parker MD, Cox GJ, Deregt D, Fitzpatrick DR, Babiuk LA 1989 Cloning and *in vitro* expression of the gene for the E3 haemagglutinin of bovine coroanvirus. J Gen Virol 70:155–164

Patel JR, Davies HA, Edington N, Laporte J, Macnaughton MR 1982 Infection of a calf with the enteric coronavirus strain Paris. Arch Virol 73:319–327

Resta S, Luby JP, Rosenfeld CR, Siegel JD 1985 Isolation and propagation of a human enteric coronavirus in stools of newborns with necrotizing enterocolitis. Science 229:978–981

Saif LJ, Wesley R 1999 Transmissible gastroenteritis virus. In: Straw BE, D'Allaire S, Mengeling WL, Taylor DJ (eds) Diseases of swine, 8th edn. Iowa State Univ Press, Ames, IO, p 295–326

Storz J, Rott R 1981 Reactivity of antibodies in human serum with antigens of an enteropathogenic bovine coronavirus. Med Microbiol Immunol 169:169–178

Tsunemitsu H, Saif LJ 1995 Antigenic and biological comparisons of bovine coronaviruses derived from neonatal calf diarrhea and winter dysentery of adult cattle. Arch Virol 140:1303–1311

Zhang XM, Kousoulas KG, Storz J 1992 The haemagglutinin/esterase gene of human coronavirus strain OC43: phylogenetic relationships to bovine and murine coronaviruses and influenza C virus. Virology 186:318–323

Zhang XM, Herbst W, Kousoulas KG, Storz J 1994 Biological and genetic characterization of a hemagglutinating coronavirus isolated from a diarrhoeic child. J Med Virol 44:152–161

Novartis 238: Gastroenteritis Viruses.
Copyright © 2001 John Wiley & Sons Ltd
Print ISBN 0-471-49663-4   eISBN 0-470-84653-4

Viruses causing diarrhoea in AIDS

Richard C. G. Pollok

Digestive Disease Research Centre, St Bartholomew's & The Royal London School of Medicine and Dentistry, Turner St, London E1 2AD, UK

Abstract. Opportunistic viral enteritis is an important gastrointestinal manifestation of HIV related disease. Cytomegalovirus (CMV) is a well established aetiological agent of disease in the gastrointestinal tract in this group. CMV enteritis may affect any region of the bowel, most commonly the colon. Diagnosis and management of these infections may be difficult. The role of other viruses in so-called 'pathogen-negative' diarrhoea remains controversial. The clinical importance of HIV-specific enteropathy is probably limited. Several viruses including astrovirus, picobirnavirus, small round structured virus and rotavirus have been implicated HIV-related diarrhoea. In addition, adenovirus has been linked to persistent diarrhoea in patients with a characteristic adenovirus colitis. The spectrum of disease morbidity and mortality amongst HIV patients has altered dramatically since the wide spread use of highly active antiretroviral therapy (HAART). Opportunistic infections, including CMV infection of the gastrointestinal tract in patients with AIDS, have diminished greatly. AIDS patients with CMV are able successfully to discontinue anti-CMV treatment without disease reactivation and with a parallel reduction in CMV viraemia following the initiation of HAART.

2001 Gastroenteritis viruses. Wiley, Chichester (Novartis Foundation Symposium 238) p 276–288

Both acute and persistent diarrhoea may occur in patients with human immunodeficiency virus (HIV). Most individuals will have a readily identifiable cause using a well established diagnostic protocol that will include stool culture and microscopy as well as histological examination of endoscopically obtained biopsies of the upper and lower gastrointestinal (GI) tract (Blanshard et al 1996). Using such a protocol the majority of 155 cases of persistent diarrhoea (82%) can be related to an identifiable bacterial, parasitic or cytomegalovirus (CMV) infection (18%). However, with the additional use of stool electron microscopy and specific immunological staining, other enteric viruses were implicated in 11% of cases. It is well established that gastrointestinal CMV infection is associated with diarrhoea but the role of enteric viral infections in HIV-related diarrhoea is controversial.

Gastrointestinal CMV infection

The pathogenic role of CMV infection is well established. Although retinitis is the most common manifestation of infection, GI infection of the oesophagus, stomach, small bowel and colon occurs in 5–15% of patients during the course of HIV infection (Jacobson & Mills 1988). Although CMV may infect any part of the GI tract the most common site of infection is the colon (Mentec et al 1994). The spectrum of symptomatology associated with CMV colitis is wide. Chronic or intermittent diarrhoea in association with abdominal pain is the most common manifestation of colonic infection. Colonic infection may also be associated with a mild or severe rectal bleeding, or abdominal pain in the absence of diarrhoea. In addition, fever is common at presentation. Pain may precede the development of toxic megacolon and intestinal perforation, in rare but clearly life threatening occurrences (Framm & Soave 1997). Colonic CMV infection may occur in association with infection elsewhere in the GI tract including the oesphagus, usually resulting in dysphagia and odynophagia, and manifesting as pain in the upper abdomen resulting from AIDS-related cholangiopathy or pancreatitis. Importantly, GI infection may also herald CMV retinitis and careful retinal assessment is therefore essential in this group.

Diagnosis of CMV infection

Definitive diagnosis of CMV enterocolitis requires intestinal biopsy. A spectrum of both upper and lower GI manifestations of CMV infection have been described. Wilcox et al (1998) prospectively evaluated 55 HIV patients by sigmoidoscopy and colonoscopy. Chronic diarrhoea and abdominal pain occurred in 80% and 50% of patients, respectively. 9% presented with lower GI bleeding with a previous history of diarrhoea. Endoscopically, appearances were heterogeneous. Three main categories were identified: colitis associated with ulceration (39%), ulceration alone (38%), or colitis alone (20%). Subepithelial haemorrhage was a common manifestation in all groups. Thirty-one patients underwent complete endoscopy to the caecum. Of these, 4 patients (9%) had disease proximal to the splenic flexure without distal involvement and therefore inaccessible by flexible sigmoidoscopy; this contrasts with early reports suggesting higher rates of right-sided colitis (Dieterich & Rahmin 1991). The same group have assessed the endoscopic appearances of CMV infection of the oesphagus (Wilcox et al 1990). Multiple ulcers were usually identified (58%), located in the middle or lower oesphagus, commonly less than 1 cm in diameter and usually superficial. The heterogeneous manifestation of CMV disease in both the colon and oesphagus makes biopsy essential for accurate diagnosis.

Histological diagnosis of CMV enterocolitis is largely dependent upon identification of characteristic cytomegalovirus inclusion bodies; the best yield is usually obtained from the base of CMV ulcers. In addition, specific immunoperoxidase staining for CMV is also useful in identifying GI disease (Culpepper-Morgan et al 1987). Positive staining is more likely from the edge of ulcers and some authors claim greater sensitivity compared to conventional histology, although it is unclear how rigorously inclusion bodies were excluded (Francis et al 1989, Theise et al 1991). The viral culture of intestinal biopsies is of limited value: it is time consuming and, in addition, CMV viraemia may occur in the absence of mucosal disease, which may lead to a false-positive diagnosis if biopsies are contaminated with blood. *In situ* hybridization has been used to assess GI CMV disease, and is both sensitive and specific, although in comparison with conventional histology it probably offers little additional benefit (Clayton et al 1989). PCR for the detection of CMV may also be more sensitive than standard histological techniques, although evidence suggests that it lacks specificity with 28% of normal gastrointestinal biopsies positive by this technique. However, as with *in situ* hybridization, there is the risk of PCR giving a false-positive in patients with viraemia (Goodgame et al 1993). Cotte et al (1996) have monitored CMV DNA levels during treatment; these levels broadly reflected clinical response although this complicated technique has not been widely adopted in the clinical management of CMV disease.

Drug treatment

Treatment of CMV enterocolitis requires parenteral therapy with either ganciclovir (5 mg/kg twice daily) or foscarnet (90 mg/kg twice daily) both of which may be associated with severe side effects. Ganciclovir may cause severe bone marrow depression with resultant anaemia and neutropaenia, and foscarnet may cause severe renal impairment, although a concomitant normal saline infusion largely seems to diminish the risk of renal damage. In an open-label randomized study comparing a 2 week course of foscarnet with ganciclovir, at the doses stated above, no significant difference in response of GI CMV disease was found between the two therapies (Blanshard et al 1995). Around 75% of patients had good clinical and endoscopic responses with disappearance of inclusion bodies as determined histologically. Relapse occurs in at least 50% of patients within around 10 weeks, survival without highly active antiretroviral therapy (HAART) is around 20 weeks. Surprisingly Blanshard et al (1995) found maintenance therapy did not increase time to relapse of GI disease or development of retinitis although numbers were small and allocation of maintenance therapy was not randomized. The use of oral ganciclovir in maintenance of GI remission has not been evaluated.

Highly active antiretroviral therapy (HAART)

Encouragingly, the advent of HAART has led to a marked reduction in mortality and morbidity amongst HIV patients (Gazzard & Moyle 1998). HAART may result in remission of previously persistent opportunistic infections, including CMV infection. However, the development of viral resistance and difficulties

TABLE 1   Rates of detection of enteric virus

Author	N	Methods	Overall prevalence in AIDS patients (%)	Viruses identified	Association with diarrhoea
Kaljot et al (1989)	23	EM, bx, culture	34	HSV	No
				CMV	No
				Adenovirus	No
Thea et al (1993)	197	EM, EIA	17	Rotavirus	No
Albrecht et al (1993)	101	EIA	19	Rotavirus	Yes
Cunningham et al (1988)	67	EM, bx, culture	7.4	Adenovirus	Yes
Grohmann et al (1993)	110	EM, EIA, PAGE	29	Astrovirus	Yes
				Picobirnavirus	—
				Calicivirus	Yes
				Adenovirus	Yes
Schmidt et al (1996)	256	EM, bx	17	Adenovirus	Yes
				Coronavirus	Yes
Thomas et al (1999)	377	EM, bx	16	Adenovirus	Yes
				Rotavirus	—
				Calicivirus	—

[1]bx, biopsy

with compliance may lead to breakthrough HIV viraemia and the re-emergence or re-acquisition of opportunistic GI infections. Unfortunately, combination antiretroviral therapy is costly and consequently unavailable to the vast majority of HIV patients world wide. Patients with stable CMV retinitis and CD4 counts of >150 cells/μl on HAART were successfully able to discontinue anti-CMV maintenance therapy without relapse of retinitis or development of extraocular disease over a mean follow-up period of 16 months (Whitcup et al 1999). Importantly immune reactivation retinitis occurred in 90% of patients started on HAART prior to discontinuation of antiCMV treatment, with substantial visual loss in the minority of patients. Macdonald et al (1998) report similar findings although they do not comment on immune re-activation retinitis and follow-up was considerably shorter. Others have found that HAART results in a significant and progressive decline in CMV viraemia in the absence of specific anti-CMV treatment (O'Sullivan et al 1999).

Adenovirus

Adenovirus has previously been reported to cause infection in other immuno-suppressed patient groups, including individuals with primary immunodeficiency and bone marrow transplant patients (Hierholzer 1992). Dionisio et al (1997) reported increasing stool carriage of subgenus F type 40 adenovirus with increasing immunosuppression amongst HIV patients. Adenovirus colitis was first described by Janoff et al (1991) in five HIV patients with diarrhoea. Adenovirus was identified by electron microscopy or culture from 67 patients being investigated for diarrhoea. Colonoscopy revealed mild inflammatory change in two of these patients. Light microscopy revealed focal necrosis and amphophilic nuclear inclusions within degenerating epithelial cells. Electron microscopy revealed characteristic hexagonal adenovirus particles within the inclusions. Maddox et al (1992) confirmed these characteristic features and found that specific immunostaining for adenovirus was both sensitive and specific for the identification of adenovirus inclusions. The pathogenic role of adenovirus remains unclear since this group of patients frequently have co-infection with other known pathogens. Thomas et al (1999) reported that adenovirus colitis was significantly more likely to be associated with chronic diarrhoea. Schmidt et al (1996) detected adenovirus only in severely immunosupressed AIDS patients with prevalence greater in patients with diarrhoea than without (10% vs. 3.3%). Both positive and negative correlations between adenovirus and diarrhoea have been reported by other groups (see Table 1) (Albrecht et al 1993, Cunningham et al 1988, Grohmann et al 1993, Kaljot et al 1989, Schmidt et al 1996, Thea et al 1993, Thomas et al 1999). Most studies indicate a strong association between adenovirus infection and co-infection with other pathogens, in particular CMV. It is therefore difficult to ascribe a pathogenic role to this virus with any certainty (Grohmann et al 1993, Schmidt et al 1996, Thomas et al 1999).

Human immunodeficiency virus

Infection of enterocytes by HIV is well documented and has been implicated as the cause of so-called HIV enteropathy, where both morphological and functional abnormalities of the gut have been described in the absence of any other detectable pathogen (Bartlett et al 1992, Ullrich et al 1989). The clinical importance of HIV enteropathy is probably limited; certainly, 'pathogen-negative' diarrhoea is comparatively short-lived and associated with a good prognosis (Blanshard & Gazzard 1995).

Other enteric viruses

Several other enteric viruses have been associated with HIV-related diarrhoea. Grohmann et al (1993) carefully examined stool specimens from patients with diarrhoea and control patients without diarrhoea. Samples were examined by electron microscopy, PAGE and enzyme immunoassay (EIA) for rotavirus, adenovirus, calicivirus and picobirnavirus. Paired sera were also analysed for antibodies to Norwalk and picobirnavirus. Overall, virus was detected in 35% of patients with diarrhoea and 12% without diarrhoea. Astrovirus, picobirnavirus, calicivirus (including small round structured virus) and adenovirus were found significantly more often in patients with diarrhoea. Unfortunately, co-infection with other known pathogens was not systematically evaluated and no information regarding the relative distribution of acute and chronic diarrhoea was provided. Schmidt et al (1996) detected virus in 17% of stool samples from 256 HIV-infected patients. Adenoviruses and coronaviruses were detected more frequently in patients with diarrhoea (10% vs. 3.3% and 15% vs. 6.6%, respectively), and both infections were associated with severe immunosupression. Thea et al (1993), working in Zaire, found no association between enteric virus shedding and diarrhoea. Overall this group found enteric virus in 17% of samples analysed including rotavirus, SSRV, coronavirus and adenovirus. They noted a trend towards increased shedding with greater immunosuppresion, a finding in common with Cunningham et al (1988).

An association of rotavirus with prolonged diarrhoea in HIV patients as detected by EIA has been reported, although other groups have not supported this finding (Albrecht et al 1993). In summary, data regarding the association of non-CMV enteric virus infection and diarrhoea are conflicting. The best evidence relates to adenovirus infection although its pathogenic role is far from certain. The impact of HAART on non-CMV enteric virus infection has not been evaluated, and warrants study. Data from selected studies that have evaluated enteric virus carriage in HIV patients are summarized in Table 1.

Conclusion

CMV enterocolitis remains an important cause of AIDS-related diarrhoea. Fortunately, the introduction of HAART has dramatically reduced the morbidity and mortality associated with this disease. The role of non-CMV enteric infection in HIV-related diarrhoea remains uncertain with the possible exception of adenovirus infection. Conclusive evidence is unlikely to become available in the post-HAART era.

Acknowledgement

Dr R.C.G. Pollok is a Wellcome Trust Research Fellow.

References

Albrecht H, Stellbrink HJ, Fenske S, Ermer M, Raedler A, Greten H 1993 Rotavirus antigen detection in patients with HIV infection and diarrhea. Scand J Gastroenterol 28:307–310
Bartlett JG, Belitsos PC, Sears CL 1992 AIDS enteropathy. Clin Infect Dis 15:726–735
Blanshard C, Gazzard BG 1995 Natural history and prognosis of diarrhoea of unknown cause in patients with acquired immunodeficiency syndrome (AIDS). Gut 36:283–286

Blanshard C, Benhamou Y, Dohin E, Lernestedt JO, Gazzard BG, Katlama C 1995 Treatment of AIDS-associated gastrointestinal cytomegalovirus infection with foscarnet and ganciclovir: a randomized comparison. J Infect Dis 172:622–628

Blanshard C, Francis N, Gazzard BG 1996 Investigation of chronic diarrhoea in acquired immunodeficiency syndrome. A prospective study of 155 patients. Gut 39:824–832

Clayton F, Klein EB, Kotler DP 1989 Correlation of *in situ* hybridization with histology and viral culture in patients with acquired immunodeficiency syndrome with cytomegalovirus colitis. Arch Pathol Lab Med 113:1124–1126

Cotte L, Drouet E, Bailly F, Vitozzi S, Denoyel G, Trepo C 1996 Cytomegalovirus DNA level on biopsy specimens during treatment of cytomegalovirus gastrointestinal disease. Gastroenterology 111:439–444

Culpepper-Morgan JA, Kotler DP, Scholes JV, Tierney AR 1987 Evaluation of diagnostic criteria for mucosal cytomegalic inclusion disease in the acquired immune deficiency syndrome. Am J Gastroenterol 82:1264–1270

Cunningham AL, Grohmann GS, Harkness J et al 1988 Gastrointestinal viral infections in homosexual men who were symptomatic and seropositive for human immunodeficiency virus. J Infect Dis 158:386–391

Dieterich DT, Rahmin M 1991 Cytomegalovirus colitis in AIDS: presentation in 44 patients and a review of the literature. J Acquir Immune Defic Syndr 4:S29–S35

Dionisio D, Arista S, Vizzi E et al 1997 Chronic intestinal infection due to subgenus F type 40 adenovirus in a patient with AIDS. Scand J Infect Dis 29:305–307

Framm SR, Soave R 1997 Agents of diarrhea. Med Clin North Am 81:427–447

Francis N, Boylston A, Roberts A, Parkin JM, Pinching AJ 1989 Cytomegalovirus infection in gastrointestinal tracts of patients infected with HIV-1 or AIDS. J Clin Pathol 42:1055–1064

Gazzard B, Moyle G 1998 1998 revision to the British HIV Association guidelines for antiretroviral treatment of HIV seropositive individuals. BHIVA Guidelines Writing Committee. Lancet 352:314–316 (erratum: 1998 Lancet 352:1394)

Goodgame RW, Genta RM, Estrada R, Demmler G, Buffone G 1993 Frequency of positive tests for cytomegalovirus in AIDS patients: endoscopic lesions compared with normal mucosa. Am J Gastroenterol 88:338–343

Grohmann GS, Glass RI, Pereira HG et al 1993 Enteric viruses and diarrhea in HIV-infected patients. Enteric Opportunistic Infections Working Group. N Engl J Med 329:14–20

Hierholzer JC 1992 Adenoviruses in the immunocompromised host. Clin Microbiol Rev 5: 262–274

Jacobson MA, Mills J 1988 Serious cytomegalovirus disease in the acquired immunodeficiency syndrome (AIDS). Clinical findings, diagnosis, and treatment. Ann Intern Med 108:585–594

Janoff EN, Orenstein JM, Manischewitz JF, Smith PD 1991 Adenovirus colitis in the acquired immunodeficiency syndrome. Gastroenterology 100:976–979

Kaljot KT, Ling JP, Gold JW et al 1989 Prevalence of acute enteric viral pathogens in acquired immunodeficiency syndrome patients with diarrhea. Gastroenterology 97:1031–1032

Macdonald JC, Torriani FJ, Morse LS, Karavellas MP, Reed JB, Freeman WR 1998 Lack of reactivation of cytomegalovirus (CMV) retinitis after stopping CMV maintenance therapy in AIDS patients with sustained elevations in CD4 T cells in response to highly active antiretroviral therapy. J Infect Dis 177:1182–1187

Maddox A, Francis N, Moss J, Blanshard C, Gazzard B 1992 Adenovirus infection of the large bowel in HIV positive patients. J Clin Pathol 45:684–688

Mentec H, Leport C, Leport J, Marche C, Harzic M, Vildé JL 1994 Cytomegalovirus colitis in HIV-1-infected patients: a prospective research in 55 patients. AIDS 8:461–467

O'Sullivan CE, Drew WL, McMullen DJ et al 1999 Decrease of cytomegalovirus replication in human immunodeficiency virus-infected patients after treatment with highly active antiretroviral therapy. J Infect Dis 180:847–849

Schmidt W, Schneider T, Heise W et al 1996 Stool viruses, coinfections, and diarrhea in HIV-infected patients. Berlin Diarrhea/Wasting Syndrome Study Group. J Acquir Immune Defic Syndr Hum Retrovirol 13:33–38

Thea DM, Glass R, Grohmann GS et al 1993 Prevalence of enteric viruses among hospital patients with AIDS in Kinshasa, Zaire. Trans R Soc Trop Med Hyg 87:263–266

Theise ND, Rotterdam H, Dieterich D 1991 Cytomegalovirus esophagitis in AIDS: diagnosis by endoscopic biopsy. Am J Gastroenterol 86:1123–1126

Thomas PD, Pollok RCG, Gazzard BG 1999 Enteric viral infections as a cause of diarrhoea in the acquired immunodeficiency syndrome. HIV Med 1:19–24

Ullrich R, Zeitz M, Heise W, L'age M, Höffken G, Riecken EO 1989 Small intestinal structure and function in patients infected with human immunodeficiency virus (HIV): evidence for HIV-induced enteropathy. Ann Intern Med 111:15–21 (erratum: 1989 Ann Intern Med 111:954)

Whitcup SM, Fortin E, Lindblad AS et al 1999 Discontinuation of anticytomegalovirus therapy in patients with HIV infection and cytomegalovirus retinitis. JAMA 282:1633–1637

Wilcox CM, Diehl DL, Cello JP, Margaretten W, Jacobson MA 1990 Cytomegalovirus esophagitis in patients with AIDS. A clinical, endoscopic, and pathologic correlation. Ann Intern Med 113:589–593

Wilcox CM, Chalasani N, Lazenby A, Schwartz DA 1998 Cytomegalovirus colitis in acquired immunodeficiency syndrome: a clinical and endoscopic study. Gastrointest Endosc 48:39–43

DISCUSSION

Estes: Where in the intestine do you see the adenovirus growing?

Pollok: In our studies we have been looking at colonic biopsies. We concurrently took biopsies from the stomach, oesophagus and duodenum, and didn't identify adenovirus in the upper GI tract. Other groups have found adenovirus in the duodenum and the liver. In immunocompromised children adenovirus has also been identified in the upper gut.

Estes: What types of adenovirus are these?

Pollok: I don't think anyone has looked systematically. Hierholzer found viruses from A, C and D subgenera.

Glass: The study by Cunningham et al (1988) found both adenovirus and rota-viruses. These adenoviruses were all enteric serotypes from 40, 41 and 42–48. These are an unusual subgroup of enteric adenoviruses. Early in the AIDS epidemic when there were a lot of oral–anal practices, it was recognized that this was a problem, and when the studies were repeated, the numbers of rotaviruses and adenoviruses came down. It is not only the setting and diagnostics, but practices in the gay community that have changed. In a study of gay men with diarrhoea conducted in Atlanta, we found picobirnaviruses which were first identified by Helio Pereira. These picobirnavaruses have been found in most AIDS populations with diarrhoea where they have been looked for. While we can't find any more of these in Atlanta because HAART treatment has decreased diarrhoea in these patients, we have a collaboration in Argentina where HAART is not used as widely. Sylvia Nates has actually documented and published about picobirnaviruses in her

AIDS populations (Giordano et al 1998). Wherever PAGE is used or a similar diagnostic, picobirnavirions have been found in HIV-infected individuals. Now that we have clones and sequences of this, these diagnostics should be more widely available for patients with HIV who have diarrhoea. The astrovirus was the number one pathogen that came out of these HIV patients in Atlanta. It is interesting that these are adults with astrovirus: we usually think of this as a childhood pathogen. In other immunocompromised patients, astrovirus is found there as well. Finally, HAART is only commonly used in western countries. In countries such as Africa, where AIDS is epidemic and diarrhoeal disease is still a major problem, there is still the opportunity to look at these bugs and figure out which ones are key.

Pollok: I believe you have published some work from Zaire (Thea et al 1993). In that study there was no association between viruses and diarrhoea.

Glass: This was an early study where we were just setting up diagnostics. With Gary Grohmann's later study we looked intensively, because it was a CDC-wide effort (Grohmann et al 1993).

Pollok: The difficulty with that is that you really need to confidently exclude all other concurrent pathogens, which is no mean undertaking, particularly in a tropical setting. This is obviously crucial if you are trying to establish causality.

Glass: In the African studies, Nigel Cunliffe and Joe Gondwe have been looking at infected children of HIV-infected parents to see at what age rotavirus became a problem (Cunliffe et al 1999). Most of those children are not yet severely immunocompromised, so they become infected with the same viruses as other Malawian children. They haven't yet finished the analysis to look and see whether those who have the worst CD4 counts in fact have either more pathogens, or pathogens that give them disease of greater severity or duration.

Bishop: Diarrhoea in children undergoing bone marrow transplantation involving immunosuppression can be associated temporarily with enteric adenovirus (type 41) infection (Blakey et al 1989).

Estes: What do you know about the mechanisms of the pathophysiology of the diarrhoea in CMV colitis?

Pollok: It is associated with an inflammatory response. Wilcox's group looked at TNFα expression in biopsies from patients with oesophageal CMV. They found them elevated, not surprisingly. I think it is an inflammatory TNFα-mediated response, but the exact mechanism of diarrhoea is not well understood.

Green: In your EM study of 60 patients, did those all have diarrhoea?

Pollok: Yes. This was a descriptive study (Thomas et al 1999). Schmidt's group had an asymptomatic control group, and they established an association of diarrhoea with adenovirus and coronavirus. What we picked up was that adenovirus-associated colitis was associated with a persistent diarrhoea. I think some of these other viruses may cause a self-limited diarrhoea even in immunosuppressed individuals.

Green: Did you do any electropherotyping of the 18% of cases that were caused by rotavirus? Do you know which rotavirus groups are responsible?

Pollok: No, this was purely a morphological study.

Koopmans: Is anything known about CMV in the gut in non-HIV-infected people?

Pollok: It does infect other immunosuppressed groups, and it rarely occurs in people without immunosuppression. Another group of patients who arguably are partially immunosuppressed are individuals with Crohn's colitis, in whom CMV colitis can rarely occur as well.

Koopmans: I am thinking about the association with adenoviruses. You saw a lot of dual infections: is there any indication that there may be reactivation of CMV by infection with adenovirus?

Pollok: Schmidt's group has suggested that adenovirus somehow makes the gut more permissive to CMV infection. But it could equally be the other way round.

Greenberg: Is the target cell type in the colon for adenovirus and CMV epithelial cells?

Pollok: As far as we know it is purely an epithelial infection.

Desselberger: You mentioned rightly that in cases of diagnosed CMV colitis you should look at the retina for CMV infection. You then explained that there was less necessity to treat against CMV. Do you have the same experience now with retinitis, that when patients are treated with HAART, less CMV-specific antiviral treatment is needed?

Pollok: There are no published data with regard to gastrointestinal infections and HAART. Obviously the priority is to diagnose CMV retinitis. This is why I showed the retinitis data.

Offit: Why do you think that some mucosal viruses, such as herpes simplex virus or CMV have the capacity to cause ulcerative disease, whereas others such as rotavirus don't?

Pollok: Many pathogens can invoke an inflammatory response, not just viruses. Some switch on production of chemokines such as interleukin (IL)-8 from the enerocytes and induce an inflammatory cascade, whereas other pathogens are more inert and don't induce the inflammatory cascade. They are probably better adapted in that sense to invading the enterocyte without inducing inflammation.

Offit: So markers of the inflammatory response are more likely to be associated with ulcerative disease?

Pollok: Yes, that is the basis of ulceration.

Greenberg: Both CMV and adenovirus have well developed machinery to avoid host immune responses, which rotaviruses and the small RNA viruses lack. They also have their own forms of chemokine analogues. They have an immense strategy to alter host immune responses. CMV can infect endothelial cells. In fact, the whole hypothesis of it having something to do with restenosis after a heart transplant is based on this tropism. It may be that it is also affecting vascular supply in the intestine as well as the epithelium.

Farthing: I would agree with that. The difference is that rotavirus is an acute self-limited infection and in general there is very little acute or chronic inflammation, whereas CMV is a persistent viral infection. When there is persistence of any cause, there is usually a progression from acute to chronic inflammation, which then involves the vasculature, causing focal ischaemia and ulceration. I would agree that CMV is not an exclusively epithelial infection. If you look at sections of bowel or oesophagus infected with CMV, there are inclusion lesions deep down in the submucosa. I think there is a vascular component which may be very important for the perpetuation of this infection.

Pollok: It is a systemic infection: many patients will have CMV viraemia for months or even years without having end organ infection.

Offit: This is like polio, where the virus will be shed for weeks or months from the intestinal tract, yet this virus doesn't cause ulceration.

Koopmans: There is no proof, even in the old literature. We have looked at this carefully. We had an experience with transgenic mice that have the polio virus receptor which we tried to use as a model (Buisman et al 2000). We wanted to induce a mucosal response so we infected them intraperitoneally. They started to shed the virus, so we have been wondering if there is a different cell type that may communicate.

Farthing: Is poliovirus found in GI tissue?

Koopmans: This has not been documented.

Farthing: It is important. I am on our national panel as a non-virological gastroenterologist with regard to the handling of body fluids and tissue specimens which potentially might be contaminated with poliovirus: we are all working towards 2005 to eradicate the disease. One of the questions that we are facing is what we should do with freezers full of faeces and other human samples. It is possible to make a risk assessment as to whether faecal samples are likely to be contaminated. But what about all the mucosal biopsies that are frozen away? Do these contain viral particles?

Koopmans: You mentioned that with CMV there were ulcers at the ileocaecal valve. I was thinking about this in connection with intussusception. Would it be conceivable that in some cases there would be latent CMV infections in children that are activated by a vaccine, setting off intussusception?

Pollok: The literature suggests that polyps function as a promoter of intussusception. It is not clear in other cases of intussusception what is the precipitant. There is a dogma about swollen Peyer's patches, and whether or not this might be promoting increased motility.

Offit: Do you see CMV colitis in children under two years of age with HIV infection?

Pollok: I have to claim ignorance because I don't look after children.

Estes: This would be an interesting thing to look at.

Greenberg: In the normal child who would get a rotavirus vaccine, if they were infected with CMV it wouldn't be latent. They would be infected at a time of high viral excretion. Most children who get infected early in life are in daycare: this is the time that they are excreting large amounts of CMV and are quite infectious.

Koopmans: What about asymptomatic congenitally infected children?

Greenberg: The CMV could still be activated, but when young children are infected with CMV it takes a year to several years to down-regulate virus replication and get it into a latent state.

Estes: If you put rotavirus in epithelial cells they signal and cause the cells to secrete IL-8. But it is surprising then that you don't see a big infiltration of inflammatory cells in children. I don't know whether or not this is because there is another regulatory molecule in the intestine that is dampening down the effect of IL-8. It was surprising when people discovered that rotavirus does induce IL-8 because this is normally what you would see in the stomach infected with *Helicobacter* or other situations where lots of inflammation is seen.

Matson: Were those studies done on late biopsies from volunteers or others infected with caliciviruses? We know that there are biopsies from the time that people were symptomatic, but were there biopsies from day four or five?

Estes: We did a kinetic study with biopsies at different times, looking more for where the virus might be replicating. The problem is that there is such a small amount of tissue to work with.

Farthing: The chemokine response to a pathogen either attaching or invading is generic. It just depends on the magnitude and duration of that response as to whether you get a major inflammatory infiltrate. I suspect that in rotavirus it is a relatively mild and short-lived response, because the invaded cells are shed and then the virus is gone.

Desselberger: You briefly mentioned enteropathy by HIV itself. Could you expand on this? There seems to be evidence in the literature that HIV can infect colonic cells.

Pollok: It is well established that HIV can infect enterocytes. This may be important for transmission. With infection of the intestinal epithelium there are documented changes including villus atrophy and crypt cell hyperplasia. It is possible to demonstrate functional changes in the infected small bowel such as impaired sugar absorbance, but I doubt that it is an important clinical entity. Christine Blanchard identified a subgroup of patients that had been investigated extensively that were pathogen negative but still had diarrhoea. She followed-up that group and found that most of those patients had a short-lived mild diarrhoeal disease that resolved within a few months.

Estes: Judy Ball has been doing some work with the peptides from the SIV glycoprotein, and some mutant peptides derived from viruses that do or don't cause diarrhoea in animal models. She thinks that this molecule can function as an enterotoxin.

Farthing: In the SIV model I think there is no question that well before the monkeys experience the effects of immunocompromise, they develop villous atrophy early in the infection. I suspect this is not typical of human disease. In our lab we tried to look at the mechanisms of HIV enteropathy, in particular to address whether it is related to T cell activation in the gut, which is the mechanism that we think explains other forms of chronic enteropathy. There are plenty of activated T cells present, but there is no difference in those with or without enteropathy. The cause of the enteropathy is still unknown. In most European and North American patients, the enteropathy is mild. In Africans, there is a much more profound effect on villous morphology. I accept what Richard Pollok says about western HIV infection, but in Africa with a much more challenged group of people it may be a factor leading to 'slim' disease, which is one of the major clinical features in that region.

References

Blakey JL, Bishop RF, Barnes GL, Ekert H 1989 Infectious diarrhea in children undergoing bone-marrow transplantation. Aust NZ J Med 19:31–36

Buisman A, Sonsma J, Kimman T, Koopmans M 2000 Mucosal and systemic immunity to poliovirus in mice transgenic for the poliovirus receptor. J Infect Dis 181:815–823

Cunliffe NA, Gondwe JS, Broadhead RL et al 1999 Rotavirus G and P types in children with acute diarrhea in Blantyre, Malawi, from 1997 to 1998: predominance of novel P[6]G8 strains. J Med Virol 57:308–312

Cunningham AL, Grohmann GS, Harkness J et al 1988 Gastrointestinal viral infections in homosexual men who were symptomatic and seropositive for human immunodeficiency virus. J Infect Dis 158:386–391

Giordano MO, Martinez LC, Rinaldi D et al 1998 Detection of picobirnavirus in HIV-infected patients with diarrhea in Argentina. J Acquir Immune Defic Syndr Hum Retrovirol 18:380–383

Grohmann GS, Glass RI, Pereira HG et al 1993 Enteric viruses and diarrhea in HIV-infected patients. N Engl J Med 329:14–20

Thea D, Glass R, Grohmann GS et al 1993 Prevalence of enteric viruses among hospital patients with AIDS in Kinshasa, Zaire. Trans R Soc Trop Med Hyg 87:263–266

Thomas PD, Pollok RC, Gazzard BG 1999 Enteric viral infection as a cause of diarrhoea in AIDS. HIV Medicine 1:19–24

Novartis 238: Gastroenteritis Viruses.
Copyright © 2001 John Wiley & Sons Ltd
Print ISBN 0-471-49663-4   eISBN 0-470-84653-4

Treatment of gastrointestinal viruses

Michael J. G. Farthing[1]

Digestive Diseases Research Centre, St Bartholomew's & The Royal London School of Medicine & Dentistry, Turner Street, London E1 2AD, UK

Abstract. The most common enteric viruses responsible for diarrhoea are rotavirus, enteric adenoviruses, caliciviruses including the Norwalk agent and astrovirus. These infections are usually mild to moderate in severity, self-limiting and of short duration and thus, specific antiviral therapy is not recommended. The standard management of these infections is restoration of fluid and electrolyte balance and then maintenance of hydration until the infection resolves. WHO oral rehydration therapy (ORT) was introduced about 30 years ago and has saved the lives of many infants and young children. During the last 10 years it has become evident that the efficacy of ORT can be increased by reducing the osmolality of the WHO oral rehydration solution (ORS) to produce a relatively hypotonic solution. Hypotonic ORS appears to be safe and effective in all forms of acute diarrhoea in childhood. Complex substrate ORS, which is also usually hypotonic, has been shown to have increased efficacy in cholera but not in other bacterial or viral diarrhoeas. Nevertheless, the scientific rationale for using rice or resistant starch as substrate in ORS is of physiological interest. Other treatments such as hyperimmune bovine colostrum, probiotics and antiviral agents are largely experimental and have not been introduced into routine clinical practice. Cytomegalovirus (CMV) infection of the gastrointestinal tract occurs mainly in the immunocompromised although it has been reported in immunocompetent individuals. CMV infects both the oesophagus and colon to produce oesophagitis, often with discrete ulcers, and colitis, respectively. Both conditions can be treated with ganciclovir or foscarnet. Failure to respond to monotherapy is an indication to use both agents concurrently.

2001 Gastroenteritis viruses. Wiley, Chichester (Novartis Foundation Symposium 238) p 289–305

Acute infectious diarrhoea continues to be a major problem throughout the world although its greatest impact is in the poor, less developed countries where more than four million pre-school children die as a result of diarrhoea each year. The vast majority of these deaths are avoidable, as dehydration and associated acidosis are the principal determinants of the high mortality of acute diarrhoeal disease. Many children suffer repeated episodes which is a major cause of protein-energy

---

[1]Present address: Faculty of Medicine, University of Glasgow, 12 South Park Terrace, Glasgow G12 8LG, UK

malnutrition, a more important factor overall than a simple lack of food. Acute infectious diarrhoea continues to be a common problem in the developed world where it has been estimated that 99 million cases of diarrhoea occur each year in the USA, causing at least 500 deaths.

Rotavirus continues to be the major cause of acute watery diarrhoea in children worldwide followed closely by enterotoxigenic *Escherichia coli*. The other gastroenteritis viruses, namely the enteric adenoviruses, caliciviruses (including the Norwalk agent) and astrovirus also contribute to the overall morbidity of acute diarrhoea. These infections are usually mild to moderate in severity and of short duration and thus antiviral therapy is not recommended. Standard management of these infections is directed towards restoration of fluid and electrolyte balance and then maintenance of hydration until the infection resolves. Other possible treatments have been evaluated in animal models of infection and in humans but these are largely experimental and have not been introduced into routine clinical practice. These include hyperimmune bovine colostrum, probiotics and antiviral agents.

Cytomegalovirus and herpes simplex virus infect the gastrointestinal tract producing oesophagitis and proctocolitis, mainly in the immunocompromised. These infections are amenable to treatment with antiviral agents.

Treatment of virus infections of the gastrointestinal tract can therefore be considered under two main categories, namely (i) supportive interventions to restore fluid and electrolyte losses without any expectations that this will modify the natural history of the infection and (ii) specific interventions aimed at inhibiting viral replication with a view to altering the natural history of the illness.

Supportive interventions in acute diarrhoea

Dehydration

Fluid requirements change dramatically during the early neonatal period and through childhood into adult life (Fig. 1). Fluid requirements (related to body weight) are greatest during infancy and thus it is this period when the child is most susceptible to fluid losses.

Dehydration is a state in which total body water is decreased and in acute diarrhoeal illnesses results from both (i) *increased fluid losses* from the gastrointestinal tract and when there is fever, increased insensible losses through the skin, and (ii) *inadequate intake* which may occur concurrently with diarrhoea when accompanied by nausea and vomiting. Whatever the mechanisms of fluid and electrolyte depletion it is vital that these are replaced promptly before large, potentially fatal deficits occur.

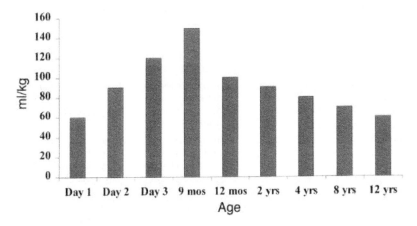

FIG. 1.   Fluid requirements in the neonate, infant and throughout childhood.

Assessment of dehydration.   During the initial clinical assessment of an infant or child with acute diarrhoea, it is essential to make an estimate of the degree of dehydration. This assessment guides the choice of the approach to rehydration (oral or intravenous) and allows an estimate to be made of the rate at which fluid should be replaced. The World Health Organization (WHO) devised a comprehensive scheme for classifying dehydration as mild, moderate and severe based on clinical parameters (Table 1). Paediatricians at Queen Elizabeth Hospital for Children in the UK developed a simplified version that enabled the severity of dehydration to be graded into four categories (Table 2).

If dehydration is severe with 10% or more body weight loss then fluid replacement should be at least 100 ml/kg, which almost inevitably must be delivered intravenously. When dehydration is mild and body weight loss does not exceed 5% fluid replacement is usually required at 50 ml/kg and can almost always be delivered orally. In the intermediate category when dehydration exceeds 5%, intravenous rehydration may be required initially, although if the infant or young child is alert and able to take oral fluid and urine output recovers rapidly then it is reasonable to pursue the oral route.

Rehydration

Oral fluid replacement remedies have been used by mothers and grandmothers for many centuries (Farthing 1988). Naturally occurring fluids such as coconut milk and other preparations containing rock salt and molasses have been described in ancient manuscripts. Formal oral rehydration therapy (ORT) began to evolve in

TABLE 1   WHO guidelines for assessment of dehydration and fluid deficit

Signs and symptoms	Mild dehydration	Moderate dehydration	Severe dehydration
General appearance and condition			
Infants & young children	Thirsty, alert, restless	Thirsty, restless, or lethargic but irritable when touched	Drowsy, limp, cold, sweaty, cyanotic extremities, may be comatose
Older children & adults	Thirsty, alert, restless	Thirsty, alert, giddiness with postural changes	Usually conscious, apprehensive, cold, sweaty cyanotic extremities, wrinkled skin of fingers and toes, muscle cramps
Radial pulse[1]	Normal rate and volume	Rapid and weak	Rapid, feeble, sometimes impalpable
Respiration	Normal	Deep, may be rapid	Deep and rapid
*Anterior fontanelle[2]	Normal	Sunken	Very sunken
*Systolic blood pressure[3]	Normal	Normal-low	Less than 10.7 kPa (80 mmHg), may be unrecordable
*Skin elasticity[4]	Pinch retracts immediately	Pinch retracts slowly	Pinch retracts very slowly (>2 seconds)
*Eyes	Normal	Sunken	Deeply sunken
Tears	Present	Absent	Absent
Mucous membranes[5]	Moist	Dry	Very dry
*Urine flow	Normal[6]	Reduced amount and dark	None passed for several hours, empty bladder
Body weight loss (%)	4–5	6–9	10% or more
Estimated fluid deficit	40–50 ml/kg	60–90 ml/kg	100–110 ml/kg

*Particularly useful in infants for assessment of dehydration and monitoring of rehydration
[1]If radial pulse cannot be felt, listen to heart with stethoscope.
[2]Useful in infants until fontanelle closes at 6–18 months or age. After closure there is a slight depression in some children.
[3]Difficult to assess in infants.
[4]Not useful in marasmic malnutrition or obesity.
[5]Dryness of mouth can be palpated with a clean finger. Mouth may always be dry in a child who habitually breaths by mouth. Mouth may be wet in a dehydrated patient due to vomiting or drinking.
[6]A marasmic baby or one receiving hypotonic fluids may pass good urine volumes in the presence of dehydration.

the 1940s largely due to the initiatives of Harold Harrison at the Baltimore City Hospital and Daniel Darrow at Yale (Darrow 1946, Harrison 1954). Chatterjee (1953) first showed that an oral rehydration solution (ORS) could rehydrate patients with cholera without the need to resort to intravenous fluids. Thus, the

TABLE 2   Simplified guidelines for assessing the severity of dehydration

% dehydration	Clinical signs
2–3%	Thirst, mild oliguria.
5%	Discernible alteration in skin tone, slightly sunken eyes, some loss of intraocular tension, thirst, oliguria. Sunken fontanelle in infants.
7–8%	Very obvious loss of skin tone and tissue turgor, sunken eyes, loss of intraocular tension, marked thirst and oliguria. Often some restlessness or apathy.
10%	All the foregoing, plus peripheral vasoconstriction, hypotension, cyanosis, and sometimes hyperpyrexia. Thirst may be lost at this stage.

practice of ORT was established but the true scientific rationale remained to be discovered.

Scientific rationale for oral rehydration therapy.   Fisher (1955) showed that glucose promoted intestinal ion transport and this observation was soon followed by the finding that sodium and glucose transport was coupled in the small intestine (Schedl & Clifton 1963). It also became evident that other solutes, such as amino acids were also absorbed by active transport, again coupled with transport of sodium ions (Fig. 2).

At the same time that these basic laboratory studies were being pursued, a US Navy Captain, Robert Phillips, working in Egypt and subsequently in the Philippines, was performing clinical rehydration studies in human cholera using glucose–electrolyte solutions. In 1961, as the seventh cholera pandemic began in the Philippines, Phillips and his team clearly showed that oral administration of glucose–salt solutions could reduce stool output in cholera and thus, could be used for oral replacement of water and electrolytes. Phillips' observations were confirmed in Dhaka (Hirschhorn et al 1968) and Calcutta (Pierce et al 1968).

Clinical developments in ORT.   ORT soon became widely used for other dehydrating diarrhoeal diseases with similar success (Farthing 1988). The WHO began a major campaign throughout the 1970s and 1980s which has successfully implemented ORT in most countries in the developing world. Subsequently, many clinical trials have been performed confirming the efficacy and feasibility of using ORT in preference to intravenous rehydration in the field setting and in particular during cholera epidemics. ORT was successfully used in cholera outbreaks in Bangladesh in 1971 (Mahalanabis et al 1973); mortality was reduced from 30% to

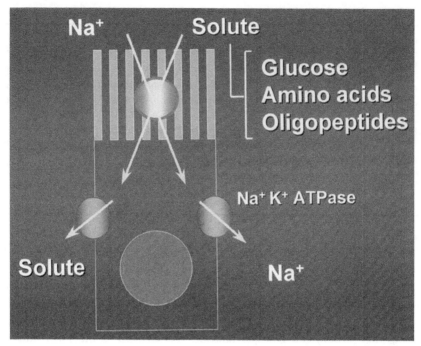

FIG. 2.   Mechanism of solute-coupled sodium co-transport in the enterocyte.

1%. Use of the WHO-ORS has been promoted widely throughout the developing world with a major decline in morbidity and mortality from acute diarrhoeal disease. ORT is safe and effective in neonates and in all except those with most severe degrees of dehydration. Clinical trials clearly show that ORT can correct both hypernatraemia and hyponatraemia and can successfully reverse acidosis in neonates and young infants.

Current controversies in ORT. The major controversies over the composition of ORS centre around the sodium and glucose concentrations and thus, osmolality, to which these components are the major contributors. Debate continues as to the necessity for including a base (bicarbonate) or base-precursor (citrate) in ORS, particularly as many other forms of metabolic acidosis such as diabetic ketoacidosis, are managed successfully by the administration of base-free fluids (Elliott et al 1987). Finally, although glucose has traditionally been the main substrate for ORS, the possibility that efficacy might be increased by using complex substrates such as cereals, resistant starch or defined glucose polymers continues to be discussed and may play an increasingly important role in future ORS formulations.

Sodium. The sodium concentration of ORS needs to be high enough to replace sodium losses and correct hyponatraemia but not so high as to cause or worsen hypernatraemia, which can itself occasionally result in death. The sodium concentration of the WHO-ORS, 90 mmol/l was probably derived from the faecal sodium concentration in adults with cholera (Molla et al 1981). Concern about widespread use of the 90 mmol/l ORS relates to hypernatraemia and periorbital oedema which occasionally occur with WHO-ORS in infants and children in the developed world fed on high solute feeds. Concerns about hypernatraemia were particularly evident in the developed world resulting in the proliferation of new ORS formulations with lower sodium concentrations (30–60 mmol/l). Part of the rationale for these developments was the observation that more than 50% of cases of acute diarrhoea in infants and young children in industrialized countries were due to rotavirus infections in which the stool sodium concentration was much lower than that of cholera. All clinical trials in well-nourished and malnourished children of all ages, including neonates and young infants in developed and developing communities have shown that ORS with sodium concentrations in the 50–60 mmol/l range are safe and effective for rehydration and maintenance therapy of mild to severe dehydration from acute non-cholera diarrhoea (Elliott et al 1989). Thus, in the developing world where bacterial gastroenteritis due to enterotoxigenic *E. coli* and cholera continues to be important, use of the 90 mmol/l WHO-ORS continues to be recommended for its safety and efficacy. However, with the increasing importance of rotavirus diarrhoea, with its associated lower sodium losses, lower sodium (50–60 mmol/l) ORS are more applicable for use in industrialized countries and are probably safe and effective in the vast majority of geographic locations in the developing world; indeed recent clinical trials would support this view.

Glucose. Glucose was the first substrate shown to be effective for ORT and is the most widely used worldwide. ORS glucose concentrations vary widely between that present in the WHO-ORS (111 mmol/l) to much higher concentrations of 200–300 mmol/l found in some of the early ORS that were produced commercially for used in industrialized countries. Recent studies in animal models of secretory diarrhoea have shown that reducing glucose concentration below that found in the WHO-ORS, does not significantly reduce glucose or sodium absorption and has in addition an important contribution by increasing water absorption, related at least in part to the lower osmolality of these solutions (Hunt et al 1991, Thillainayagam et al 1998). Recent clinical studies confirm that low glucose (70–100 mmol/l), hypotonic ORS reduce stool volume in children with acute gastroenteritis (Rautanen et al 1993, International Study Group on Reduced-Osmolality ORS solutions 1995).

ORS osmolality and complex substrates.   Until several years ago, the WHO-ORS and the majority of commercially available ORS were isotonic or moderately hypertonic, because of the relatively high concentrations of sodium and/or glucose. There is now evidence that high glucose ORS may increase stool volume, because of monosaccharide intolerance, and high sodium ORS, particularly if administered without *ad libitum* water in the maintenance phase, can produce hypernatraemia.

The discovery that rice powder and other cereals could replace glucose and improve efficacy of ORT in the early 1980s had an important impact on our thinking, both regarding the physiological principles of ORT and also its practical implementation (Gore et al 1992, Thillainayagam et al 1998). One important aspect of these solutions is that it is possible to deliver an increased amount of substrate without increasing the overall osmolality, because glucose is present in the form of starch, a high molecular weight molecule. It has been difficult to demonstrate increased substrate absorption in human disease states and studies in animal models have failed to show that this was the explanation for their increased efficacy. However, it is clear that the osmolality of the cereal-based solutions is extremely low, usually in the range of 150–170 mOsm/kg.

In recent years, we and others examined the hypothesis that reducing ORS osmolality is the major determinant for improving water absorption from both simple and complex carbohydrate-based ORS. We were able to show that reducing osmolality of standard glucose–electrolyte ORS resulted in improved water absorption in all of the models described. The majority of ORS now used in the UK are hypotonic (Table 3). Thus, these studies with complex carbohydrate ORS and the previous work with low osmolality glucose ORS suggest that osmolality is an important determinant of ORS efficacy (Thillainayagam et al 1998).

Rice/starch based ORS has been shown to be superior to WHO-ORS in adults with cholera and in infants with acute diarrhoea, the majority of whom had rotavirus infection. The major benefit accrued from these ORS relates to reduced faecal losses because of increased absorption of fluid and electrolytes.

The concept of using complex carbohydrate in ORS has recently been developed further with the incorporation of amylase-resistant starch in place of glucose or rice starch (Ramakrishna et al 2000). Resistant starch, such as that found in certain varieties of high-amylose maize starch, is poorly digested in the small intestine such that 50–70% of this starch passes into the colon and is fermented to short chain fatty acids (SCFAs). SCFAs promote sodium and fluid absorption in the colon and therefore might enhance the pro-absorptive capacity of ORS. This proposal has been evaluated in a randomized controlled trial in cholera which compared WHO-ORS with rice starch ORS and a resistant starch ORS. The resistant starch ORS significantly reduced faecal losses and the duration of the diarrhoea compared to the other two ORS. It remains to be established whether

TABLE 3 Composition (mmol/l) of oral rehydration solutions available in the UK in 2000

ORS	Na	K	Cl	HCO₃	Citrate	Glucose	Osmolality (calculated)
Powders							
Oral rehydration salts BP							
WHO	90	20	80	—	10	111	311
Diocalm Junior	60	20	50	—	10	111	251
Dioralyte	60	25	45	—	20	90	240
Dioralyte Relief	60	20	50	—	10	—⁺	
Electrolade	50	20	40	30	—	111	251
Rehidrat	50	20	50	20	9	91*	336
Effervescent tablets							
Dioralyte	60	25	45	—	20	90	240

Data from *British National Formulary*, March 1999.
⁺Contains cooked rice powder 6 g/sachet (30 g/l).
*Also contains sucrose 94 mmol/l and fructose 1–2 mmol/l.

resistant starch ORS is also more effective in other forms of acute infective diarrhoea.

Specific interventions for gastrointestinal virus infections

A variety of approaches have been used to try and reduce the duration and severity of gastrointestinal virus infections with the aim of changing the natural history of the infection. These interventions include the use of antiviral agents and other forms of antimicrobial chemotherapy, oral administration of immunoglobulins, probiotics and oral administration of growth factors.

Antiviral agents

Viral oesophagitis due to infection with herpes simplex virus (HSV) or cytomegalovirus (CMV) and CMV colitis are found most commonly in individuals with HIV infection. These infections in the immunocompromised host require treatment with antiviral agents. In severely symptomatic patients with HSV oesophagitis, aciclovir 5 mg/kg should be given intravenously every 8 hours for 7–10 days (Genereau et al 1996). In these patients oral maintenance therapy with 400 mg aciclovir orally twice daily should probably also be given. Milder infections may respond to oral aciclovir. When HSV is resistant to aciclovir an alternative therapy is foscarnet 40–60 mg/kg intravenously every 8 hours for 2–3 weeks.

CMV oesophagitis and colitis should be treated with ganciclovir 5 mg/kg intravenously twice daily for 3–6 weeks (Dieterich et al 1988, Nelson et al 1991). Maintenance therapy with oral ganciclovir 1000 mg orally three times daily may also be considered. An alternative drug is foscarnet.

Currently no antiviral agent is recommended for the treatment of viral gastroenteritis. However, human interferon α (IFNα) has been evaluated in a pig model of rotavirus infection (Lecce et al 1990). IFNα reduced virus excretion and mortality and improved weight gain compared to controls. The cysteine protease inhibitor E-64-c decreased diarrhoea and resulted in more rapid resolution of small intestinal changes in suckling mice infected with a human rotavirus strain (Ebina & Tsukada 1991). These findings are clearly of interest, but it is unlikely that these agents will find a place in the routine management of this infection.

Immunoglobulins

Attempts have been made to reduce the duration and severity of rotavirus infection by the oral administration of anti-rotavirus immunoglobulin with the aim of reducing intraluminal viral load. Initial experiments were performed in children which showed that orally administered human serum immunoglobulin could survive passage through the gastrointestinal tract (Losonsky et al 1985). Cows were then immunized with rotavirus to produce hyperimmune bovine colostrum. Several clinical trials have shown that colostrum-treated children had reduced stool weight and frequency, required less ORS, cleared rotavirus more rapidly from the stool and had a shorter duration of illness (Hilpert et al 1987, Guarino et al 1994, Mitra et al 1995, Sarker et al 1998). Despite these promising results hyperimmune colostrum has as yet not found a place in the management of this infection.

Probiotics

The concept of feeding innocuous bacteria to treat or prevent intestinal infection is not new and was considered by Louis Pasteur at the end of the last century. Several strains of lactobacilli have been evaluated as adjunctive therapy in children with rotavirus infection and preliminary studies indicate that early administration reduces the duration of diarrhoea compared to controls (Kaila et al 1992, 1995, Isolauri et al 1994, Majamaa et al 1995, Shornikova et al 1997). In addition treatment with lactobacilli may also enhance the specific antibody response to rotavirus infection. Further work is required to confirm these findings before implementation can be widely recommended.

Growth factors

Growth factors such as epidermal growth factor (EGF) and transforming growth factor α (TGFα) are known to promote epithelial cell growth in the small intestine.

Both growth factors have been evaluated in a pig model of rotavirus infection. Orally administered EGF at supraphysiological doses increased villus height and lactase activity in the small intestine but did not speed recovery from diarrhoea (Zijlstra et al 1994). TGFα, again administered orally, promoted mucosal recovery and improved epithelial barrier function but did not affect the functional capacity of the small intestine (Rhoads et al 1995). These are interesting mechanistic studies showing the potential of naturally occurring growth factors to promote tissue recovery, but as yet there is no indication that they have a role in the management of human infection.

References

Chatterjee HN 1953 Control of vomiting in cholera and oral replacement of fluid. Lancet 2:1063

Darrow DC 1946 The retention of electrolyte during recovery from severe dehydration due to diarrhea. J Pediatr 28:515

Dieterich DT, Chachoua A, Lafleur F, Worrell C 1988 Ganciclovir treatment of gastrointestinal infections caused by cytomegalovirus in patients with AIDS. Rev Infect Dis 10 (Suppl 3):S532–S537

Ebina T, Tsukada K 1991 Protease inhibitors prevent the development of human rotavirus-induced diarrhea in suckling mice. Microbiol Immunol 35:583–588

Elliott EJ, Walker-Smith JA, Farthing MJG 1987 The role of bicarbonate and base precursors in the treatment of acute gastroenteritis. Arch Dis Child 62:91–95

Elliott EJ, Cunha-Ferreira R, Walker-Smith JA, Farthing MJG 1989 Sodium content of oral rehydration solutions: a reappraisal. Gut 30:1610–1621

Farthing MJG 1988 History and rationale of oral rehydration and recent developments in formulating an optimal solution. Drugs 36:80–90

Fisher RB 1955 The absorption of water and of some small solute molecules from the isolated small intestine of the rat. J Physiol (Lond) 130:655–664

Genereau T, Lortholary O, Bouchaud O et al 1996 Herpes simplex esophagitis in patients with AIDS: report of 34 cases. The Cooperative Study Group on Herpetic Esophagitis in HIV Infection. Clin Infect Dis 22:926–931

Gore SM, Fontaine O, Pierce NF 1992 Impact of rice-based oral rehydration solution on stool output and duration of diarrhoea: meta-analysis of 13 clinical trials. Br Med J 304:287–291

Guarino A, Canani RB, Russo S et al 1994 Oral immunoglobulins for treatment of acute rotaviral gastroenteritis. Pediatrics 93:12–16

Harrison HE 1954 The treatment of diarrhoea in infancy. Pediatr Clin N Am 1:335–348

Hilpert H, Brüssow H, Mietens C, Sidoti J, Lerner L, Werchau H 1987 Use of bovine milk concentrate containing antibody to rotavirus to treat rotavirus gastroenteritis in infants. J Infect Dis 156:158–166

Hirschhorn N, Kinzie JL, Sachar DB et al 1968 Decrease in net stool output in cholera during intestinal perfusion with glucose-containing solutions. N Engl J Med 279:176–181

Hunt JB, Elliott EJ, Farthing MJG 1991 Comparison of rat and human intestinal perfusion models for assessing efficacy of oral rehydration solutions. Aliment Pharmacol Ther 5:49–59

International Study Group on Reduced-Osmolality ORS solutions 1995 Multicentre evaluation of reduced-osmolality oral rehydration salts solution. Lancet 346:282–285

Isolauri E, Kaila M, Mykkanen H, Ling WH, Salminen S 1994 Oral bacteriotherapy for viral gastroenteritis. Dig Dis Sci 39:2595–2600

Kaila M, Isolauri E, Soppi E, Virtanen E, Laine S, Arvilommi H 1992 Enhancement of the circulating antibody secreting cell response in human diarrhoea by a human lactobacillus strain. Pediatr Res 32:141–144

Kaila M, Isolauri E, Saxelin M, Arvilommi H, Vesikari T 1995 Viable versus inactivated lactobacillus strain GG in acute rotavirus diarrhoea. Arch Dis Child 72:51–53

Lecce JG, Cummins JM, Richards AB 1990 Treatment of rotavirus infection in neonate and weanling pigs using natural human interferon alpha. Mol Biother 2:212–216

Losonsky GA, Johnson JP, Winkelstein JA, Yolken RH 1985 Oral administration of human serum immunoglobulin in immunodeficient patients with viral gastroenteritis. A pharmacokinetic and functional analysis. J Clin Invest 76:2362–2367

Mahalanabis D, Choudhuri AB, Bagchi NG et al 1973 Oral fluid therapy of cholera among Bangladesh refugees. Johns Hopkins Med J 132:197–205

Majamaa H, Isolauri E, Saxelin M, Vesikari T 1995 Lactic acid bacteria in the treatment of acute rotavirus gastroenteritis. J Pediatr Gastroenterol Nutr 2:333–338

Mitra AK, Mahalanabis D, Ashraf H, Unicomb L, Eeckels R, Tzipori S 1995 Hyperimmune cow colostrum reduces diarrhoea due to rotavirus: a double-blind, controlled clinical trial. Acta Paediatr 84:996–1001

Molla MA, Rahman M, Sarker A et al 1981 Stool electrolyte content and purging rates in diarrhoea caused by rotavirus, enterotoxigenic E. coli and V. cholerae in children. J Pediatr 98:835–838

Nelson MR, Connolly GM, Hawkins DA, Gazzard BG 1991 Foscarnet in the treatment of cytomegalovirus infection of the esophagus and colon in patients with acquired immune deficiency syndrome. Am J Gastroenterol 86:876–881

Pierce NF, Banwell JG, Mitra RC et al 1968 Effect of intragastric glucose-electrolyte infusion upon water and electrolyte balance in Asiatic cholera. Gastroenterology 55:333–343

Ramakrishna BS, Venkataraman S, Srinivasan P, Dash P, Young GP, Binder HJ 2000 Amylase-resistant starch plus oral rehydration solution for cholera. N Engl J Med 342:308–313

Rautanen T, el-Radhi S, Vesikari T 1993 Clinical experience with a hypotonic oral rehydration solution in acute diarrhoea. Acta Paediatr 82:52–54

Rhoads JM, Ulshen MH, Keku EO et al 1995 Oral transforming growth factor-alpha enhances jejunal mucosal recovery and electrical resistance in piglet rotavirus enteritis. Pediatr Res 38:173–181

Sarker SA, Casswall TH, Mahalanabis D et al 1998 Successful treatment of rotavirus diarrhea in children with immunoglobulin from immunized bovine colostrum. Pediatr Infect Dis J 17:1149–1154

Schedl HP, Clifton JA 1963 Solute and water absorption by human small intestine. Nature 199:1264–1267

Shornikova AV, Casas IA, Mykkanen H, Salo E, Vesikari T 1997 Bacteriotherapy with Lactobacillus reuteri in rotavirus gastroenteritis. Pediatr Infect Dis J 16:1103–1107

Thillainayagam AV, Hunt JB, Farthing MJG 1998 Enhancing clinical efficacy of oral rehydration therapy: is low osmolality the key? Gastroenterology 114:197–210

Zijlstra RT, Odle J, Hall WF, Petschow BW, Gelberg HB, Litov RE 1994 Effect of orally administered epidermal growth factor on intestinal recovery of neonatal pigs infected with rotavirus. J Pediatr Gastroenterol Nutr 19:382–390

DISCUSSION

Greenberg: Where do we stand with WHO recommendations for the appropriate type of ORS?

Farthing: There has been considerable discussion as to whether a change should be made. The WHO has sponsored some very important studies in this area, but there is a concern that by changing the recommendation we will derail the whole programme. There is also still concern that the lower sodium solutions may not be as effective as the WHO solutions in severe cholera. At the moment, the WHO solution is used worldwide and can be used in all forms of acute diarrhoea, and is used by infants and adults alike. This is its great strength. In Europe and many developed countries, the industry has moved us towards hypotonic solutions. In the UK all the solutions available are of this hypotonic variety.

Vesikari: I don't think much progress has really been made since the December 1994 meeting about this subject in Bangladesh. The excuse is that there are a couple of cases of severe cholera in which patients may have had a hyponatraemia following treatment with hypotonic solutions. The real reason that the composition of ORS has not changed is logistical, I suspect. Resistance to change has been tremendous, but there is no real scientific reason for not changing.

Farthing: This has to be balanced against the deaths that have occurred with the WHO solution. This is always conveniently forgotten. There was a most devastating paper published just three or four years ago, where the mothers had made up the solutions incorrectly and gave concentrated WHO solution with fatal results. The problem with the WHO solution is that once you go into the maintenance phase, it has to be given diluted 2:1 with water. Everyone forgets this. I think it is simpler to have a simple solution that is taken all the way through and is safe.

Offitt: In the USA we are not very good at rehydrating children orally with moderate diarrhoea. We bring them into the hospital and give them intravenous fluids. Have you had more success with oral rehydration in the UK? If so, what leads to this success?

Farthing: The best example I quote in this context is John Walker-Smith's experience at the Queen Elizabeth Hospital in Hackney, which is a deprived, multiracial area in the east of London. In the 1970s when John first came to London, he had a gastroenteritis unit at the hospital. They had initiated an oral rehydration programme and would treat many children as in-patients, teaching the mothers and discharging the children often the same day. This unit closed in the late 1980s because there were no patients. We can no longer do studies on acute diarrhoea in this country because there are so few admissions. Mothers in the UK are now well informed and many will keep ORS sachets at home. Even in these relatively deprived areas it is quite unusual to find children being rehydrated intravenously.

Vesikari: Intravenous rehydration is not as good as oral. We did a study in the mid 1980s in which we randomized children to i.v. and to oral rehydration. The end result was that the duration of diarrhoea in the orally rehydrated group was approximately 1 day shorter (Vesikari et al 1987).

Glass: One thing you didn't mention that we put in our MMWR recommendations for management of diarrhoea patients in the USA was breast feeding. Have you got any thoughts on feeding?

Farthing: The principles are that breast feeding continues throughout the illness and children should eat as soon as they want to. Disaccharidase deficiency is a real phenomenon in severe villous damage. We know from animal models of rotavirus infection that recovery does take some days. It is not surprising that some children do not handle disaccharides well in the first 10 days after disease.

Glass: We often get calls from patients with chronic diarrhoea who are immunocompromised. Are any of these probiotics or globulins of specific use for chronic diarrhoea caused by rotavirus, astrovirus or calicivirus?

Farthing: There is no doubt that immunoglobulin has been useful in some settings where there is chronic infection, particularly in immunocompromised individuals. In this unusual situation, when there is persistent infection, it is a reasonable intervention to try. I do not know about probiotics in this setting.

Glass: We have looked at infections with Norwalk-like virus (NLV) in soldiers in the field. We found much seroconversion in American soldiers who went to Thailand. None of these people had diarrhoea, and we were quite surprised. It turned out they had all received γ-globulin beforehand for the prevention of hepatitis. Now the military is introducing the hepatitis A vaccine instead of the γ-globulin. We suspect that γ-globulin might have protected against NLV diarrhoea. The military has experienced outbreaks on aircraft carriers, and the naval forces get no γ-globulin. The marines that travel on these ships all get γ-globulin. What we need to watch out for is an outbreak of NLV on an aircraft carrier where the marines are protected by γ-globulin but the naval forces become ill because they haven't received γ-globulin.

Farthing: Have you looked at anti-NLV titres in the standard immunoglobulin populations?

Glass: It is there. We also looked for rotavirus antibody titres, and these soldiers all had high titres of rotavirus antibody. We thought this was perhaps from the γ-globulin.

Koopmans: I have a bit of a problem with the probiotic story because of some animal experiments that I am aware of. Depending on which strain of *Lactobacillus* is used, you can either get a complete Th1 shift or a Th2 shift of cytokine responses (Maassen et al 2000). There are very different effects on the immune system here. I recall a paper in which there was neonatal death in immunodeficient mice with *Lactobacillus* strains (Wagner et al 1997). This to me was pretty shocking and tells me to be cautious about using these preparations.

Vesikari: There are certainly differences between *Lactobacillus* strains: some of them work and others don't. I don't know whether they are dangerous in healthy children; I doubt it. We have worked with two strains: *Lactobacillus reuteri* and *Lactobacillus GG*, both of which clearly have an effect on rotavirus diarrhoea and shorten the duration of diarrhoea by approximately 1 day (Shornikova et al 1997a,b). Whatever you buy in the health food store may not work. It is easy to get such products on the shelf because there is no requirement of proof of efficacy.

Bishop: I just want to throw in as an argument a rather complex mechanism by which lactobacilli might work. This goes back to some very early work, prior to the description of rotavirus. By culturing the upper intestinal contents of children with acute gastroenteritis we observed an overgrowth of *Candida albicans* in the upper small intestine of many children (Barnes et al 1974). This overgrowth was associated with disaccharidase diffusion, and we could reproduce lactase depression in the small intestine of infant rabbits by inoculation of *C. albicans* (Bishop & Barnes 1974). Lactobacilli are antagonistic to *C. albicans*. It may be that the mechanism by which lactobacilli shorten the duration of diarrhoea following acute rotavirus disease is by preventing *C. albicans* overgrowth and consequent sustained disaccharidase damage in the upper small intestine.

Matson: One of the things about different hosts and different pathogens is the varying extent of basal membrane injury. What role does transudation of sodium and water have in diarrhoea?

Farthing: It probably has quite a large role, but has not been adequately studied in this setting. Mary Estes' data on tight junction function are important. We know that *Vibrio cholerae* produces a toxin that specifically loosens tight junctions. It is an unexplored area. There is no doubt that the upper part of the gut is already a leaky organ. Any infection or injury in that area is likely to make it leakier. Passive transudation is likely to be important, but it is not something that we have been able to study easily in human disease.

Matson: Are there any published data on prebiotics: compounds that adjust the gut flora that might alter susceptibility to diarrhoea?

Farthing: The concept is there; experiments have been done in adults. The difficulty with them is that you have to eat large quantities of foods containing oligofructoses such as onions, garlic and carrots. If you are vomiting and not feeling too good, this is quite a challenge! I have not seen any large, well controlled clinical trials in this area as yet.

Bishop: I can't see how they'd work in preventing upper small intestinal infection, where there is normally no resident flora.

Saif: I wanted to revisit the issue of immunoglobulin (IgG) antibody protection against rotavirus. In our pig model, we have found that IgG antibodies can protect in a passive way (Hodgins et al 1999, Parreno et al 1999, Schaller et al 1992). We can give circulating maternal antibodies that are mostly IgG that are derived from the serum of sows. If we administer these intraperitoneally, they get into the neonatal pig's circulation and presumably transudate back into the intestine in a passive manner. We can also passively protect if we orally administer colostrum and milk rotavirus antibodies (Hodgins et al 1999, Parreno et al 1999, Schaller et al 1999). There are also studies that Japanese investigators have initiated where they immunize chickens with rotavirus and get egg yolk antibodies that protect calves passively. In all these scenarios IgG antibodies can passively protect against rotavirus infections in the neonate. In the neonate IgG antibodies can also get back into the intestinal tract. When we immunized pigs by parenteral immunization with inactivated human rotavirus, we got high titres of IgG, but at challenge (34 weeks post-immunization) we couldn't detect IgG antibodies in the intestine (transudated from serum or locally produced) and we didn't get protection against rotavirus diarrhoea after challenge (Yuan et al 1998, To et al 1998).

Estes: It is different in different animal models. It is clear in the rabbit model that IgG protects, and it can protect in the mouse model in certain circumstances.

Saif: It also protects passively in the neonatal pig model.

Farthing: Have you used it as a treatment in the pig model? In the study I showed in humans it had been used as a treatment for active acute infection.

Saif: We didn't try it that way. We have always administered it the day before we give rotavirus.

Vesikari: So far we have talked about the treatment of acute diarrhoea. The passive administration of IgG or even lactobacilli may work, but this treatment always comes too late when the worst of the episode has already happened. Such treatments shorten diarrhoea, but don't take care of the acute problem that needs to be dealt with oral rehydration. What can be done prophylactically? Michael was right that you can immunize all the cows in Switzerland to produce this wonderful hyperimmune milk, but you will never be able to immunize enough cows to produce passive antibody for all the children in the world. In this sense this approach, as a general prophylactic measure, is out, even if it might be feasible when directed at certain target groups. Lactobacilli, on the other hand, can be grown in large quantities, and administration of such probiotics might be a feasible preventive therapy and even a competitor to the vaccine approach.

Kapikian: What about the use of bismuth salicylate, which has been shown in a volunteer study to reduce the severity and duration of abdominal cramps after Norwalk virus challenge (Steinhoff et al 1980)?

Farthing: It is effective, but only modestly. There are concerns about giving bismuth compounds to the very young age group because of retention of bismuth.

Kapikian: What do you use when you travel?

Farthing: I take a single large dose of quinolone, and if I still have trouble four hours later I take another dose.

Glass: Earlier on you described the mechanisms of vomiting. We see a lot of outbreaks on cruise ships where vomiting is a key component and where the virus is thought to spread through vomitus. You didn't mention a single drug or treatment for vomiting.

Farthing: I agree; that was an omission. Many travellers and pharmacies on cruise ships will carry the classic anti-emetic drugs. They are of modest efficacy in this situation. I am not aware that they have been subjected to rigorous clinical trials during acute gastrointestinal infection. It might also be worth evaluating the role of a 5-HT$_3$ receptor antagonist. The protocol I would choose would be to try large doses early on in the illness. However, it would have to be a serotonin-related form of vomiting for this to work.

References

Barnes GL, Bishop RF, Townley RRW 1974 Microbial flora and disaccharidase depression in infantile gastroenteritis. Acta Paed Scand 63:423–426

Bishop RIF, Barnes GL 1974 Depression of lactase in the small intestine of infant rabbits by *Candida albicans.* J Med Microbiol 7:259–263

Hodgins DC, Kang S-Y, deArriba L et al 1999 Effects of maternal antibodies on protection and the development of antibody responses to human rotavirus in gnotobiotic pigs. J Virol 73:186–197

Maassen CB, van Holten-Neelen C, Balk F et al 2000 Strain-dependent induction of cytokine profiles in the gut by orally administered lactobacillus strains. Vaccine 18:2613–2623

Parreno V, de Arriba L, Kang S et al 1999 Serum and intestinal isotype antibody responses to Wa human rotavirus in gnotobiotic pigs are modulated by maternal antibodies. J Gen Virol 80:1417–1428

Schaller JP, Saif L J, Cordle CT, Candler E, Winship TR, Smith KL 1992 Prevention of human rotavirus induced diarrhea in gnotobiotic piglets using bovine antibody. J Infect Dis 165:623–630

Shornikova AV, Isolauri E, Burkanova L, Lukovnikova S, Vesikari T 1997a A trial in the Karelian Republic of oral rehydration and *Lactobacillus GG* for treatment of acute diarrhoea. Acta Paediatr 86:460–465

Shornikova AV, Casas IA, Isolauri E, Mykkanen H, Vesikari T 1997b *Lactobacillus reuteri* as a therapeutic agent in acute diarrhea in young children. J Pediatr Gastroenterol Nutr 24:399–404

Steinhoff MC, Douglas RG Jr, Greenberg HB, Callahan DR 1980 Bismuth subsalicylate therapy of viral gastroenteritis. Gastroenterology 78:1495–1499

To TL, Yuan L, Ward LA, Gadfield K, Saif L J 1998 Serum and intestinal isotype antibody responses and correlates of protective immunity to human rotavirus in a gnotobiotic pig model of disease. J Gen Virol 79:2661–2672

Vesikari T, Isolauri E, Baer M 1987 A comparative trial of rapid oral and intravenous rehydration in acute diarrhoea. Acta Paediatr Scand 76:300–305

Wagner R, Warner T, Roberts L, Farmer J, Balish E 1997 Colonization of congenitally immunodeficient mice with probiotic bacteria. Infect Immun 65:3345–3351

Yuan L, Kang S-Y, Ward LA, To TL, Saif L J 1998 Antibody-secreting cell responses and protective immunity assessed in gnotobiotic pigs inoculated orally or intramuscularly with inactivated human rotavirus. J Virol 72:330–338

Summing-up

Mary K. Estes

Department of Molecular Virology and Microbiology, Baylor College of Medicine, 1 Baylor Plaza, Houston TX 77030, USA

We have had a stimulating meeting that has provided a comprehensive review of gastroenteritis viruses. Developments in electron cryomicroscopy and X-ray crystallography and the combined use of these techniques to probe viruses have enhanced the ability of structural data to provide us with a molecular understanding of virus function. New structural approaches are leading to the elucidation of the contribution of different viral proteins to different parts of particle structure and are also revealing details of replication functions. For example, comparisons of transcription inactive and active subviral particles of rotavirus are beginning to provide a dynamic structure-based view of the virus replication process. In the future, these kinds of data should lead us to new information about antigenic determinants and perhaps antivirals.

There has been enormous progress in the identification of receptors for rotavirus, and we are beginning to understand early events in virus replication. Rotavirus RNA replication depends crucially on the 3′ and 5′ terminal sequences of the viral RNA and on the interaction of the RNA with several virus-encoded, non-structural proteins made in infected cells. Sequences at the 3′ terminus of non-polyadenylated rotavirus mRNAs are also important for the initiation and enhancement of translation of viral proteins and the concomitant shut-off of host cellular protein synthesis. But many open questions with regard to genome replication, genome packaging, and viral assembly remain. Despite progress, there is a continuing search for reverse genetic systems for many of these viruses. It was exciting to hear that apparently the coronaviruses have broken this barrier, but we still have these challenges for the rotaviruses and the human caliciviruses. Progress with the feline calicivirus and astrovirus systems, that are using reverse genetic systems that are still in their infancy, are beginning to highlight the power of these techniques. This is certainly known from other viruses where reverse genetic systems are available. The further development and exploitation of these systems is going to lead rapidly to a more detailed understanding of the mechanisms of replication and of genes important in virulence.

There has been good progress in demonstrating a role of IgA as a correlate of protection for rotavirus, although there is controversy as to whether IgG is also important. An important remaining question is which antibodies against which of the rotavirus proteins are most important in protection. There are still big gaps in our understanding of the immunology of other gastrointestinal virus infections. In particular, whether a correlation exists between protection and the presence of antibody against caliciviruses remains unclear.

Knowledge about the aetiology and epidemiology of acute gastroenteritis has been enhanced by the development of new diagnostic assays over the last several years. New assays have helped to fill what Tom Flewett called the 'diagnostic gap' (Flewett et al 1987) and now almost all outbreaks of disease that are investigated carefully are associated with a known etiologic agent. We have seen that the combined use of new diagnostics with cogent clinical observations has helped to focus the clinical significance of many of the gastroenteritis viruses. There is still a need for development and a wider use of more simple assays, particularly in the clinical and community setting. We have learned the importance of epidemio- logical studies that consist of a mixture of both active and passive surveillance. It is clear from the diagnostic progress that rotaviruses remain the single most important cause of life-threatening diarrhoeal disease in young children. However, the use of new assays is also changing the epidemiology of some of the other gastroenteritis viruses: human caliciviruses are becoming increasingly detected as important pathogens. The clinical significance of the other agents remains less well defined, and more information is needed. The Norwalk-like viruses are clearly the key pathogens in food- and water-transmitted disease.

We now have good phenomenological information on virus diversity, although the biological significance of this diversity remains rather unclear. Studies of rotavirus circulation in many countries have shown that rotaviruses of different serotypes co-circulate at any one time, and these co-circulating viruses interact genetically by forming *in vivo* reassortants. In addition, evidence is accumulating that some of the rotaviruses infecting man may originate from domestic animals. Multiple, genetically diverse strains of caliciviruses also may co-circulate, and new calicivirus strains may arise by recombination. It is not known whether these strains represent biologically relevant distinct serotypes. We have a better understanding of potential mechanisms of virus evolution than we do of transmission dynamics. Future studies will need to determine the impact of changing virus serotypes on vaccination strategies and disease pathogenesis.

There has also been progress in understanding the rotavirus genes involved in virus virulence. Many rotavirus genes (RNAs 3, 4, 5, 7, 8 and 10) have been implicated in viral pathogenesis. However, recent attention has focused on the product of gene segment 10, a protein called NSP4 that has been shown to function as the first described viral enterotoxin. New data support a model whereby this protein is released from virus-infected cells and diarrhoea results from the activation of a signal-transduction cascade in secretory cells that affects calcium and chloride homeostasis and leads to an efflux of ions and water. In an animal model, antibodies to this enterotoxin also protect against virus-induced disease. Rotavirus infection may also be pathogenic by affecting the enteric autonomous nervous system. This work has stimulated new ideas about how gastrointestinal viruses cause disease, and future work will discover if other gastrointestinal viruses also produce enterotoxins. Future treatments for gastroenteritis could target secretory processes as well as interfere with the enteric nervous system and be used to counteract newly recognized common mechanisms of pathogenesis for both viral and bacterial-induced disease.

The unexpected difficulties into which the first licensed rotavirus vaccine has run in the last year have been disappointing for researchers and physicians in both developed and developing countries. It is hoped that many remaining questions about the relative risk and pathogenesis of intussusception can be answered clearly and quickly. There is a clear need for a rotavirus vaccine, particularly in developing countries. This is undiminished by the events over the last year, and a safe vaccine is everybody's goal. Several other candidate rotavirus vaccines are on the horizon.

There are increasing numbers of people in the world with immune deficiencies due to cancer treatment, human immunodeficiency virus (HIV) infection and transplantation. We have heard about the different spectrum of opportunistic viral infections in such patients. Infected, immunocompromised people may be a further source for viral evolution and spread. This is an area that hasn't been explored or exploited extensively. Fortunately, with the advent of highly active antiretroviral therapy (HAART) against HIV infection, the clinical need to treat HCMV colitis has decreased dramatically, presumably because of enhanced immune function under HAART treatment.

We have heard compelling molecular evidence that viruses may be transmitted from animals to humans, but further work is required to prove this. Finally, I think it remains critical that we remember an idea that was first mentioned in my introduction and that was discussed throughout this meeting. While most of the viruses we have talked about infect cells in the epithelial layer of the intestinal villi, the outcome of infection is often not simply a consequence of killing these epithelial cells; rather we need to think more globally, and try to understand the epithelial cell response to infection and how that response and signalling may affect other cells within the intestinal villi as well as at possible systemic sites.

I would like to end the meeting by thanking all the participants for their imaginative and provocative contributions. I think the book will be both interesting and stimulating to others inside and outside the fields of basic and clinical virology, infectious diseases, gastroenterology, and cell and molecular biology.

Reference

Flewett TH, Beards GM, Brown DWG, Sanders RC 1987 The diagnostic gap in diarrhoeal aetiology. In: Novel diarrhoea viruses. Wiley, Chichester (Ciba Found Symp 128) p 238–249

Index of contributors

Non-participating co-authors are indicated by asterisks. Entries in bold indicate papers; other entries refer to discussion contributions.

Subject index